KEY ASPECTS OF COMFORT
Management of Pain, Fatigue, and Nausea

Sandra G. Funk, Ph.D., is an Associate Professor and Director of the Research Support Center (RSC) at the School of Nursing, the University of North Carolina at Chapel Hill. A faculty member of the School of Nursing for over 12 years, she served as coordinator of the graduate research sequence, teaching graduate research methods, statistics, and computer applications, for nine years, and has been Director of the RSC for the past three. She has served as research and statistical advisor to nursing faculty and graduate students in several universities, and, for five years, was research advisor to the Robert Wood Johnson fellows in general pediatrics at Duke University. She has served as principal and co-investigator of numerous grants and has published in the areas of preschool developmental screening, research utilization, decision making, scaling, and cluster analysis.

Elizabeth M. Tornquist, M.A., is a former journalist and free-lance writer; she has been a member of the faculty of the School of Nursing at the University of North Carolina at Chapel Hill for 14 years, where she teaches writing to graduate students and serves as editor in residence. Ms. Tornquist is also on the faculty of the Curriculum of Public Health Nursing at the University of North Carolina at Chapel Hill. She is the author of *From Proposal to Publication: An Informal Guide to Writing about Nursing Research* as well as numerous articles on writing.

Mary T. Champagne, Ph.D., R.N., is Assistant Professor and Chairperson of the Faculty at the School of Nursing, the University of North Carolina at Chapel Hill. She is also on-site principal investigator of a multi-site study designed to establish the validity of the Braden Scale in predicting risk of pressure sore development in hospitalized, nursing home, and home care patients, and co-principal investigator of a 5-year study which will test interventions to prevent the development of acute confusion in hospitalized elderly patients. She is currently National Nurse Advisor for Humana Heart Institute International in Louisville, KY.

Laurel Archer Copp, Ph.D., R.N., is Dean and Professor at the School of Nursing, the University of North Carolina at Chapel Hill. Dr. Copp is an authority on management of pain and author of *Perspectives in Pain;* she has also published numerous articles and book chapters reporting her research on coping with pain. She is currently editor of the *Journal of Professional Nursing*.

Ruth A. Wiese, M.S.N., R.N., a former faculty member of the University of Nebraska College of Nursing and an inservice instructor and coordinator of staff development in a clinical setting, is currently Research Associate and Project Manager for "Disseminating Nursing Research: A Focused Conference/Monograph Series" at the School of Nursing, University of North Carolina at Chapel Hill.

Management of Pain, Fatigue and Nausea

Edited by

Sandra G. Funk, Ph.D.

Elizabeth M. Tornquist, M.A.

Mary T. Champagne, Ph.D., R.N.

Laurel Archer Copp, Ph.D., R.N., F.A.A.N.

Ruth A. Wiese, M.S.N., R.N.

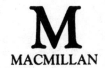

MACMILLAN

First published in 1989 by
Springer Publishing Company, Inc.
536 Broadway
New York NY 10012

This edition first published 1994 by
THE MACMILLAN PRESS LTD
Houndmills, Basingstoke, Hampshire RG21 2XS
and London
Companies and representatives
throughout the world

ISBN 0–333–60798–8

A catalogue record for this book is available from the British Library.

Printed in Great Britain by
Mackays of Chatham PLC
Chatham, Kent

The Disseminating Nursing Research Project

ADVISORY COMMITTEE

Chair:

Carolyn A. Williams, Ph.D., R.N., F.A.A.N.
Dean and Professor, School of Nursing
University of Kentucky

Members:

Norma M. Lang, Ph.D., R.N., F.A.A.N.
Dean and Professor, School of Nursing
University of Wisconsin-Milwaukee

Ora L. Strickland, Ph.D., R.N., F.A.A.N.
Professor, School of Nursing, University of Maryland

Linda R. Cronenwett, Ph.D., R.N., F.A.A.N.
Director of Nursing Research
Dartmouth-Hitchcock Medical Center

INVESTIGATORS

Principal
Investigator:

Sandra G. Funk, Ph.D.
Associate Professor and Director, Research Support
Center, School of Nursing
University of North Carolina at Chapel Hill

Co-Investigators:

Mary T. Champagne, Ph.D., R.N.
Assistant Professor

Laurel Archer Copp, Ph.D., R.N., F.A.A.N.
Dean and Professor

Elizabeth M. Tornquist, M.A.
Lecturer

"Disseminating Nursing Research: A Focused Conference/Monograph Series" is funded by the National Center for Nursing Research, National Institutes of Health, Grant #R18 NR01357.

Contents

Part III. Fatigue

Part IV. Nausea

Part V. Comfort

Part VI. Research Utilization

Acknowledgments

Support for this project was provided by a research utilization grant (#R18 NR01357), "Disseminating Nursing Research: A Focused Conference/Monograph Series," awarded to the School of Nursing, the University of North Carolina at Chapel Hill, from the National Center for Nursing Research at the National Institutes of Health. We are most appreciative of the support provided by the National Center for Nursing Research for this project and of the thoughtful direction and guidance provided by our Advisory Committee: Dr. Carolyn A. Williams, Dr. Norma M. Lang, Dr. Ora L. Strickland, and Dr. Linda R. Cronenwett. For our first conference and monograph, Dr. Laurel Archer Copp, Co-Investigator on the project, also served as the pain expert on the Advisory Committee, and Dr. Patricia H. Cotanch, Assistant Professor of Psychiatry, School of Medicine, Duke University Medical Center, and Barbara F. Piper, Doctoral Candidate, School of Nursing, University of California, San Francisco, joined the Advisory Committee to provide content expertise in the areas of nausea and fatigue, respectively; we are grateful for their contributions. Heartfelt thanks are extended to our project secretary, Stacy, S. Miller, for her work on this volume; to S. Page Davis and Reneé N. Lambert, who assisted her; to Patience Vanderbush, Gillian Floren, and Claire Viadro, who worked with the editors in developing conference materials and preparing this volume; and to Marie Gangemi, who provided consultation on various aspects of publication.

For those wishing to contact our information center or receive copies of the newsletter, *Nursing Research/Nursing Practice Connection*, call or write to: Ruth Wiese, Project Manager, School of Nursing, CB# 7460 Carrington Hall, University of North Carolina at Chapel Hill, Chapel Hill, NC 27599-7460; telephone: (919) 966-2263.

S.G.F.

Contributors

Janet E. Angus, M.Sc.N., R.N.
Tutor, Faculty of Nursing, University of Toronto, Toronto, Canada

Neils C. Beck, Ph.D.
Associate Professor, Department of Psychiatry, University of Missouri-Columbia

Jeanne Q. Benoliel, D.N.Sc., R.N., F.A.A.N.
Professor, School of Nursing, University of Washington, Seattle

Judith E. Beyer, Ph.D., R.N.
Associate Professor, School of Nursing, University of Colorado Health Sciences
  Center, Denver

Melinda Calhoon, M.S.N., R.N.
Clinical Instructor, School of Nursing, The University of North Carolina at Chapel
  Hill

Felissa L. Cohen, Ph.D., R.N., F.A.A.N.
Professor of Medical Surgical Nursing, College of Nursing, University of Illinois,
  Chicago

Douglas Conner, Ph.D.
Research Fellow, School of Nursing, University of Colorado Health Sciences
  Center, Denver

Patricia H. Cotanch, Ph.D., R.N.
Assistant Professor of Psychiatry, School of Medicine, Duke University Medical
  Center, Durham, North Carolina

Linda R. Cronenwett, Ph.D., R.N., F.A.A.N.
Director, Nursing Research, Dartmouth-Hitchcock Medical Center, Hanover,
  New Hampshire

Leanna J. Crosby, D.N.Sc.
Assistant Professor, College of Nursing, University of Arizona, Tucson

Diane Holditch Davis, Ph.D., R.N.
Assistant Professor, School of Nursing, The University of North Carolina at Chapel Hill

Colleen K. DiIorio, Ph.D., R.N.
Associate Professor and Director, Center for Nursing Research, School of Nursing, Emory University, Atlanta

Marylin J. Dodd, Ph.D., R.N., F.A.A.N.
Associate Professor and Chairperson, Department of Physiological Nursing, School of Nursing, University of California, San Francisco

Marilee I. Donovan, Ph.D., R.N.
Chairperson, Medical Nursing, Rush-Presbyterian-St. Luke's Medical Center, Chicago

Pamela Duchene, D.N.Sc., R.N.
Associate Chairperson, Gerontological Nursing, Rush-Presbyterian-St. Luke's Medical Center, Chicago

Theresa P. Dulski, M.S., R.N.
Lecturer, College of Nursing, The University of North Carolina at Charlotte

Joann M. Eland, Ph.D., R.N.
Associate Professor, College of Nursing, The University of Iowa, Iowa City

Sandra Faux, Ph.D., R.N.
Assistant Professor and Coordinator, Graduate Program, The University of Western Ontario, London, Ontario, Canada

Sandra Ferketich, Ph.D., R.N.
Associate Professor and Head, Division of Family and Community Health Nursing, College of Nursing, University of Arizona, Tucson

Roxie L. Foster, M.S., R.N.
Doctoral Candidate in Nursing, School of Nursing, University of Colorado Health Sciences Center, Denver

Barbara F. Fuller, Ph.D., R.N.
Professor, School of Nursing, University of Colorado Health Sciences Center, Denver

Fotini Georgiadou, Ph.D.
Research Associate, School of Nursing, University of Washington, Seattle

Joan Hamilton, M.Sc.(A), R.N.
Palliative Care Nurse Coordinator, Hamilton General Hospital, Hamilton, Ontario, Canada

Sally B. Hardin, Ph.D., R.N.
Professor of Psychiatric Nursing, College of Nursing, University of South Carolina, Columbia

Nancy Olson Hester, Ph.D., R.N.
Assistant Professor and Senior Faculty Associate, Center for Nursing Research, School of Nursing, University of Colorado Health Sciences Center, Denver

William L. Holzemer, Ph.D., R.N., F.A.A.N.
Professor, Physiological Nursing, Director, Office of Research, Evaluation and Computer Resources, School of Nursing, University of California, San Francisco

Yoshiyuki Horii, Ph.D.
Professor, Department of Communication Disorders and Speech Science, University of Colorado, Boulder

Ada K. Jacox, Ph.D., R.N.
Professor and Director, Center for Nursing and Health Services Research, School of Nursing, University of Maryland, Baltimore

Susan Christensen Jamar, M.S., R.N., O.C.N.
Hospice Coordinator, Arrowhead Alternative Services, Eveleth, Minnesota

Melinda L. Jenkins, M.S., R.N.C.
Family Nurse Practioner, Community Health Center, Middletown, Connecticut

Mary H. Johnson, M.N., R.N.
Clinical Nurse II in Adult Oncology, Division of Nursing, University of Missouri Hospitals and Clinics, Columbia

Nancy J. Krokosky, M.N.C.S., R.N.
Cardiovascular Clinical Nurse Specialist, Veterans' Administration Medical Center, Pittsburgh

Joanne M. Laframboise, M.Sc.N., R.N.
Lecturer, Faculty of Nursing, The University of Western Ontario, London, Ontario, Canada

Ada M. Lindsey, Ph.D., R.N., F.A.A.N.
Professor and Dean, School of Nursing, University of California, Los Angeles

Nancy Lovejoy, D.S.N., R.N.
Assistant Professor, Department of Physiological Nursing, School of Nursing, University of California, San Francisco

Richard W. Madsen, Ph.D.
Associate Professor, Department of Statistics, University of Missouri-Columbia

Ruth McCorkle, Ph.D., R.N., F.A.A.N.
Professor, School of Nursing, University of Pennsylvania, Philadelphia

Margaret Shandor Miles, Ph.D., R.N., F.A.A.N.
Professor, School of Nursing, The University of North Carolina at Chapel Hill

Nancy M. Mills, Ph.D., R.N.
Assistant Professor, School of Nursing, University of Missouri-Kansas City

Kathleen J. Moran, M.S.N, R.N., C.C.R.N., C.N.R.N.
Pain Clinical Nurse Specialist, Department of Nursing Consultation and Research and Department of Neurology, University of Cincinnati Medical Center

Marlene A. Moyer, M.S.N, R.N.
Nurse Manager, Burn Center, Hermann Hospital, Houston

Virginia J. Neelon, Ph.D., R.N.
Associate Professor, School of Nursing, The University of North Carolina at Chapel Hill

Terry S. Nelson, M.S.N., R.N.
Clinical Nurse, The Johns Hopkins Hospital, Baltimore

Ann M. Newman, M.S.N., R.N.
Assistant Professor, College of Nursing, The University of North Carolina at Charlotte

Steven M. Paul, Ph.D.
Instructor, Department of Physiological Nursing, School of Nursing, University of California, San Francisco

Barbara F. Piper, M.S., R.N.
Doctoral Candidate, Department of Physiological Nursing, School of Nursing, University of California, San Francisco

Norann Y. Planchock, Ph.D., R.N.
Associate Professor and Department Head, Graduate Studies and Research in Nursing, Northwestern State University, Shreveport, Louisiana

Laura E. Pole, M.S.N., R.N., O.C.N.
Oncology Clinical Nurse Specialist, Lewis-Gale Hospital, Salem, Virginia

Kathleen Potempa, D.N.Sc.
Assistant Professor, College of Nursing, University of Illinois, Chicago

Richard C. Reardon, Ph.D.
Staff Psychologist, Veterans' Administration Medical Center, Pittsburgh

Verna A. Rhodes, Ed.S., R.N.
Associate Professor, School of Nursing, University of Missouri-Columbia

Bradley M. Rodgers, M.D.
Chief, Division of Pediatric Surgery, University of Virginia Children's Medical Center, Charlottesville

Eileen A. Ryan, M.S.N., R.N.
Clinical Instructor/Lecturer, School of Nursing, University of Pennsylvania, Philadelphia

Marilyn C. Savedra, D.N.S., R.N.
Associate Professor, Department of Family Health Care Nursing, School of Nursing, University of California, San Francisco

Charles E. Schunior, M.A., R.N.
Assistant Head Nurse, Duke University Medical Center, Durham, North Carolina

Barbara J. Shelton, Ph.D., R.N.
Associate Professor, School of Nursing, University of Missouri-Columbia

Rani Hajela Srivastava, M.Sc.N., R.N.
Assistant Professor, School of Nursing, Memorial University of Newfoundland, St. John's, Newfoundland, Canada

Debra A. Stergios, M.S.N., R.N.
Administrative Head Nurse, University of Virginia Children's Medical Center, Charlottesville

Mary D. Tesler, M.S., R.N.
Clinical Professor, Department of Family Health Care Nursing, School of Nursing, University of California, San Francisco

Donna J. van Lier, Ph.D., C.N.M.
Certified Nurse-Midwife, Atlanta OB-GYN Associates, Northwest Medical Center, Atlanta

Judith Ann Ward, M.S., R.N.
Assistant Clinical Professor, Department of Family Health Care Nursing, School of Nursing, University of California, San Francisco

Phyllis M. Watson, Ph.D., R.N.
Vice President for Nursing, Lakeland Regional Medical Center, Lakeland, Florida

Catherine J. Webb, M.A., R.N.
Assistant Professor/Pediatric Clinical Nurse Specialist, School of Nursing and Children's Medical Center, University of Virginia, Charlottesville

Steve Weller, M.D.
Radiation Therapist, Mills-Peninsula Hospitals, Burlingame, California

Diana J. Wilkie, M.S., R.N.
Doctoral Candidate, Department of Family Health Care Nursing, School of Nursing, University of California, San Francisco

KEY ASPECTS OF COMFORT
Management of Pain, Fatigue, and Nausea

Part I

INTRODUCTION

[1]

Patient Comfort: From Research to Practice

Sandra G. Funk and Elizabeth M. Tornquist

Nurses are constantly faced with the need to provide comfort for patients in acute and long-term settings, in ambulatory settings, and in the home. Though the meanings of "comfort" are personal and individual, all nurses know generally what comfort is, and they know its opposite—suffering. Three of the problems that cause most human suffering are pain, fatigue, and nausea. They are seen in postoperative patients, patients with a variety of acute conditions, the chronically ill, and the terminally ill.

They occur in the tiny infant undergoing lifesaving procedures, in the adolescent with terminal cancer, in burn patients, in those struck by catastrophic illness, in the elderly with arthritis, and in patients of all ages who are receiving heavy doses of chemotherapy for cancer. Pain, fatigue, and nausea frequently occur as a triad. Any one of them has a profoundly distressing effect; together they create almost insurmountable difficulties.

Management of pain, fatigue, and nausea is complicated by the fact that all three share a common inexpressibility. As Scarry (1985) notes, pain is so certainly present for the person experiencing it that it is undeniable, but it is easy to "remain wholly unaware of its existence" in another person (p. 4). In part this is because pain is so difficult to describe. Scarry adds, "Physical pain does not simply resist language but actively destroys it, bringing about an immediate reversion to a state anterior to language, to the sounds and cries a human being makes before language is learned" (p. 4).

Though fatigue and nausea are perhaps less overwhelming than

3

pain, they too remain private, subjective experiences isolating the sufferer. Nurses are the people best equipped to confront this isolation and bring comfort to the suffering. To do so, they must have an understanding of the experience of suffering, the skills to assess its characteristics, and the tools to effectively reduce it—to provide comfort. Research can offer guidance in each of these areas. Yet, in spite of the existence of important and critical research in these areas, by and large practitioners are not using the research to enhance their practice (Kirchhoff, 1982; Brett, 1987).

Many explanations for this situation have been proposed—including barriers in the practice setting, lack of access to research reports and time to read them, and inadequate research skills and values of practitioners—but nearly all explanations include the notion that our current means for getting research information to practicing nurses are not adequate (Bohannon & LeVeau, 1986; Hunt, 1981; King, Barnard, & Hoehn, 1981; Kirchhoff, 1983; Miller & Messenger, 1978).

The two major channels for communicating research results are nursing journals and research conferences. Only a small portion of the nursing research conducted is ever published in journals, there is usually a sizeable time lag before publication, and the research is almost always published in "research" journals, which, as Chin and Jacobs (1983) note, are read mainly by researchers. Practitioners tend to read more practice-oriented journals. In addition, research on a particular topic may be scattered through several journals so that even those who read research consistently may have difficulty assessing the overall state of the research and its readiness for practice.

There are further problems. Researchers tend to write for other researchers. Bohannon and LeVeau (1986) and King et al. (1981) note that research articles are often presented in too technical a fashion for practitioners. Research "jargon" is the norm, findings are stated probabilistically, conclusions are couched in tentativeness, implications typically focus on further research rather than application, and the meaning of the knowledge for nursing practice is often ignored.

The research conferences that have sprung up around the country in the last few years represent a beginning effort to increase communication between researchers and clinicians, but often such conferences are rather fragmented, with presentations on widely varying topics so that it is difficult for the practitioner to come away with a coherent view of any one area. Frequently there has been no prior evaluation of scientific merit of the research presented, so the practitioner has to rely on his or her own skills to evaluate its quality. There is little focus on application, and, as with journals, the research is usually presented in a technical fashion most appropriate for other researchers. Further, conferences reach a rather narrow audience, and published proceedings, which reach a larger audience, usually parallel the conference and share its same shortcomings. Thus, as King et al. (1981) concluded several years ago, changes in both the kind of information disseminated and the medium of communication are needed.

This volume is one part of a multifaceted approach to improving the dissemination of nursing research. Our goal is to encourage the use of research in nursing practice through broad dissemination of research findings that are relevant and ready for use, in a form understandable to practicing nurses, with suggestions for implementation and further clinical evaluation, and with support and consultation during the implementation phase. There are three major components to the model: (1) topic-focused, practice oriented research conferences; (2) related, broadly distributed, carefully edited volumes based on the conference presentations; and (3) an information center to provide ongoing dialogue and consultation.

The first conference, in March 1988, was on key aspects of comfort— management of pain, fatigue, and nausea. This topic was selected because of its importance to the practice of nursing, its applicability to a broad range of settings, the availability of ongoing research in the area, the ability of nurses to control interventions, and the perceived gap between knowledge and practice. Researchers were invited through a national call to submit their research for presentation at the conference. Over 130 submissions were received. They were reviewed by a panel of 10 individuals with practice and research expertise in the areas of pain, fatigue, or nausea, or with methodological or statistical expertise. Papers were selected based on scientific merit, significance, and readiness for practice. The conference was structured to include information on the current bases for practice, the selected research papers, discussion sessions led by both clinicians and researchers that focused on moving the research into practice, strategies for implementation, and demonstration sessions.

This volume stems from the conference; its purpose is to provide a wider audience of practicing nurses with the most current research on pain, fatigue, and nausea—research that describes the occurrence and characteristics of these symptoms, research that presents instruments to measure their existence and qualities, and research that tests nursing-based interventions for their relief. Since the purpose of the volume is to present the latest in nursing research, the selected papers necessarily reflect the scope and focus of research today. However, descriptive, assessment, and intervention foci are balanced where possible. Negative findings are included when they are felt to illustrate important points. Replicated findings were preferred, but unreplicated research is also included if aspects of the findings are ready for informal use or clinical trials. Collectively, these works provide the clinician with the knowledge and means to enhance practice and improve patient comfort.

Each chapter has been edited extensively with the clinical audience in mind. Each study is presented as a full research report, but technical language is minimized, only directly relevant literature is cited, research methods are presented directly and simply, results sections focus on describing the major findings rather than the statistics, and discussion sections detail implications for practice. Separate sections on pain, fatigue, nausea, and general comfort are included. Introductory chapters describe the current bases for nursing practice in these areas. New research studies follow. A discussion of this new research, emphasizing implications for practice and directions for further research, concludes each section. There is also a comprehensive reference list at the end of each section.

This book represents an effort to effectively communicate research findings to clinicians. As such it is only one—though we think crucial—step in the process of moving from the conduct of research to its use in practice. The final chapter in the book describes strategies for using research in practice. As outlined in that concluding chapter, it is hoped that the clinician reading this book will take note of particularly relevant findings and begin to use the new knowlege in practice—whether informally through viewing patients' pain, fatigue, and nausea in a new light or formally through making changes in patient care. Always, the clinician should evaluate the impact of such changes.

To assist clinicians with this process, to allow them to share their implementation experiences with one another, and to afford clinicians and researchers an opportunity for dialogue, we have established an information center and a newsletter, *Nursing Research/Nursing Practice Connection*, which will provide a mechanism for such communication. Clinicians are invited and encouraged to share their implementation experiences with others through the center and its newsletter; researchers are invited to share their latest findings and updates of research on pain, fatigue, and nausea. Through an ongoing exchange of ideas and experiences of researchers and clinicians, patient care will truly be enhanced.

References

Bohannon, R. W., & LeVeau, B. F. (1986). Clinicians' use of research findings: A review of literature with implications for physical therapists. *Physical Therapy, 66,* 45–50.

Brett, J. L. (1987). Use of nursing practice research findings. *Nursing Research, 36,* 344–349.

Chin, P. L., & Jacobs, M. K. (1983). *Theory and nursing: A systematic approach.* St. Louis: The C. V. Mosby Co.

Hunt, J. (1981). Indicators for nursing practice: The use of research findings. *Journal of Advanced Nursing, 6,* 189–194.

King, D., Barnard, K. E., & Hoehn, R. (1981). Disseminating the results of nursing research. *Nursing Outlook, 29,* 164–169.

Kirchhoff, K. T. (1982). A diffusion survey of coronary precautions. *Nursing Research, 31,* 196–201.

Kirchhoff, K. T. (1983). Using research in practice: Should staff nurses be expected to use research? *Western Journal of Nursing Research, 5,* 245– 247.

Miller, J. R., & Messenger, S. R. (1978). Obstacles to applying nursing research findings. *American Journal of Nursing, 78,* 632–634.

Scarry, E. (1985). *The body in pain: The making and unmaking of the world.* New York: Oxford University Press.

[2]

Key Aspects of Comfort

Ada K. Jacox

The choice of comfort as the umbrella concept for a volume on research for nursing practice seems particularly appropriate. The idea that nursing is concerned with providing comfort is well accepted, and the aspects of comfort considered here—pain, fatigue, and nausea— are phenomena commonly experienced by patients and managed by nurses.

The chapters represent a broad spectrum of concerns and contain a wealth of information useful to clinicians. Volumes that focus on making research findings useful to clinicians are needed by our profession as a way of translating research and disseminating the findings so that they can be used in practice. It is encouraging to see this kind of development in nursing and it is one more indication that nursing is coming of age.

Only a few decades ago, there was only one journal concerned primarily with nursing research. Now, there are half a dozen, but just as important, many of the specialty journals regularly publish research-based articles and have research columns. Additionally, national, regional, and local conferences of nurses commonly include presentations of research relevant to practice. We have moved beyond the stage of advocating research-based practice to implementing it, although clearly there is considerable research yet needed.

Nurses' commitment to research also is reflected in the establishment of the National Center for Nursing Research within the National Institutes of Health (NIH) in 1986. This was a remarkable achievement for nursing. It required the concerted efforts of the major nursing organizations and of nurse researchers, administrators, and clinicians to make it clear that the public will be better served if nursing practice is firmly based on research and nursing will be better served if its research programs are part of the broader scientific community. The National Center for Nursing Research is concerned not only with the support of research projects, but also with dissemination of research results. This volume and the conference on which it is based represent one expression of the latter function.

The importance of the key aspects of comfort discussed in this volume was underlined by an invitational conference held by the National Center for Nursing Research in January 1988 to begin defining a national nursing research agenda. The preliminary priorities identified included nursing interventions to prevent or minimize complications associated with hospitalization or treatment, particularly infection, nausea and vomiting due to chemotherapy, falls, and pressure sores; and nursing interventions to prevent or minimize the pain resulting from aversive procedures or pathophysiological conditions. Pain was identified by one group of participants as one of the five highest priorities for nursing research, because nurses are responsible for managing pain; because it is universal, cuts across all acute illnesses, and affects cognitive, sensory, and biologic functions; and because there are nursing interventions directed at pain. The conference also identified maintenance of physiological and psychological integrity, including promotion of comfort, as a priority for the chronically ill. Thus, high priority was placed on research dealing with pain, comfort, nausea and vomiting, and similar concepts at this initial conference.

THEORETICAL CONSIDERATIONS

Pain, nausea, and fatigue represent dimensions of the broader concept of comfort; other dimensions include depression, anxiety, insomnia, and dyspnea. All of these concepts are multidimensional; that is, they include both biological and behavioral aspects and they are also related to one another. It is quite common, for example, to find that unrelieved pain leads to fatigue, which in turn makes the pain even more difficult to tolerate. It is also at times hard to distinguish between these phenomena, making it difficult to know whether a patient is experiencing anxiety, pain, nausea, some combination of them, or something else. These and related concepts are overlapping and interactive, reflecting the complex nature of many of the phenomena with which nurses deal.

The complexity must be taken into account in several ways. First, the complexity is important in the theoretical connections among these concepts and in their connections to other concepts important for intervention or management. Second, the complexity affects research, which must be planned to either control for some of the complexity or take it into account in other ways. Finally, the question of how these phenomena can be managed successfully in patients is made more difficult by their complexity, in part because we do not yet understand them well enough.

Let us consider first how to organize the concepts in relation to one another, or how to specify a theoretical framework that will be useful for practice. There is nothing so practical as a good theory that adequately reflects clinical reality and provides the clinician with guidelines for patient care. I'm not referring to the global, broad nursing theories, although those are useful for certain purposes. Rather, I am talking about the usefulness of specifying more precisely how concepts are related to one another. This can be done in a number of ways: I will discuss two of them to illustrate the kinds of activities that clinicians and researchers must undertake together to produce clinically useful research.

One way to organize concepts is through nursing diagnoses, first referred to by McManus in 1950. During the past 15 years, a considerable amount of work has been done in the development of nursing diagnoses. Although they are becoming increasingly useful in helping nurses think about their practice in different ways, there remain considerable difficulties with them. This is true in part because of the atheoretical and eclectic nature of the process used to identify nursing diagnoses and in part because of the political problems in trying to identify phenomena that are not already in the domain of medicine.

At the First National Conference for Classification of Nursing Diagnoses in 1973, participants were asked to identify "health problems or health states diagnosed by nurses and treated by means of nursing intervention" (Gebbie & Lavin, 1975, p. 1). Subsequent revisions resulted in a list of 50 diagnostic concepts accepted by the North American Nursing Diagnosis Association (NANDA) for clinical testing (Gordon, 1985). There is consensus that the NANDA list, which is perhaps the most widely used, is incomplete and not yet sufficiently validated (Gordon, 1985). For example, with regard to the concepts discussed in this volume, pain is viewed as a nursing diagnosis, fatigue has been accepted as one of approximately 20 diagnoses to be tested, but nausea and vomiting are not yet on the list. Their absence reflects both the incomplete nature of the list and the problems in trying to identify nursing phenomena that are separate from medical phenomena.

Several years ago, I was requested to speak at a conference on nursing diagnoses about the research that I had done on discomfort. I said that I had not done research on discomfort but on pain. I was told that pain was a medical term and not a nursing diagnosis. I said that I had studied pain, that the patients knew that I was studying pain, that nurses with whom I discussed my research understood that I had studied pain, and that it was confusing to call it something else.

This illustrates some of the difficulty in trying to define nursing phenomena as if there were no overlap with medical phenomena. Nursing and medicine are different disciplines, but there is considerable overlap between the sorts of things that nurses and physicians are concerned with, and it is not useful to patients or to clinicians to try to call them by different names. While the phenomena may be the same, disciplines often deal with them differently, however. When I was studying pain, I was struck by the difference between the way physicians use the concept and the way nurses use it. In medical textbooks, discussion of pain usually is limited to how various aspects of pain can be used in diagnosing a disease or injury. Little attention is given, except in pharmacology books, to ways to deal with patients' pain. Nurses, on the other hand, are interested in what is causing the pain, but their primary focus is on how to assess and manage it. This is true of a number of the other symptoms that are of interest to both physicians and nurses, but for different reasons. This is not said in a critical way, but only to distinguish between the use that the two professions make of the same concepts.

We must name concepts in ways that are meaningful to patients as well as to nurses and other health professionals. Concepts such as pain, fatigue, nausea and vomiting, depression, anxiety, insomnia, and dyspnea have well understood meanings. Furthermore, all are within the purview of nursing to diagnose and manage. The notion that nursing diagnoses must be totally distinct from medical diagnoses or conditions can lead to the notion that the interventions ought also to be separate, as should the patient outcomes; both of these ideas are potentially misleading and overly constrictive of nursing practice. The intent here is not to argue that we should not develop nursing diagnoses, but simply to say that they should make clinical as well as political sense, and that we must recognize their very early stage of development. Further, those who are developing nursing diagnoses understand the early stage of development and their tentativeness. They invite the testing and submission of new diagnoses.

A second way of grouping concepts is that developed by Catherine Norris, who, in a book published in 1982 titled Concept Clarification, proposed the umbrella concept of protection. Norris chose her concepts in an eclectic way and ended with a theoretical synthesis. She selected concepts that are common human problems, are classified at lower levels in hierarchies of need, occur frequently, and are phenomena that nurses are expected to do something about. She also tried to eliminate medical phenomena as much as possible. "For example," she said, "the understanding of myocardial infarct is necessary to medicine. It is interesting to nurses, but nurses do not work with it. Concepts necessary to nursing in this context might be dyspnea, restlessness, and nausea. Physicians are interested in these behaviors, but their real focus is on the treatment of the infarction" (Norris, 1982, p. xvii). The concepts included in Norris's book are long-term itching, nausea and vomiting, thirst, hunger, shivering, fatigue, insomnia, disorientation, immobilization, and pressure sores. These are interesting concepts and clearly of relevance to nursing. Norris claims that these concepts and the following five belong to nursing: diarrhea, constipation, flatulence, urinary frequency, and perspiration. She describes these phenomena as basic physiologic protective mechanisms that fit under the umbrella concept of protection. In the thoughtfully analytic manner characteristic of her writing, she concludes that "all of the phenomena . . . are related. Taken as a whole, they reflect a comprehensive mechanism for survival—cellular adjustment and cellular repair—in terms of threat to an organism's total integrity. These protective mechanisms originate at precortical or subcortical levels as reflex actions or, in some cases (e.g., hunger and thirst) as drives" (Norris, 1982, p. 402). While Norris certainly does not exclude psychosocial phenomena from nursing's concern, she focuses on physiological mechanisms because of her belief that they have not received adequate attention in the development of nursing's knowledge base.

While Norris's formulations are due considerable respect, I am not suggesting that they, any more than nursing diagnoses, be adopted in their entirety by nursing. These two ways of organizing nursing concepts are described simply to suggest the beginning and tentative nature of the work underway that is attempting to systematically organize and study phenomena that have long histories in nursing. In doing this it is important that we recognize the early stage, not of nursing certainly, but of nursing's attempt to identify, organize, and study its concepts. In doing this, we must not shy away from claiming domains that are also claimed by others. Our practice clearly overlaps with that of physicians and others, and we must not pretend or be persuaded otherwise. Nurses must be free to identify, label, and study those phenomena with which they are most concerned. This is no easy task and it is important that we not come to premature closure in accepting any one set of concepts as nursing's.

In identifying those concepts of greatest relevance for nursing practice, we also should pay more attention to phenomena that are important to patients and that cause them discomfort or distress. When a patient, for example, I experienced rather distressing phenomena that the physicians and nurses did not know about except in a general way, and had little or no knowledge of how to manage. In a related vein, Copp (1974) observed that patients in her study who had tried various methods to relieve pain were reluctant to try them in a hospital because they were afraid that their coping behaviors might be against the rules or laughed at as not scientific. There are probably numerous other experiences that patients have that are not acknowledged or studied by health professionals. In identifying and studying relevant nursing concepts and methods for relieving discomfort, we need to be sensitive to phenomena that have not yet been named, whether they are to be named by clinicians or by patients.

THE CONCEPT OF COMFORT

Let us now turn to the key concept for this volume—comfort, a concept closely identified with nursing. The noun *comfort* is defined as "a state or feeling of having relief, encouragement, or consolation . . . physical or mental well being, especially in freedom from want, anxiety, pain, or trouble . . . something that gives or brings comfort . . . "; as a verb it means "to make strong, strengthen, encourage; make secure; invigorate . . . assist, help, . . . to impart strength and hope . . . to relieve especially of mental distress . . . to make comfortable" (*Webster's*, 1959, p. 454). The concept of comfort is a broad one that encompasses physical, biological, and psychosocial aspects. It is multidimensional and encompasses numerous other concepts.

Interestingly, little research has been done on the concept of comfort, except for its subcomponents, such as pain, nausea and vomiting, and fatigue. The word is widely used in the nursing literature, but usually without definition, since the meaning of comfort seems to be so universally understood. Comfort measures are identified in nursing texts; for example, the following list is given by Beland (cited in Watson, 1979, p. 90):

1. Removing noxious stimuli from the external environment (e.g., bright lights, loud or sudden noises, inadequate heating and ventilation, and untidy surroundings).
2. Giving attention to the position of the patient and frequently changing her or his position.

3. Making the bed comfortable.
4. Relieving muscle tension by range-of-motion exercises, a back rub, or a therapeutic massage.
5. Performing therapeutic procedures (e.g., applying warm, moist packs, giving a warm bath, administering prescribed pain-relieving medications, inhalation exercises and treatment, relaxation, and meditation exercises).
6. Identifying the implications of illness for the patient and the use of the available resources for support or protection. Preparing the patient for what to expect and what is expected while maximizing the patient's control, choices, and alternatives.
7. Modifying approaches to the patient in relation to the severity, extent, and phase of care.

The list reflects a wide range of activities designed to promote comfort.

In Chapter 35, Hamilton explores how the chronically ill hospitalized elderly define comfort. She notes five recurring themes: comfort as related to hospital life, the approach and attitudes of staff, self esteem, the disease process, and positioning. These findings show the broad scope of the concept of comfort.

A number of years ago I became interested in what patients meant when they said they were experiencing discomfort, because it was apparent that, when questioned about the amount of pain they were experiencing, patients' understanding of what they were being asked about differed from what the interviewers thought they were questioning them about.

At the beginning of each interview, patients were asked if they were currently in pain. Ten or fifteen minutes later, they were given a six-point pain scale to complete. Zero indicated no pain; 1, mild pain; 2, discomforting; 3, distressing; 4, horrible; and 5, excruciating. Twenty-five percent of the patients who said they were not in pain at the beginning of the interview later checked 1 or 2 on the pain scale, indicating that they were experiencing mild or discomforting pain. Some patients did not identify what they were experiencing as pain if it was only mild or discomforting. The question raised by this finding was, "If it was not pain, what was it?" (Jacox, 1979).

We asked patients to describe the kinds of experiences they considered to be painful events and the kinds of experience they considered to produce discomfort. From their responses, 30 events or conditions were listed; 200 additional patients were then asked to classify each condition in terms of whether or not they had ever experienced it, and if they had, whether they characterized it as pain, discomfort, or neither. The event that most people agreed was painful was slamming a finger in the door. Ninety-six percent of the patients identified this as painful and four percent as uncomfortable. The highest agreement among patients on what constituted discomfort was itching. Eighty percent defined it as producing discomfort, seven percent as painful, and thirteen percent as neither.

In general, those experiences defined as painful included primarily sharp, throbbing, or acute physical sensations. The experiences defined as producing discomfort had to do with psychosocial situations such as lack of kindness or waiting for a new procedure to be done. Sensations defined as producing discomfort generally were those producing pressure or associated with dullness or aching.

This illustrates the overlap between the concepts of discomfort and pain, but the same kind of overlap exists in all of the concepts considered in this volume. The concepts are overlapping in that they share some common elements. Additionally, as we have seen, what one person defines as pain, another will define as discomfort, and another as neither.

Sometimes, for the purpose of measuring concepts, attempts are made to define them in mutually exclusive ways, so that behaviors categorized in one category cannot also be categorized in another. While it may be possible to separate some of these concepts analytically, in practice they are frequently seen together, and the attempt to define them in mutually exclusive ways is not useful for clinical purposes.

In addition to overlapping, the concepts are interactive: they tend to influence each other. For example, someone who is very anxious may interpret a noxious stimulus as being very painful, and then in turn become more anxious. There often is a cycle that occurs among these and other concepts. Norris (1982, pp. 394–397) gives the following illustrations: "Fatigue may accompany nausea . . . fatigue may follow vomiting . . . fatigue may precede, accompany, or follow disorientation." And so forth. Additionally, "Insomnia often precedes or accompanies disorientation . . . insomnia may accompany or be preceded by fatigue . . . insomnia often accompanies itching . . . insomnia may precede or accompany bedsores . . . . Nausea often accompanies pain and also may occur in immobilization and bedsores." We know that extreme pain may produce fatigue, that anxiety may increase pain, and that each of these may be related to depression and dyspnea. In research reported in this volume, for example, Crosby shows that pain and depression are related in a group of patients with rheumatoid arthritis.

Thus far we have considered some of the problems involved in identifying, naming, and organizing concepts of relevance to nursing, and some of the research reporting their overlapping and interactive nature. Let us now turn briefly to some methodological issues, including the kinds of research and research approaches needed.

METHODOLOGICAL CONSIDERATIONS

It is clear that we still don't know very much about the incidence of many of these phenomena, and there is need for a great deal of descriptive research documenting the circumstances under which the phenomena are present singly or in combination. At an NIH consensus conference on the management of pain held in May 1986, one of the recommendations was to conduct epidemiological studies of the incidence and prevalence of pain. We don't know what constitutes an average course of pain for patients experiencing different conditions and treatments. We don't even know the peak periods of pain for patients undergoing many surgical procedures. Norris (1982) points to the absence of research on nausea and vomiting and notes that the vast majority of the studies that have been reported deal with nausea related to drugs under research. While there is some research related to vomiting in selected pathologies, she found only seven published articles related to nausea from 1965 to 1980, and only three of these were research reports. Some articles reported on nausea and vomiting in cancer patients, which seems to be nursing's current focus of interest in the study of nausea and vomiting.

Similar observations were made by Hart and Freel with regard to fatigue: "While the occurrence of fatigue is expected to accompany and, at times, be a precursor to most pathological conditions, few attempts have been made to describe the phenomenon, its expected duration, or its course as it is related to pathological change" (1982, p. 259). We need careful and detailed descriptions of the incidence and patterns of pain, nausea, fatigue, and other discomforts commonly experienced by patients.

In addition to descriptive studies of the phenomena related to comfort, we need experimental studies that test the effectiveness of nursing interventions in relieving the distressing symptoms of pain, nausea, fatigue, depression, and anxiety. Just as both psychosocial and biological factors play a role in the etiology of these phenomena, so must the interventions reflect both behavioral and biological dimensions. Perhaps partly in response to medicine's clear dominance over interventions that are biologically, anatomically, or chemically based, nurses have tended to develop and use interventions which are more psychosocially based. While this is understandable and promotes the development of research complementary to medical research, it is also important that nurses develop and study interventions that are biologically, anatomically, chemically, and even electronically based, since many such interventions can be safely and effectively used by nurses.

Some representative nursing interventions described by Bulecheck and McCloskey, in *Nursing Interventions: Treatments for Nursing Diagnoses* (1985), illustrates this emphasis on testing psychosocially based nursing interventions. The interventions include relaxation training (actually a combination of biological and psychological components), cognitive reappraisal, music therapy, patient contracting, counseling, nutritional counseling, sexual counseling, reminiscence therapy, patient teaching, exercise (with both biological and psychological components), group psychotherapy, preparatory sensory information, and active listening. This is not an exhaustive list but it does represent the kinds of interventions included in the book. The observation that these are primarily psychosocial is not a criticism of the book, for the book reflects nursing research and practice. Beland's list of comfort measures discussed earlier in this chapter included such interventions as frequently changing the patient's position, relieving muscle tension by range of motion exercises, a back rub or a therapeutic massage, applying warm moist packs, and so forth. Much of what nurses do for patients requires biological or a combination of biological and psychosocial knowledge, and interventions must be designed to include both aspects. This echoes Norris's concern that nursing have a balanced focus in the development of its knowledge base, and it is pleasing to see such a combination of interventions reflected in the chapters in this volume.

The phenomena associated with comfort should not be studied in isolation from each other, since they so commonly occur together in patients. While it may be necessary in the beginning to isolate one or two phenomena for study, such as the relationship between pain and anxiety, more complex studies are needed to understand how these phenomena influence each other and are influenced by other factors as well. There is a need to study the inter-relationships among phenomena in both descriptive and experimental studies. This represents the necessary next step in our understanding of these complex phenomena.

Still another methodological issue is the type of research approach to use. One measure of how far we have progressed in recent years is that it is now unnecessary to spend much time urging an emphasis on qualitative as well as quantitative approaches in our research. While there is still some lingering bias among the logical positivists who believe that nothing is really scientific unless it is quantitatively measured, there is considerably more acceptance of the validity of the qualitative approach, and of combined quantitative and qualitative approaches. We have moved beyond the need to advocate the use of qualitative methods. The acceptance of qualitative as well as quantitative research in the study of nursing problems is much more consistent with nursing's holistic philosophy than was the more constrictive logical positivism that dominated science into the 1960s.

There are still some problems remaining. We need more research in more settings and larger samples; we also need to recognize the value of case studies along with instrument development, descriptive, and experimental studies. Earlier in nursing, case studies were used almost exclusively in describing patient problems, and they acquired a bad reputation. Perhaps we've all grown up enough now to see the value in well done case studies that provide insights into phenomena that can then be explored more systematically.

Moving from a concern with research approaches, I would note the need for replication of research. The research done in nursing is impressive in scope and depth, as illustrated in the *Annual Review of Nursing Research*, an ongoing series initiated by Harriet Werley and Joyce Fitzpatrick, of which six volumes have been published (1983–1988). One of the striking things about the research summarized and synthesized in those volumes is the lack of replication of studies. The same situation was noted in a major research utilization project called the Conduct and Utilization of Research in Nursing (1982), carried out in Michigan in the 1970s. This project tried to recommend for practice only research that had been replicated, but precious little of it was found. Serious attention needs to be given to identifying promising descriptive and experimental studies conducted in one setting and with one population, and repeating these in other settings with other populations. In our emphasis on doing an original piece of work, we have tended to overlook the value of careful replication.

Finally, we must become more involved in interdisciplinary teams conducting research. Nurses' involvement should not be merely as collectors of data or performers of the intervention, but as coinvestigators who are involved in the planning, implementation, analysis, and publication of the research findings. Just as a nursing perspective adds to the overall value of the treatment team, so can that perspective increase the value of the research conducted. The NIH consensus conference on pain mentioned earlier involved quite a number of nurses both in the conference planning and the presentation of research findings. Nursing research was acknowledged as important, and the role of the nurse in managing pain and on the interdisciplinary team dealing with pain was emphasized. The same kind of involvement by nurses needs to occur in interdisciplinary research on nausea, fatigue, insomnia, dyspnea, and other phenomena that cross disciplines. Don't be afraid to join an interdisciplinary team as a fully participating member. Your perspective is a valuable one and you will contribute to the significance of the research.

PRACTICE CONSIDERATIONS

To conclude, let us consider briefly some practice issues. At times, nursing is criticized as being overly routinized, because it often is. There is great need for nurses to use creative and thoughtful approaches in dealing with complex clinical problems. Such approaches require the ability to understand and evaluate the knowledge available for practice. Any nurse graduating from a baccalaureate degree program or above has at least a basic understanding of research. The dissemination of research findings will be further facilitated by the insistence that those doing the research translate it into language understandable to nonresearchers and publish it in general and specialty journals. In this volume, for example, authors have been encouraged to emphasize the findings of research and the implications for clinical practice. Making research understandable in this way will promote its dissemination and implementation in practice.

As we would expect, a number of the chapters in this volume report studies of the development of measurement instruments, or are descriptive in nature. There are more experimental studies in adult pain than in children's pain, and that is a reflection of the fact that there has been substantially more work done generally in the field of adult pain, and thus nurses have more to draw on. In contrast, nurses have provided the leadership in studying children's pain, both in assessment and now in moving to interventions. In fatigue and nausea, we see some of the same beginning focus on developing measurement instruments and assessing and describing the phenomena, with relatively few experiments—that's to be expected. These areas of study will have the same sort of developmental course that has occurred in adult pain. This volume reflects where we are in nursing research generally, and it shows good progress.

The interventions presented here are both biologically and behaviorally based, with nurses doing pioneering work in testing the behavioral interventions, particularly for patients experiencing pain. There is evidence that assessment instruments and interventions are being used in practice. There are numerous pain flow charts in use, and a handy visual analogue scale that patients can use to indicate their pain. Pain audits are being done to determine whether or not pain is being adequately managed.

To give a brief historical perspective on pain research, 20 years ago, when I first became interested in the study of pain, there was virtually no nursing research in the literature. Wanda McDowell at Ohio State University had published a little red book on how to assess patients' pain that I carried around for years. A few years later Dorothy Crowley wrote a monograph on pain that was very useful. And then in the early 1970s Jean Johnson and I separately began to publish in the area, then Laurel Copp and Margo McCaffery. We now have moved to the point where there is a third generation of researchers.

We should see similar occurrences in the study of fatigue, nausea, and other phenomena involved in comfort. That is how professions evolve into maturity, and that is what nursing is doing. There has been tremendous growth in clinical practice. There are research programs of individual nurses and teams of researchers, and the research is becoming cumulative. We can be pleased by the amount and quality of the research presented here. The designs and analyses reflect increased sophistication in those areas. We have the beginnings of a community of scholars, and that is an important milestone in nursing's development.

In translation of research findings into practice, we clearly have a good bit of work to do. There is need for increased attention to research and development in clinical agencies; any major nursing service in 1988 is incomplete without a program of research and development. More and more agencies are employing nurse researchers to carry out studies and to help practicing nurses learn how to implement the results of those and other studies—and we need a great deal more of that.

Nurse clinicians need to be creative in trying some of the numerous interventions suggested in our research literature. This is not to say that findings from a single study can be immediately applied in all situations. It is possible, however, to take the ideas that work in one setting and with one group of patients and try them in preliminary work with other patients. This, of course, requires a knowledge of the intervention, how to use it, and how to evaluate its effectiveness. Some of this preliminary and exploratory work will lead to the development of more systematic research.

It is true that in many settings nursing is highly routinized, and in such settings creative use of new knowledge is neither required nor perhaps even tolerated. This climate is responsible for much of the frustration and dissatisfaction with practice that have long been expressed by nurses. For this to change, nurses must be more aggressive in insisting on the ability to practice professional nursing. This means having the freedom and expectation that patient problems will be carefully evaluated by nurses, who will then use whatever knowledge is available to deal with them. This kind of reflective practice based on research findings as well as other experience is required if nurses are to deal successfully with the many patient care problems confronting them. Researchers, therefore, should take very seriously their work in developing the knowledge base for practice, and clinicians should be creative, thoughtful, and assertive in using this knowledge in the interest of patients.

References

Bulecheck, G. M., & McCloskey, J. C. (1985). *Nursing interventions: Treatments for nursing diagnoses.* Philadelphia: W.B. Saunders Co.

Conduct and Utilization of Research in Nursing (CURN) Project. Using Research to Improve Nursing Practice. (1982). New York: Grune & Stratton, Inc. 11 volumes, 1548 pages.

Copp, L. A. (1974). The spectrum of suffering. *American Journal of Nursing, 74,* 491–495.

Fitzpatrick, J. J., & Taunton, R. L. (Eds.). (1987). *Annual Review of Nursing Research, 5.*

Fitzpatrick, J. J., Taunton, R. L., & Benoliel, J. Q. (Eds.). (1988). *Annual Review of Nursing Research, 6.*

Gebbie, K. M., & Lavin, M. A. (Eds.). (1975). *Classification of nursing diagnoses: Proceedings of the first national conference.* St. Louis: The C. V. Mosby Co.

Gordon, M. (1985). Nursing diagnosis. *Annual Review of Nursing Research, 3,* 131.

Hart, L. K., & Freel, M. I. (1982). Fatigue. In C. M. Norris (Ed.), *Concept clarification,* (pp. 251–261). Rockville, MD: Aspen Systems Corporation.

Jacox, A. K. (1979). Pain assessment. *American Journal of Nursing, 79,* 895–900.

McManus, L. (1950). Assumptions of functions in nursing. In Teachers College, Division of Nursing Education, *Regional planning for nursing and nursing education.* New York: Teachers College Press.

Norris, C. M. (1982). *Concept clarification.* Rockville, MD: Aspens Systems Corporation.

National Institutes of Health. (1986). *Consensus development conference statement. The integrated approach to the management of pain, USHHS, 6* (3), (document no. 491–292; 41148).

Watson, J. (1979). *Nursing: The philosophy and science of caring.* Boston: Little, Brown, & Co.

Webster's third new international dictionary of the English language unabridged, Vol. 1, A-G. (1959). Chicago: Encyclopedia Britannica, Inc.

Werley, H. H., & Fitzpatrick, J. J. (Eds.). (1983–1985). *Annual Review of Nursing Research, 1–3.*

Werley, H. H., Fitzpatrick, J. J., & Taunton, R. L. (Eds.). (1986). *Annual Review of Nursing Research, 4.*

Part II

PAIN

[3]

Relieving Pain: The Current Bases for Practice

Marilee I. Donovan

Current practice in the management of pain represents a collage of reactions to a conception of pain that has evolved over thousands of years. Only a small percentage of what we do to manage pain is grounded in research.

Aristotle, in the 4th century B.C., believed that pain was an emotion. Today there are still those who practice, study, and publish in a manner that suggests that they believe pain is primarily an emotional reaction that can be conquered by willpower. For instance, the *Time-Life* science series published in the early 1970s mentioned pain in only two sections: "The Mind" and "Health and Disease," under emotions.

In the Middle Ages, pain was viewed as possession by demons, punishment for sins, and the will of God. Our Puritan heritage is woefully evident today in statements such as "You'll have to wait another hour. It isn't time for your pain medication yet." "A little pain won't hurt you." "Grin and bear it." "Just a few seconds longer . . . you can take it . . . ." Research reported by Rankin and Snyder (1984), by my colleagues and myself (Donovan & Dillon, 1987; Donovan, Dillon, & McGuire, 1987), and by Halvorson and Page (1988) demonstrates that caregivers do not have the goal of total relief of pain for patients. John Kilwein, a pharmacist in Pittsburgh, proposes that our culture long ago embraced the philosophical notion that pain has some redeeming value and says that Puritanism, disguised as medical science, leads to undermedication of patients in pain. Pain is viewed as a moral weakness; caregivers are unwilling to give doses of analgesics that are adequate to provide relief; fears of addiction are exaggerated and patients suffer needlessly (Kilwein, 1983).

In the 19th century, the role of the nervous system in the transmission of pain was discovered, and thus began our romance with neurosurgery and anesthesia. It was acceptable to sever or block a nerve's transmission (perceived as removing the pain), even while it was a sign of weakness or a breach of morality to treat or medicate the pain (cover it up). These beliefs are still evident among patients, family members, and caregivers. They often act in a way that reflects the beliefs that freedom from pain is bad, that covering up pain is dangerous, and that suffering has merit. In our research, we asked caregivers what they would do if a patient who was receiving morphine 12 mg q4 hours reported total pain relief and some feelings of mild euphoria. One third of those responding said they would reduce the dose of the narcotic because of the euphoria.

Here is another example my staff reported to me: A young adult patient suffering the pain of stomatitis during the process of bone marrow transplantation was receiving meperidine intravenous push q3h prn. He confided that sometimes he wasn't really experiencing that much pain but he liked the feelings he got from the meperidine.

I suspect that the majority of us like the feelings associated with wine and cocktails. Do we deserve those feelings more than a 19-year-old whose life is in danger and who has been isolated for weeks? I do not condone the use of intravenous meperidine to improve a patient's feelings about life; for that I would suggest hypnosis to capture the state of euphoria and relaxation. However, the judgments made about this patient, the punitive approaches taken by some of his caregivers, and the conclusion that the patient was an addict are unacceptable, unfounded, a violation of the contract with the patient, and possibly bordering on abuse.

Most caregivers have had some exposure to the delaying tactics of physicians and nurses who do not administer analgesics because they cover up pain. The implication is that the existence of pain is essential for diagnostic purposes. But how often is pain really used for diagnosis? How many myocardial infarcts are treated without EKG and laboratory confirmation? How many fractures are cast without an x-ray? How much surgery is attempted without x-ray, laboratory, or biopsy indications? Fifty years ago, symptoms were the determinants of treatment. However, contemporary medicine treats objective findings on a chart, not subjective findings such as pain.

Why do rational physicians and nurses respond to patients' pain in the ways we have described?

Patients themselves may hold beliefs that lead to undertreatment of pain. They don't expect total pain relief, they fear "covering up" pain, and they want to be "good" patients who don't complain and don't take too much medication.

It wasn't until Melzack and Wall (1965) proposed the Gate Control Theory of pain that we gained a more integrated view of pain and pain management. The most significant additions made by Melzack and Wall to the understanding of pain were their identifications of (1) the gating mechanism by which painful impulses are modulated in the dorsal horn of the spinal cord before ascending to the thalamus and cortex, where they are recognized as pain; and (2) the interacting effects of cognitive and emotional processes within the cerebral cortex and midbrain on the transmission of painful impulses. The Gate Control Theory acknowledges that emotional states (moods), learning, knowledge, and thought processes help to determine whether the gating mechanism in the spinal cord allows or stops the transmission of pain impulses.

This suggestion of a link between cortical processes and pain transmission reactivated interest in the relationships between psychological states and pain perception. Indeed, the Gate Control Theory of pain stimulated the development of a new field in psychology. The resulting interest in the effects of cognitive, emotional, and cultural variables on the pain experience is evident in several of the chapters in this volume. Depression, anxiety, mood in general, and temperament are commonly investigated. Patients' perceptions and the methods by which patients cope with pain are also considered important areas for research.

In the decade that followed Melzack and Wall's work, new methods of pain assessment and management began to be used and tested. Multidimensional pain assessments became essential. The McGill Pain Questionnaire (MPQ) (Melzack, 1975), a tool to quantify the sensory, affective, and evaluative components of the pain experience, became the most widely accepted method of describing and quantifying pain. If the MPQ wasn't appropriate, wasn't sensitive enough, or could not be completed by the patient, there was little available to assist the clinician assessing a patient's pain.

However, we cannot blame the lack of sophisticated assessment tools for the poor treatment of pain reported in our acute care institutions (Donovan, Dillon, & McGuire, 1987; Marks & Sachar, 1973). Our current research indicates that many physicians and nurses do not even ask patients, "Are you in pain?" or seek to quantify the intensity of the pain using a simple verbal scale ("If 0 is no pain and 10 is the worst pain imaginable, how much pain do you have right now?") (Donovan, Slack, & Wright, 1988).

Melzack and Wall's view that the dorsal horn, the brain stem, and the cortex play essential roles in enhancing, modulating, and integrating the pain experience brought a more holistic view of pain than earlier theories of pain had allowed. But the view that pain was an individual experience was inaugurated by nurses like Laurel Copp (1974) and Margo McCaffery (1972).

Soon a variety of new techniques for pain management emerged. Many of these are discussed in the pages that follow. Hypnosis, imagery, distraction, music therapy, laughter, and sensory information can be broadly classified as behavioral or cognitive approaches to the management of pain. The rationale for their use comes from the Gate Control Theory, which links cognitive and emotional functioning with the transmission and perception of pain.

Cutaneous stimulation (i.e., the application of heat, cold, massage), acupuncture, transcutaneous electrical nerve stimulation (TENS), and implanted electrical stimulation of the dorsal horn and thalamus have also become increasingly common in practice. Cutaneous stimulation techniques interfere with the transmission of pain impulses, lessening the perception of pain. Biofeedback is both a distraction technique that modulates incoming painful stimuli and a method of reducing the muscle activity that may be contributing to the pain. Patients' use and evaluation of many of these techniques are explored in the chapters in this volume.

In the mid–1970s endogenous opiates were discovered (Pert & Snyder, 1973), which drew attention to epidural analgesia. Nonnarcotic analgesics were considered the panacea of the early 1980s. However, the hoped-for therapy (epidural analgesia or nonnarcotic analgesic) that would be simple, universally effective, nonaddicting, without side effects, and inexpensive, and that did not lead to patients' developing a tolerance, met every patient's needs, and required little nursing time was elusive. Nonnarcotic analgesics were often as addicting as narcotics; epidural analgesia produced greater side effects than expected, and tolerance developed rapidly in some patients. Some patients even develop tolerance to the effects of TENS units. Interventions that require large expenditures of nursing time have become less acceptable as a result of prospective reimbursement and the nursing shortage. Even the intervention that seems to be most effective, patient-controlled analgesia (PCA), is not embraced by all patients. Thus, there is still no panacea for pain.

And twenty years of information from hospice programs in the United States and England have done little to correct the misconceptions and practices of caregivers. It is still commonly, but erroneously, believed that tolerance inevitably develops if a patient is given narcotics on a regular basis. The fear of addiction remains common among patients, family members, physicians, and nurses despite large studies indicating a risk of less than 1% (Porter & Jick, 1980). The erroneous belief that morphine commonly produces life-threatening respiratory depression has been reinforced most effectively by the notorious *Journal of the American Medical Association* article, "It's Over, Debbie" (1988). The result of this belief is that patients are undermedicated. Our most recent study found that the average dose of narcotic ordered for 102 medical inpatients was still below therapeutic levels, and that the average dose taken by the patient was 1/4 to 1/3 of that ordered. This confirms the earlier findings of Marks and Sachar (1973) and Donovan, Dillon, and McGuire (1987).

We now have the ability to modulate or reduce pain at four points: (1) At the peripheral site of pain, nonnarcotic analgesics, the application of heat and cold, and local anesthetics can alter the release of nociceptive substances and decrease accompanying muscle spasm response; (2) in the spinal cord, stimulation of large nerve fibers (by direct electrical stimulation, massage, application of heat or cold, and therapeutic touch), epidural analgesics, and neurosurgical procedures can interfere with the transmission of pain impulses; (3) in the brainstem, electrical stimulation, acupuncture, treatment of the emotional reaction component, narcotic analgesics and neurosurgical procedures can effectively reduce or eliminate the transmission of pain impulses; and (4) in the cortex, cognitive techniques (hypnosis, imagery, music therapy, relaxation), behavioral training, narcotic and narcotic antagonist analgesics, and tricyclic antidepressants provide additional methods to control the pain experience. With all of these interventions available, one would expect that pain would usually be adequately controlled.

However, that is not the case. In 1986 the NIH-sponsored consensus conference on pain concluded that despite all of the resources and therapies available, acute pain and cancer pain are significantly undertreated and chronic pain is often overmedicated. The assessment and treatment of children are significantly worse than the care of adults with pain (National Institutes of Health, 1986).

The following model of pain may help to explain why this is occurring and what we could do to correct the situation. The Gate Control Theory of pain has established that pain is a complex, multidimensional experience. Loesser (1986) has suggested a different way of viewing this multidimensional phenomenon (see Figure 3.1). According to Loesser, the biochemical and neurological activity that is the basis of the Gate Control Theory is only the inner core of the pain phenomenon. The perception of pain surrounds this essential core and is

FIGURE 3.1.   The model of pain assessment.

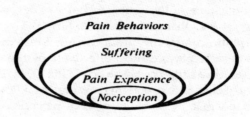

in part a response to it. This perception is in turn encircled by the personal experience of suffering. The clinician has direct access to none of these layers of the experience of pain. Only the pain behaviors (those that are observed and self-reported perceptions) constituting the outer layer of the model are available to the clinician or to the researcher.

Even this model may not adequately explain the phenomenon of pain. This multilayered, complex, multidimensional experience exists within a system that responds to and is affected by the patient (see Figure 3.2). The only references to the impact of organizations and organizational policies or procedures on pain and pain control found in the literature are in three publications arising from work by Fagerhaugh, Strauss, and Glaser in the early 1970s (Fagerhaugh, 1974, 1977; Strauss, Fagerhaugh, & Glaser, 1974).

Yet consider these four examples of patients about whom the author was consulted:

1. Mr. L. is dying. His physician has promised him that he will not suffer. However, over the months of his illness, Mr. L. has developed tolerance and requires morphine 10mg qlh by continuous intravenous infusion. The intern has just read the *JAMA* article "It's Over, Debbie" and refuses to participate in "killing this patient with a lethal dose of morphine." The primary nurse spends 4 hours finding the attending

FIGURE 3.2.   Factors affecting expression and control of pain.

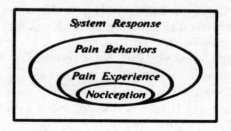

physician to obtain the necessary order. Mr. L. suffers intensely in the interval.

2. Mrs. P. has had a hysterectomy. Postoperatively, she was ordered morphine 10mg q4–6 hours prn. Kay, the nurse caring for Mrs. P. on the evening shift, had a hysterectomy several years ago. Kay remembered having had very little pain. She also disliked the feelings associated with receiving a narcotic. Kay doesn't ask Mrs. P. about her pain, nor does she tell Mrs. P. that she will have to ask for an analgesic if she needs one.

3. Mr. T. is suffering from intense pain from diabetic neuropathy. He tells no one because when he was hospitalized three months ago someone told him there was nothing that could be done about it.

4. Mr. S. has metastatic prostatic cancer. Following radiation his pain has been well controlled with round-the-clock doses of liquid morphine 8mg q4h. Three days after he is discharged, the nurse receives a phone call from Mrs. S. Mr. S. is unable to get out of bed, is withdrawn, and refuses to eat. As the nurse tries to elicit information on what has changed, she discovers that Mrs. S. thought Mr. S. was taking too much medication, so she hid the liquid morphine on the morning after he returned home.

Clearly none of these failures to control pain were the result of nociception, pain perception, suffering, or pain behaviors. In each situation, there was an appropriate and effective method available to control the pain. It wasn't used. A patient can't get relief from an intervention that isn't employed.

Fagerhaugh (1977) cautioned us that "interactions between staff and patient, and among staff members themselves, are immensely important to the management of pain." We have ignored this message, and the result is that undertreatment of pain in children and of acute and cancer pain in adults is a major health problem in this country despite an array of approaches to the assessment and treatment of pain that would seem to assure success (Bonica, 1986). While some are developing and testing new interventions and more efficient and sensitive assessments, I hope that some of us will examine the factors that prevent us from using the knowledge we have, so that patients can truly benefit from our improved scientific basis of practice.

References for this chapter appear in the reference list for the section on Pain in Adults.

Section A

PAIN IN INFANTS AND CHILDREN

[4]

Do Preterm Infants Show Behavioral Responses to Painful Procedures?

Diane Holditch Davis and Melinda Calhoon

The extent to which preterms experience pain is a controversial question for nurses and physicians. Since neonates can neither verbalize pain nor remember early pain when they are old enough to speak, it may be easier for clinicians to conduct the painful procedures necessary for the survival of these infants if they deny that preterms experience pain. As a result, a large number of painful procedures, including surgery, are conducted on preterms without analgesia or anesthesia (Shearer, 1986; Stevens, Hunsberger, & Browne, 1987). Support for the belief that preterm infants do not feel pain is provided by the neurobiological evidence that their brains are immature and myelination is incomplete (Volpe, 1987). In addition, early studies found that even fullterm neonates either lacked a response to painful stimuli or had only a corticate reflex (McGraw, 1941; Peiper, 1963).

However, the idea that preterms do not experience pain is now being questioned. Pain impulses are known to be transmitted by unmye-

We wish to thank Dr. Sandra Funk for statistical consultation and Mark C. Davis, Charlene Garrett, and Greg Samsa for technical assistance. This research was supported by a 1986 Sigma Theta Tau Research Grant; a 1986 NAACOG Research Grant; BSRG 507 RR07073 fron the Biomedical Research Support Program, Division of Research Resources, NIH; IBM Fund Junior Faculty Development Award from the University of North Carolina at Chapel Hill; a University of North Carolina at Chapel Hill Research Council Grant; and a University of North Carolina at Chapel Hill School of Nursing Summer Research Award.

linated fibers as well as myelinated ones (Price & Dubner, 1977). Clinicians, especially nurses, have long described pain behaviors in preterms (D'Apolito, 1984). Recent research has demonstrated that full-term neonates show behavioral and physiological responses to a variety of painful stimuli, including blood drawing and circumcision (Anders & Chalemian, 1974; Emde, Harmon, Metcalf, Koenig, & Wagonfeld, 1971; Franck, 1986; Owens & Todt, 1984; Porter, Miller, & Marshall, 1986). Studies of preterm infants undergoing surgery have demonstrated that they experience a marked physiological stress response that can be inhibited by the use of deep anesthesia (Anand & Hickey, 1987).

Only a few studies have investigated pain in preterms during the minor but painful procedures commonly performed in the neonatal intensive care unit. Porter, Miller, and Marshall (1987) found that when preterm infants received local anesthesia for lumbar punctures, they experienced less deterioration in oxygenation and a smaller increase in heart rate. Two other studies found physiological and behavioral changes in preterm infants in response to heel sticks (Beaver, 1987; Field & Goldson, 1984).

It has been suggested that physiological distress in preterms during common procedures is the result of overstimulation from handling, rather than pain. Painful procedures involve much handling, and studies have found physiological deterioration in preterms as a result of a variety of nursing procedures, nonpainful as well as painful (Gottfried, 1985; Norris, Campbell, & Brenkert, 1982). In addition, a study of one preterm found that the behavioral and physiological distress the infant exhibited in response to chest physiotherapy—an uncomfortable procedure—was similar to that exhibited in response to social interaction (Gorski, Hole, Leonard, & Martin, 1983). That study has been widely interpreted as indicating that handling is the principal cause of distress in preterms. As a result, when clinicians write about pain in preterms, they usually also discuss overstimulation (e.g., D'Apolito, 1984).

The purposes of this study, therefore, were first to determine whether preterms exhibit behavioral responses to painful procedures that differ from their behaviors during routine handling and, if so, to identify behaviors that practicing nurses could use for assessment of pain. In addition, the extent to which nurses respond to infant pain behaviors was explored.

METHOD

Subjects

The subjects for the study were 12 preterm infants who were part of a larger longitudinal study of behavioral development during the preterm period. Subjects were selected from a tertiary care hospital in the southeastern United States and enrolled in the larger study as soon as their medical condition was no longer critical and consent could be obtained from their parents. Infants were observed weekly from 7 to 11 P.M. until they reached 40 weeks gestational age or were discharged from the hospital. During the observations, infant sleep-wake states, infant behaviors, and caregiver behaviors were recorded every 10 seconds. The end of the 10 seconds was signaled audibly through an earphone from an electronic timer on an event recorder. Nursing and medical care and parental visitation continued as though the observer were not there.

All infants who experienced painful or uncomfortable procedures, such as routine bloodwork, during their observations were included in the present study. These procedures were relatively uncommon because the observations were conducted in the evening, and bloodwork was usually done during the day. Two subjects underwent painful procedures during three different observations and the other 10 subjects experienced such procedures once. Since the infant behaviors changed from week to week due to changes in developmental status, medical condition, and the nursing staff, each observation was analyzed individually. Thus, a total of 16 observations were available for analysis.

The 12 subjects (5 females and 7 males) formed a typical neonatal intensive care sample. Birth weights averaged 1180 gm (SD 363) and mean gestational age at birth was 29 weeks (SD 2.7). The age of the infants at the time of the observations for this study ranged from 29 to 39 weeks gestational age with a mean of 33.6 weeks (SD 3.0). All subjects had been mechanically ventilated, 8 had neurological complications (intraventricular hemorrhage, abnormal EEG, and/or birth asphyxia), and 4 had major surgery. None of the infants were critically ill at the time of the observations, but most still had medical complications. On 10 of the 16 observations, the infant was receiving oxygen: 1 by nasal CPAP, 7 by oxygen hood, and 2 by nasal cannula. During 7 observations, infants experienced pathologic apnea, and during only 2 observations did the infants receive bottle feedings. During the rest of the observations, the infant was either NPO (3) or fed by gavage (10) or gastrostomy tube (1).

Variables and Their Measurement

For data analysis, each observation was divided into three mutually exclusive contexts: painful care, routine care, and baby alone. Painful care began whenever the infant experienced a painful or uncomfortable procedure—needle sticks, suctioning, or tape removal—that lasted at least 30 seconds and ended when the nurse left the baby alone or resumed routine care by taking vital signs, feeding, changing, or performing another procedure. Thus, the period of painful care also included the time after the procedure that the nurse spent comforting and repositioning the infant. All care that was not classified as painful care was considered to be routine care. Observation time when the infant was not receiving care was considered baby alone time.

Two recovery contexts within baby alone time were defined: the first 5 minutes alone after painful care was called pain recovery, and the first 5 minutes alone after routine care was called routine recovery. The time span of 5 minutes was chosen arbitrarily, based on expected recovery time. If more than one pain recovery or routine recovery period occurred during an observation, data were combined and the total time was considered to be the recovery period. It was possible for a recovery period to be shorter than 5 minutes if the nurse intervened with the baby before 5 minutes were up. There was no pain recovery time during 6 observations because the nurses provided routine care immediately after the painful procedure. Thus, analyses of behaviors during recovery time were conducted on 10 observations.

Ten infant behaviors were examined in this study—four infant sleep-wake states and six infant activity behaviors. The sleep-wake states, judged on the basis of muscle tone, motor activity, respiration, eye-opening, and eye movement (Davis & Thoman, 1987; Thoman, 1985; Thoman, Davis, & Denenberg, 1987) were:

1. Waking. One of the following states: alertness, nonalert waking activity, fussing, or crying. The infant may or may not show motor activity during waking.
2. Drowse or Transition. Transition between waking and sleeping. If the infant's level of motor activity is low, the eyes are either "heavylidded," opening and closing slowly, or open but dazed in appearance. If there is generalized motor activity, the infant's eyes are typically closed but may open and close rapidly.
3. Active Sleep. The infant's eyes are closed. Respiration is uneven and primarily costal in nature. Sporadic motor movements occur, but muscle tone is low between these movements. REMs occur intermittently.

4. Quiet Sleep. The infant's eyes are closed, and respiration is relatively slow and abdominal in nature. A tonic level of motor tone is maintained, and motor activity is limited to occasional startles, sighs, or other brief discharges.

The six infant activity behaviors were selected either because these behaviors were known to signal distress or because other researchers had suggested that they might (Gorski et al., 1983). The behaviors were:

1. Negative Facial Expression. A cry face or a frown; this expression may be isolated or may occur with crying.
2. Jitter. A rhythmic movement of at least three cycles; it may involve only part of an extremity or as much as the entire body.
3. Startle. A sudden infant movement involving at least one whole extremity, though it may involve the entire body, as in a Moro reflex.
4. Hiccup.
5. Spit-Up or Gag. Drools, regurgitation, coughs, sneezes, or gags.
6. Large Movement. A movement involving the extremities and the trunk.

Finally, two caregiver behaviors were examined because these behaviors could be used as comfort measures:

1. Talk. Talking to the infant.
2. Positive Touch. Positive or affectionate touching of the infant (e.g., stroking or kissing the infant, giving a pacifier).

The infant behaviors were measured as percentages of the two care contexts (painful procedures and routine handling), baby alone time, and the two recovery contexts. The comfort behaviors were measured only as percentages of the care contexts because they did not occur when the infant was alone. These percentages were calculated by dividing the number of 10-second periods in which each behavior occurred during each context by the number of periods in the context. Thus, if painful care occurred for 4 minutes (24 10-second periods) and the baby was awake for 3 minutes (18 periods) during this context, waking was said to occur during 75% of painful care.

RESULTS

Contexts as Percent of the Total Observation

The five contexts were measured as percentages of the 16 4-hour observations. Painful care averaged 3.9% of the total (9 min.), and routine care averaged 16.4% (39 min.). Painful care included chest physiotherapy (5 instances), IV removals and restarts (2), nasopharyngeal suctioning (3), bloodwork (3), changing cardiac leads (2), and dressing changes (2). One infant experienced 2 different painful procedures during the same observation. The baby alone time averaged 79.7% of the total observation time (191 min.). The time spent in pain recovery averaged 1.1% (3 min.) of the 16 observations, and 1.8% (4 min.) of the 10 pain recovery observations. Routine recovery averaged 9.0% (22 min.) of the 10 observations during which pain recovery occurred.

Infant Behaviors During Care Contexts

Table 4.1 presents the infant behaviors during the two care contexts. The patterning of sleep-wake states during painful care differed significantly from that during routine care [$F(3, 45) = 7.05$, $p < .001$; two factor (context by state) repeated measures analysis of variance]. Correlated t-tests indicated that during painful care the percentage of waking was significantly greater (34.4% vs. 17.0% for routine care), and active sleep (32.8% vs. 56.6%) and quiet sleep (0% vs. 2.4%) occurred less. Two of the infant activity behaviors were significantly more frequent during painful care: negative facial expressions (38.9% vs. 17.4%) and large moves (69.2% vs. 45.4%). The percentages of drowse or transition, jitters, startles, hiccups, and spit- ups did not differ in these two contexts.

It is clear, therefore, that preterm infants as young as 29 weeks gestational age exhibit behavioral responses to painful and uncomfortable procedures that differ from their behaviors during routine care. Overstimulation from handling is unlikely to explain the distress preterms experience during these procedures. The behavioral responses observed indicate increased arousal as evidenced by increased waking, less sleep, and a greater number of large moves. These infants also showed an emotional response, an increase in negative facial expressions.

Infant behaviors during painful care differed in intensity and quantity, rather than quality, from those during routine care. No behavior, except the absence of quiet sleep, was unequivocally associated with pain, and the absence of quiet sleep has limited value for assessment since half of the routine care periods also lacked quiet sleep. This find-

TABLE 4.1 The Mean Amounts (and Standard Deviation) of Each Infant Behavior and Nursing Comfort Measure as Percentages of Painful and Routine Care[a]

Infant Behavior	Painful Care		Routine Care	
	Mean	(SD)	Mean	(SD)
Waking	34.4	(36.2)	17.0	(25.3)**
Drowse or Transition	32.8	(32.3)	23.9	(17.5)
Active Sleep	32.8	(36.8)	56.6	(29.7)**
Quiet Sleep	0.0	(0.0)	2.4	(3.4)*
Negative Facial Expression	38.9	(32.9)	17.4	(20.9)**
Jitter	7.2	(13.8)	5.8	(5.5)
Startle	1.2	(2.6)	1.9	(2.4)
Hiccup	1.2	(5.0)	1.2	(3.1)
Spit or Gag	2.6	(8.3)	0.8	(1.2)
Large Movement	69.2	(22.5)	45.4	(10.7)***
Nurse Talk	8.9	(6.9)	9.8	(7.4)
Nurse Positive Touch	4.1	(9.5)	9.9	(11.2)

[a]Due to sample size and distribution considerations, nonparametric Wilcoxen tests were performed in addition to the correlated t-tests. All significant t-tests were replicated with significant Wilcoxen results.
*Correlated t-tests indicate significant differences between the two care contexts, $p < .05$.
**Correlated t-tests indicate significant differences between the two care contexts, $p < .01$.
***Correlated t-tests indicate significant differences between the two care contexts, $p < .001$.

ing is not surprising since routine care involves stressful handling and also a fair amount of discomfort for preterms. Discomfort during routine care differs from painful procedures primarily in length and intensity.

Despite the lack of qualitative differences in behaviors during the two care periods, experienced neonatal nurses who are familiar with the typical behavioral repertoires of their preterm infants should have no difficulty in recognizing the increased arousal and negative affect associated with pain. In fact, nurses already use changes in infant behavior and activity for assessment. The two behavioral signs of pain used most commonly by practicing nurses are crying (which includes a negative facial expression) and activity (Franck, 1987); both are pain behaviors identified in this study. Thus, these findings provide empirical support for the clinical judgment of neonatal nurses.

Once preterms experiencing pain are identified, nursing interventions to reduce or eliminate pain are needed. The American Academy of Pediatrics (1987) and several investigators (Anand & Hickey, 1987; Yaster, 1987) have recommended that analgesia and anesthesia be used with preterm infants whenever their use would be appropriate for older children and adults. However, using drugs for the minor procedures in this study would not be practical. Comfort measures are the most promising nursing interventions for preterms experiencing minor painful or uncomfortable procedures. Therefore, we examined the comfort measures nurses used with the infants in this study.

Nursing Comfort Measures

The percentages of talk and positive touch did not differ during painful and routine care (see Table 4.1). For two infants, however, the percentage of positive touch during painful care was much greater than during routine care. For these two infants, nurses were probably using positive touch as a comfort measure. Yet when the sleep-wake states and infant activity behaviors of these infants were compared with those of the rest of the group, they did not appear to differ.

Thus, despite the infants' behavioral distress during painful procedures, nurses did not appear to utilize comfort measures. Talking serves many purposes besides comfort, so it may be that the amount of talking nurses did for comfort was obscured by other talking. Positive touches, however, are only performed to indicate affection or to comfort the infant. Thus, the lack of difference in the amount of positive touch clearly indicates that nurses were not using comfort measures consistently.

Additional research is needed to determine why nurses do not perform the nursing intervention most likely to reduce behavioral distress during painful procedures. One possible explanation is that nurses have learned that comfort measures are ineffective with preterm infants. For example, the behaviors of the two infants who received comfort measures did not appear to differ from those of infants without comfort measures. Two studies of the use of comfort measures with preterm infants indicate that these interventions have questionable effectiveness in reducing the negative effects of painful procedures. Field and Goldson (1984) found that giving infants pacifiers reduced the behavioral, but not physiological, effects of heel sticks. Beaver (1987) found that stroking the leg of a preterm actually increased physiological deterioration during heel sticks.

Yet it is more likely that the lack of difference between the behaviors of infants receiving comfort measures and those not receiving comfort in this study resulted from the fact that the nurses used comfort measures to reduce distress to an acceptable level, rather than to eliminate it. The two infants who received comfort measures may have experienced a reduction in distress that was acceptable to their nurses. However, a goal of reducing, rather than eliminating behavioral responses to pain in preterm infants is neither humane nor in line with the current goals of pain relief in older children and adults.

Comfort measures remain the only practical method of reducing the pain associated with minor procedures in preterm infants. Neonatal nurses report using at least nine different comfort measures to manage pain in preterms (Franck, 1987). Yet to date, only two different comfort measures, pacifiers and stroking, have been studied with only one painful procedure, heel sticks (Beaver, 1987; Field & Goldson, 1987). Ways to vary the timing of the comfort measure or to combine different interventions have not been studied, and the effectiveness of different comfort measures has not been examined. Until research on these different comfort measures is available, practicing nurses must rely on their clinical judgment and utilize comfort measures that appear to be most effective in eliminating both the physiological and behavioral responses to painful procedures.

Infant Behaviors During the Recovery Periods

Comparison of the behaviors of preterm infants during the two recovery periods, pain recovery and routine recovery (see Table 4.2), indicated that wake states did not differ during these periods [$F(3, 27) = 0.42$, $p > .05$; two factor (context by state) repeated measures analysis of variance]. In addition, none of the percentages of infant activity behaviors differed significantly between these two contexts. Therefore, the percentages of each infant state and activity behavior were averaged over the two recovery periods and compared with the percentage of the variable during the total baby alone time. Four variables differed significantly. During recovery periods, infants exhibited more drowse or transition, less active sleep, less quiet sleep, and more large movements than during their total alone time.

These findings indicate that behavioral responses to minor painful procedures last only as long as the infant is experiencing painful stimuli. The behaviors of infants are indistinguishable during the recovery period after painful procedures and after routine care, at least with our limited sample. However, preterms are more aroused after both types of care than during their overall time alone, as evidenced by increased drowse or transition, decreased sleep, and increased activity levels. Thus, it is likely that preterm infants would benefit from interventions after nursing care that decrease arousal and promote sleep.

These findings provide additional evidence that jitters, startles, hiccups, and spitting-up are not signs of pain in preterm infants. The amounts of these behaviors did not differ between the two care contexts or between the recovery contexts and the overall alone time. Other authors have suggested that hiccups and spitting-up are strong

TABLE 4.2 The Mean Amounts (and Standard Deviation) of Each Infant Behavior as Percentages of Painful and Routine Recovery and Baby Alone Time.[a,b]

Infant Behavior	Pain Recovery		Routine Recovery		Baby Alone	
	Mean	(SD)	Mean	(SD)	Mean	(SD)
Waking	21.1	(36.0)	9.8	(12.4)	4.0	(5.3)
Drowse or Transition	23.0	(30.8)	28.3	(29.8)	9.4	(6.8)*
Active Sleep	55.8	(42.1)	53.7	(34.8)	72.2	(11.5)*
Quiet Sleep	0.0	(0.0)	8.2	(10.5)	14.4	(8.3)*
Negative Facial Expression	26.5	(41.4)	13.0	(19.0)	9.3	(7.2)
Jitter	16.3	(2.0)	7.4	(5.9)	10.8	(7.0)
Startle	2.3	(4.5)	1.9	(118)	2.9	(1.4)
Hiccup	1.3	(4.2)	2.0	(6.3)	3.1	(2.8)
Spit or Gag	0.0	(0.0)	0.5	(0.9)	0.4	(0.6)
Large Movement	54.2	(39.6)	31.4	(14.6)	25.6	(9.0)*

[a]Correlated t-tests showed no significant differences between the two recovering contexts.
[b]Due to sample size and distribution considerations, nonparametric Wilcoxen tests were performed in addition to the correlated t-tests. All significant t-tests were replicated with significant Wilcoxen results.
*Correlated t-tests indicate significant differences between the two recovery contexts and baby alone time, $p < .05$.

indicators of infant stress (D'Apolito, 1984; Gorski et al., 1983). Certainly there are many clinical examples of associations between these behaviors and infant distress; in the present study, one infant began an episode of hiccups during a painful procedure. Our overall findings, however, indicate that most episodes of jitters, startles, hiccups, and spitting-up are spontaneous behaviors that have no particular significance. Thus, nurses do not need to intervene just because an infant displays one of these behaviors.

DISCUSSION

Clearly preterm infants as young as 29 weeks gestational age respond to painful and uncomfortable procedures with a greater increase in arousal and more negative facial expressions than during routine care. After painful procedures, their behaviors are similar to those after routine care, but the infants continue to be more aroused than during their overall alone time. In view of these findings and others showing reduced physiological deterioration in infants receiving anesthesia for painful procedures (Porter et al., 1987), the failure of nurses and other health professionals to intervene to reduce or prevent pain in preterm infants is ethically indefensible. Nurses can ensure that preterms receive analgesia and anesthesia for major procedures, such as surgery, circumcision, and chest tube insertion, except when these drugs would cause life-threatening complications. For minor painful procedures, including needle sticks, tape removal, and chest physiotherapy, nursing comfort measures can be used.

The findings also indicate that nurses can use changes in arousal and the amount of negative facial expressions to identify infants in need of intervention and to evaluate the effectiveness of interventions with infants in pain. However, practicing nurses need to be aware that these behavioral signs have only been validated for use in the assessment of relatively brief periods of pain during minor procedures. The behaviors of infants experiencing prolonged pain, such as after surgery, may differ. For example, studies of fullterm infants after circumcision have shown that these infants exhibit decreased arousal and increased amounts of quiet sleep (Anders & Chalemian, 1974; Emde et al., 1971). One infant in the authors' larger longitudinal study exhibited a marked increase in quiet sleep, from 24% of the observation to 42%, after an inguinal hernia repair. Identification of behavioral cues appropriate for the assessment of prolonged pain awaits additional research and clinical observations.

Finally, although this study found that preterm infants respond behaviorally to painful procedures, much additional research is needed to clarify this response. A number of variables, including the maturity of the infant, the infant's medical condition, the type of procedure, and the length of painful stimulation, undoubtedly affect the infant's behaviors. The relationship between behavioral and physiological distress in preterms needs clarification. Research is also needed to examine the timing, selection, and effectiveness of comfort measures. Altogether, this research will provide a strong empirical foundation for the relief of pain in preterm infants.

[5]

Vocal Measures of Infant Pain

Barbara F. Fuller, Yoshiyuki Horii, and Douglas Conner

Infant pain is difficult to assess because of the lack of tools to measure infant behavior quantitatively and the fact that preverbal children cannot self report pain. This problem has recently received increased attention (Levine & Gordon, 1982; Owens, 1984). Facial expression (Izard & Dougherty, 1982), heart rate, respiratory rate and transcutaneous oxygen levels, body movement (Owens, 1984), and vocal behavior (Fuller & Horii, in press-a) have been explored as potential indicators of infant distress. All except vocal behavior, however, either cannot be satisfactorily ranked on a numerical scale or are influenced by factors other than the infant's distress. Acoustic measures are promising for two reasons. First, the cry draws the caretaker's attention to the infant, influencing infant-caretaker interactions, and second, it involves complex neurophysiological mechanisms (Bosma, Truby, & Lind, 1965) that provide subtle information about the infant's biological status.

Early research on infant crying used acoustic features of pain-induced cries to identify neurological damage in newborns (Koivisto, Michelsson, Sirvio, & Wasz-Hockert, 1974; Michelsson, 1971; Michelsson, Sirvio, & Wasz-Hockert, 1977; Zeskind & Lester, 1978). One landmark study (Wasz-Hockert, Lind, Vuorenkoski, Partanen, & Valanne, 1968) identified an acoustic variable (tenseness) that differentiated pain-induced cries from hunger-induced cries, but this method only generated nominal data which does not reflect magnitude or amount. Pitch, a ratio-level variable that does reflect magnitude, has recently been reported to increase during circumcision (Porter, Miller, & Marshall, 1986). Unfortunately, pitch by itself cannot be used to assess infant pain because changes in the pitch of infant cries can also be caused by neurological or metabolic disturbances such as hyperbilirubinemia, brain damage, or hypoxemia (Koivisto, 1987; Michelsson, Sirvio, & Wasz-Hockert, 1977).

Several potentially useful acoustic measures of adult speech seem to be influenced by stress arousal. Because stress arousal increases striated muscle tension, the rate and depth of breathing, and airway diameter, it elevates voice intensity, pitch, and "tenseness" (Laver, 1980; Levi, 1975; Scherer, 1981; Williams & Stevens, 1972). Most people are familiar with the ideas of intensity and pitch, though not necessarily with tenseness. A tense voice is one that has relatively more energy in the higher frequencies of the sound spectrum than a relaxed voice.

Some research indicates that stress arousal may also alter jitter and shimmer of adult voices (Brenner, Shipp, & Doherty, 1983; Hollien, Michel, & Doherty, 1973; Williams & Stevens, 1972), but these have not been studied in infant vocalizations. Shimmer is a technical term describing fluctuations in the amplitude of the vocal cord vibrations that generate pitch. Jitter is a technical term referring to fluctuations in the duration of individual cycles of the vocal cord vibrations that produce pitch.

In a two-phase research project, we explored the potential for using these acoustic variables, either singly or in combination, as clinical measures of infant distress/pain.

PHASE ONE

The purpose of the first phase was to ascertain if any variables could differentiate between "pain-induced" cries and other situationally defined cries and cooing.

Method

Vocalizations of 13 2-month-old, 15 4-month-old, and 13 6-month-old healthy infants were recorded. Four types of vocalizations performed by each infant were then compared: (a)pain-induced crying evoked in a previously noncrying infant by a routine DPT immunization; (b) hungry cries that spontaneously occurred with a short delay in the infant's usual feeding time; (c) fussy cries spontaneously occurring about the time of the infant's usual naptime; and (d) cooing produced in response to maternal en face soft sounds and fondling. Sample vocalizations were collected in the mother's presence in both clinic and infant home settings. All vocalizations were classified by both the mother and pediatric nurse data collector at the time of audiotaping as being a pain, fussy, or hungry cry or cooing. Vocalizations not falling into one of these categories were not audiotaped.

One-hundred and nine recorded vocalizations were analyzed using valid and reliable computer programs written by Dr. Horii (Horii, 1979; Horii & Hughes, 1972). One measured pitch, jitter, and shimmer. The other calculated the energy in decibels for each 20 Hz segment of audio frequency from the lowest to the highest (5,000 Hz) frequencies in the sound spectrum. The mean value of the relative spectral energy (RMSE) for each sample was considered the degree of tenseness; the closer the frequency was to zero, the more tense the vocalization was considered to be.

Results

Of all the measures (pitch, jitter, shimmer, and tenseness as reflected by RMSE), only two differed significantly among the four types of vocalizations. These were pitch [F (3,93) = 9.82, $p < .001$] and tenseness [$F(3, 108) = 11.36$, $p < .001$]. However, instead of differentiating pain-induced cries from other types of cries, pitch only differentiated hungry cries from the other cries and from cooing (Fuller & Horii, in press-a). Since the pain stimulus was brief and the infants were held in their mothers' arms while it occurred, there may have been more discomfort associated with some of the hunger cries than with some of the pain-induced ones. Tenseness, however, differentiated pain cries from all other types of vocalizations. Pain-induced cries were significantly more tense than the other two types of cries and all cries were significantly more tense than cooing (Fuller & Horii, in press-b). This suggested that tenseness might be a promising infant pain assessment measure.

PHASE TWO

The second phase of our research followed up this discovery and was designed to ascertain whether tenseness, alone or in combination with other variables such as pitch, could differentiate between: (1) cries induced by physically traumatic and presumably painful stimuli and noxious nontraumatic stimuli and (2) cries associated with presumed differing levels of pain.

Method

Data on pitch, loudness, and tenseness of cries were collected on 16 1–2 day old healthy infants who were undergoing circumcision. All infants met the following criteria: (a)normal vaginal delivery requiring only local maternal anesthetic, (b)full-term (>37 wks) gestation, (c)birth weight >5 lbs, (d)5-minute Apgar >7, (e)Gomco circumcision, (f)parental informed consent, (g)physician approval, and (h)a ponderal index between 2.20 and 2.92. The last criterion ensured elimination of any infants at risk for neuro-developmental impairment, a factor known to alter the pitch of cries (Zeskind & Lester, 1981).

Cries were recorded 30–60 minutes before the infant was placed on the "circ board" (Situation 1—S1), during betadine swabbing of the area to be circumcised (this is noxiously arousing but not physically damaging and thus presumed to be a nonpainful stimulus) (S2), during placement of the Gomco clamp (S3), during cutting of the foreskin (S4), after the procedure was finished but while the Gomco clamp was still attached (S5), after the clamp was removed but the infant was still restrained on the board (S6), and 30–60 minutes after the infant was removed from the board (S7). Cries were elicited in Situations 1 and 7 by placing an uninflated blood pressure cuff on the infant's arm, by partially uncovering the infant, or by predischarge photography.

Two to four samples of each infant's cries during each situation were subsequently computerized, and measures of pitch, loudness, and tenseness were obtained using the same computer analysis as in Phase 1. Since various persons have proposed different cutoff points for distinguishing between high and low frequencies, we used six different mathematical measures of the spectral energy reflecting tenseness. One was relative mean spectral energy (RMSE). The five other measures reflected various ratios of energy in different portions of the spectrum. One measure (F1) reported the frequency (Hz) at which the sound energy (dB) was equally distributed above and below the frequency. Another measure (F2) reported the frequency (Hz) at which the sound energy (dB) distributed above the frequency was double that found below it. A third measure (F5) was the frequency (Hz) at which the sound energy (dB) found above the frequency was half that found below it. On these three measures, increased tenseness is reflected in a shift to higher frequencies. Two other measures reported the ratios of voice energy at 1000 Hz (R1) and 2000 Hz (R2). These ratios were determined by dividing the total relative sound energy above a particular frequency by the total relative sound energy below that frequency. A cry with increased tenseness will have a higher ratio at these frequencies than one that is less tense.

Results

Only pitch and tenseness differed significantly among the seven situations (see Table 5.1). Loudness did not differ. Pitch was significantly

TABLE 5.1 Mean Values of Acoustic Variables of Cries Among the Seven Situations

Acoustic Variables	Situations				
	S1 Pre- Circumcision	S2 Cleansing	S3-4 Clamping Cutting	S5-6 Restrained	S7 Post- Circumcision
Pitch*	457	484	489	481	511
RMSE**	28	22	20	25	25

* S1 significantly different from S7 ($p < .001$).
** S2 significantly different from S1, S5–6 ($p < .001$); S3–4 significantly different from S1, S5, S7 ($p < .01$).

higher 30–60 minutes following circumcision (S7) than beforehand (S1). Pitch also increased with restraint and betadine cleansing (S2) and during the actual clamping and cutting (S3 and S4); however, these differences from pitch levels before any procedure was done (S1) were not significant.

With restraint and betadine cleansing (S2), tenseness increased markedly and significantly from preprocedure levels (S1). Then it stayed at the same high level during clamping and cutting (S3 and S4), which involved the most physical trauma. After clamp removal (S5), when the infant was still restrained (S6), the tenseness of cries decreased significantly but it did not return to preprocedural levels even 30–60 minutes afterward (S7).

These results indicate that circumcision procedures (S2–S4) progressively increase vocal tenseness and for at least 30–60 minutes afterwards this tenseness continues, albeit at somewhat reduced levels. The fact that tenseness did not increase significantly from betadine cleansing to clamping and cutting (from S2 to S3 and S4) or decrease significantly for 60 minutes after the procedure is probably a result of the small sample size.

Since human auditory discrimination uses combinations of acoustic variables rather than a single measure, we also used Discriminant Function Analysis to compare combinations of acoustic variables—pitch and the same six measures of tenseness (RMSE, R1, R2, F5, F1, and F2)—with infants' cries during different situations. The aim was to discover whether these combinations of variables would correctly identify a cry as belonging to a particular situation.

The results indicate that, indeed, infants' cries from various situations can be differentiated using combinations of pitch and tenseness. The major differences follow:

S2 crying was more tense than S1 crying.

S3/4 crying was similar in tenseness but had a higher pitch than S2 cries.

S3/4 crying had a higher pitch and was more tense than S1 cries.

S5, S6, and S7 cries were less tense than S3/4 crying but had a similar pitch.

S6 and S7 cries did not differ.

S6/7 cries were more tense and higher in pitch than S1 cries.

Thus, it is possible, on the basis of combinations of tenseness and pitch, to discriminate between arousal due to nonphysically traumatic stimuli (restraint and betadine cleansing—S2) and arousal due to physically traumatic and presumably painful stimuli (the actual clamping and cutting of circumcision—S3 and S4) and between crying before a pain-provoking situation has occurred and crying up to an hour afterward. Crying associated with arousal without physical trauma (betadine cleansing of restrained infant) is characterized only by increased tenseness, whereas crying associated with arousal due to physical trauma (clamping and cutting) is characterized by increases in both tenseness and pitch. Because cries 30–60 minutes following circumcision (S7) were of higher pitch and more tense than S1, this suggests that the effects of physically traumatic arousal may still remain.

DISCUSSION

Differences in such acoustic variables as pitch and tenseness can be discriminated by persons trained in phonetics or acoustics. Trained listeners can distinguish the cries of healthy and high-risk newborns based on acoustic variables such as pitch (Zeskind & Lester, 1978). Even untrained listeners can differentiate the "urgency" in cries during clamping and cutting from precircumcision cries based on pitch and certain nonacoustic crying variables (Porter, Miller, & Marshall, 1986). Hence, it is conceivable that pediatric nurses could be trained to auditorially distinguish between combinations of tenseness and perhaps intensity, pitch, or other variables in infant cries and use these distinctions in infant pain assessments. Indeed, perhaps many have already intuitively trained themselves to do this.

In the near future we intend to explore the feasibility of training nursing students and nurses to use combinations of these acoustic variables in the assessment of acute pain states among infants.

[6]

Acute Pain Behavior in Infants and Toddlers

Nancy M. Mills

Assessment and management of pain in children three years of age and under is difficult for even the most experienced pediatric nurses. Lack of communication skills hampers infants' and toddlers' ability to describe pain to caregivers, and few pain assessment tools have been developed for this group. Further, few systematic observations of infants and toddlers experiencing prolonged pain have been conducted to provide a guide to others, and changes in acute pain behavior at different developmental stages have had limited study.

The purposes of this study were to describe the behaviors of infants and toddlers in prolonged acute pain and to examine differences in those behaviors across a three-year age span.

METHOD

Thirty-two infants and toddlers who were inpatients in a private children's hospital and who had experienced tissue trauma from surgery, burns, or fractures were studied. Only children who had experienced tissue trauma within 24 hours of the first observation, who were normal in development as determined by the patient record, and who had not had an analgesic within four hours of the observations were included in the study. Informed consent was obtained from parents or guardians.

A 30-minute observation form, a parent interview guide, and a patient record information form developed in a pilot study of the pain behaviors of 50 children aged birth to 12 years were used to collect data. The infants and toddlers in the current study were observed on three occasions for 30 minutes, or a total of 90 minutes. Where possible, observations were scheduled throughout the day so as to include morning, afternoon, and evening hours. Interviews to explore parents' perceptions of the pain behaviors displayed by their children followed the observations. Additionally, parents were asked to indicate how they distinguished pain behavior from well and ill behavior. Observations and interviews were recorded in narrative and audiorecordings. Demographic data and notes written by nurses and physicians describing the child's pain behavior were collected from the records.

RESULTS

Five types of behaviors associated with prolonged acute pain in infants and toddlers were identified: motor movements, communications, facial expressions, changes in interactions, and efforts toward self-consolation. As would be expected, the children's maturation and development were reflected in the behaviors in each category; new behaviors for each age level are reported in Table 6.1 and Table 6.2. The most *common* behaviors are summarized in the narrative below.

Infants: Birth to 3 Months

Motor movements included physical extremity movements; the general body responses of jerking—a response somewhat like a startle; and splinting, or drawing the legs up to the abdomen more than normal flexion posture. Physical extremity movements ranged from mild wiggling and kicking of arms and legs to flailing, thrashing, and hard kicking associated with loud crying. Clenched fists were frequently seen, and in some of the infants, jerking occurred every 15 minutes.

Infants' communications ranged from brief, mild crying and grunting to sustained, intense crying. Neonates cried 15 to 30 seconds and quieted. By two months of age, crying lasted as long as three minutes. Crying was considered by parents to be associated with both hunger and pain; they used contextual cues to determine when the cry was a pain cry. For example, quiet infants would cry out when picked up and parents called this a pain cry.

Facial expressions in this group ranged from neutral to frowning or grimacing. Sometimes the infants appeared to be frowning in sleep. Grimacing was often associated with physical movement.

The infants interacted less with parents than did children not in pain.

TABLE 6.1 New Infant Pain Behaviors[a]

0-3 Months	3-6 Months	6-9 Months	9-12 Months
Motor Movements			
Kick/flail		Kick/aggress	Push hands away
Wiggle/thrash		Pull away/arch	Elevate limb
Jerk		Wring hands	Limb control
Splint		Bite/pinch self	
Clench fists		Rub/roll body	
		Log roll	
		Hunch body part	
Communication			
Intermittent	Sustained Cry	Antic. crying	Language: mommy
cry	Moan/whimper	Fear cry	Receptive language
Facial Expressions			
Frown/grimace	Serious	Fear	Anger
Clenched jaw	Surprise	Sadness	
	"O" mouth	Flinch	
Interactions			
Sleep disturbed	Fear		
Interact less	Cling		Jerk away
Shut down more	No play		
Self-Consolation			
Lie still	Pacifier	Repetitive move.	Elevate limb
	Move/turn	Seek escape/resist	
	slowly	Self-bite/pinch	
		Change position	

[a]The table displays only new behaviors observed at each age. In each category behaviors observed at younger ages continue to be seen at each older age, but usually in a more refined or controlled manner.

Some babies slept more, while others' sleep was lighter and intermittent. Many parents noted that their children were sleep disturbed.

Self-consolation behaviors were defined as behaviors initiated by infants to decrease pain or increase comfort. Parents felt infants even at one month of age learned to lie still. After surgery, the babies would move fairly normally a few times, and their movement was associated with crying out. Parents said that after those experiences the infants moved less often than usual.

Infants: 3 to 6 Months

Physical extremity movements within this group were the same as those noted in younger infants, although generally there was greater

TABLE 6.2 New Toddler Pain Behaviors[a]

12-18 Months	18-24 Months	24-30 Months	30-36 Months
Motor Movements			
Grab to resist		Walk on toes	
Tremors			
Jump			
Communication			
	"ow," "hurt"	Pain talk	Tell what hurts
	"burn"	Express wants	
	Ask for parents	Resist	
	Vocal play	Question	
	Followed instructions	Plead	
Facial Expressions			
Vigilance			Pout
Interactions			
Aggression towards care providers	Avoid eye contact	Stall Play	Anger at parents Aggression at parents
Self-Consolation			
Seek comfort			
Bite a towel			

[a]The table displays only new behaviors observed at each age. In each category behaviors observed at younger ages continue to be seen at each older age, but usually in a more refined or controlled manner.

control of body movements. General body responses included squirming, writhing, and frequent jerking. For example, one child jerked and cried out 14 times in one 30-minute observation. The intensity of jerking varied from mild movements to intense jerks that turned two infants from their sides to their backs. Whimpering or crying out was usually associated with jerking. Parents reported that jerking kept the children from sleeping well at night. Pain medicine reduced the frequency of jerking but did not stop it. Splinting involved moving slowly to turn over. Infants with abdominal wounds kept one leg flexed up and moved the other leg when kicking.

Infants' communications consisted of moans, whimpers, and cries, usually restrained. They sometimes went from restrained crying to vigorous crying when moved suddenly. Crying was sustained as long as five minutes. On three occasions an infant who had had cardiac surgery went limp after crying, as though exhausted. Infants whimpered when they were not moving. Vigorous cries were associated with coughing, jerking, turning, and touching the surgical wound.

Parents thought their infants had more serious expressions than usual. Expressions included surprise and the mouth puckered to an "O" shape; these occurred with sudden movements and were followed by crying.

Three changes in interactions were recorded for this age group. The infants did not want to play, and one mother thought her infant was more inclined to cling, while another mother said her infant was aware of strangers and was fearful when approached.

Infants 3 to 6 months old were able to self-console by putting a pacifier in their own mouths. They also more obviously limited movement of body parts adjacent to their wounds. When pain was intense, the infants lost control and parent efforts to console were also not effective at that point.

Infants: 6 to 9 Months

New motor movements among the 6- to 9-month-old infants included hand wringing, pinching or biting themselves, and rubbing body parts. In addition, repetitive movements such as rolling side to side or rolling the head side to side were observed. General body movement was more controlled. Log rolling to keep the trunk splinted was reported. Children with burns arched and twisted to attempt to escape burn debridement. Hunching a painful body part was also observed.

Children with burns screamed during dressing changes. Crying lasted up to five minutes. Additionally, children cried with nonpainful events such as being moved to the treatment room, seeing nurses with masks, or seeing parents leave. Facial flinching was observed with sudden motor movements.

In a number of observations, infants played with toys for a few seconds, but play alternated with whimpering and looking about. Play may have been momentarily distracting. This age group changed positions often, and parents thought these were efforts to seek a more comfortable position. Efforts to escape pain and aggressive behavior toward caregivers doing nonpainful procedures were observed.

Infants: 9 to 12 Months

Two refinements in behavior occurred among the infants in this age group. One infant tried to remove the nurse's hands holding him during dressing changes. And one child with burns was frequently observed to hold his arm up in the air over his head. This seemed to be a position of comfort and he resisted the therapist's efforts to lower the arm.

Crying within this group was sustained as long as nine minutes. Some children cried out for mommy during procedures, and one child shook his head "no, no" over and over during painful procedures. Burned infants seemed to listen to verbal cues from nurses: the magic words were "almost done" or "all done." The infants quieted then and watched the face of the nurse. If the nurse was not truly done, the infant resumed crying.

One new expression became apparent with this group: some children wore angry expressions and reacted aggressively to hurtful procedures.

Toddlers: 12 to 18 Months

Young toddlers were more sophisticated in their resistance to painful procedures. One child fought to take the wash rag from his nurse and pushed at her to move her away. Jumping during painful dressing changes was observed. General body tremors were reported during burn treatments and when the children were in their cribs.

Toddlers cried at the sight of their own blood, when they saw syringes or scissors, when ointment was applied, when wounds were checked, and when temperatures were taken rectally. Vocalizations were like those in older infants. One toddler mouthed "no no" over and over in his sleep.

Parents were sure their child was angry on occasion. Facial expressions did not differ from those of older infants, but toddlers with burns were even more wary and vigilant than that group. The memory of previous burn treatments and cues which meant that treatments were beginning seemed to contribute to this. The treatment room was adjacent to the patient rooms, and nurses entered it through patient rooms, wearing masks. Before the children were taken to the treatment area, the whirlpool tub was turned on and the sound was clearly audible in their rooms. As soon as the whirlpool sound came on and nurses entered in masks, the children became vigilant. They stopped eating, watching television, and interacting. They silently watched the actions of the nurses. If a sound occurred behind a child, he turned quickly and tracked the movement of that person as well. Thus, a significant amount of anxiety was generated by the awareness of what was about to happen. When more than one child had dressing changes, the children watched each child carried into the treatment room and then heard all the crying and screaming as he experienced dressing changes.

Toddlers resisted the nurses doing their treatments by kicking them. However, they clung to other nurses as though seeking adult protection from being placed in the tubs for dressing changes. Two burned children alternated playing with toys in the water with crying.

Toddlers: 18 to 24 Months

The major changes in toddlers 18 to 24 months of age were in their communications and interactions. New terms used included "ow," "hurts," and "burns." Some toddlers used sentences, and one boy with bladder spasms alternated sing-song vocal play with crying. On three occasions, toddlers complied with verbal instructions from nurses or parents: "Put your hand in the water—hold still."

Some toddlers in this age group avoided eye contact with strangers but did not cry when approached. Three children played with parents, but their play was interrupted by cries from muscle spasms (fractures, bladder).

Toddlers: 24 to 30 Months

One child in this group walked on his toes to keep from straightening his burned thigh. These toddlers communicated more clearly with nurses. They expressed pain by saying "Yes, it hurts," "my hurt," "ear hurt." One child expressed his feelings by saying "I'm mad." Verbal resistance occurred: "No off, no bath." They asked for information such as: "Are you done?" "Why?" They stalled: "I want to go to bed."

Toddlers: 30 to 36 Months

There were few changes in the behaviors observed in toddlers 30 to 36 months old. Language skills increased. One girl refused to get out of bed or turn, saying "I too sick." According to her mother, "sick" was the word the girl used for pain. Two toddlers had pouting facial expressions when asked to move. Interactions were similar to those in the previous age group. However, anger and aggression at parents as well as nurses were observed. Self-consolation efforts were also similar to those of other toddlers. One child asked to have her stomach rubbed above her abdominal wound. The parent lightly stroked the child's abdomen in the place where the child placed her hand. This went on for hours. If the parent stopped rubbing the area, the child roused, cried, and said "No, rub it." When this child was to get up or turn she refused help from her parents or nurses and told them, "No! You hurt me!"

Symptoms

Heart rate, respiratory rate, color, and diaphoresis were recorded for each subject once per 30-minute observation. Heart rate and respiratory rate were sometimes above average for age but were within normal ranges. A number of confounding factors influenced the rates that we recorded, such as fear, fever, and abdominal distension. Pallor was only observed twice in 75 observation periods. Diaphoresis was not reported.

DISCUSSION

Nursing textbooks often do not distinguish between pain behaviors associated with short-term insults, such as injections, and prolonged pain, such as postsurgical pain; and in fact, most of the information on pain behaviors is based on research with brief pain. There is some evidence that physiological and behavioral adaptations occur with prolonged pain. As a consequence, we may not recognize pain behavior if it is associated with a prolonged stimulus.

The information provided by this study may help nurses to recognize long-term pain behaviors. The study may also sensitize nurses to the environmental or contextual aspects of pain. We may be able to reduce the impact of anxiety on pain and reduce the influence of modeling other children's responses. Additionally, nurses can support efforts to self-console. Play may be viewed as distracting rather than an indication of the absence of pain.

In this study parents often depended on nurses or physicians to tell them what to expect when the child was in pain. Parents became uncomfortable when behaviors of their infant seemed to indicate pain, especially if they had been told the child would not have pain or that pain would be minimal. Many parents did not report pain to nurses when nurses came in to assess the child. Nurses rarely asked parents if the child was in pain.

Parents need to be taught about nonverbal pain behaviors in children under three so that they recognize these behaviors and can distinguish them from behaviors that indicate disease.

[7]

Children's Words for Pain

Mary D. Tesler, Marilyn C. Savedra, Judith Ann Ward, William L. Holzemer, and Diana J. Wilkie

The value of patients' verbal reports for the assessment and management of pain has been documented (Bailey & Davidson, 1976; Craig, 1980; Fabrega & Tyma, 1976; Gaston-Johansson, 1984). Melzack and Torgerson (1971) developed a list of words to describe the sensory, affective, and evaluative dimensions of pain, and their work led to the McGill Pain Questionnaire, a useful tool to assess pain in adults. However, no similar tool exists for children. This chapter describes the first stage of a program of research to develop and test a tool for assessing the quality, intensity, and location of pain in children aged 8 to 17 years.

Pain words appear early in children's vocabulary. Nelson (1973) reports the use of "hot" in a child's vocabulary as early as 13 months and "hurt" at 24 months. Ross and Ross (1984a) interviewed 994 school-age children and reported that the children used colorful and discrete descriptors along with many similes to describe their pain. K. L. Thompson and J. W. Varni (personal communication, July, 1986) used a word list in an instrument to assess pediatric pain though the source of these words was not reported. The authors asked children 9–12 years old (Savedra, Gibbons, Tesler, Ward, & Wegner, 1982; Tesler,

This project was supported by the American Cancer Society, Northern California Division, and the National Institutes of Health, National Center for Nursing Research (1 R01 NU 01045–01). A fuller description of the work reported here appears in Dubner, R., Gerhert, G. F., & Bond, M. R. (Eds.) Pain research and clinical management: Vol. 3, Proceedings of the Vth World Congress on Pain. Amsterdam: Elsevier, 1988 (pp. 348–352).

Ward, Savedra, Wegner, & Gibbons, 1983) and, later, 13–17 years old (Savedra, Tesler, Ward, & Wegner, 1988), to list words that described their pain experience, and these words provided the basis for the present study.

While all the studies provide evidence that children use words to describe pain, it is not clear whether there are sex, age, ethnic, or other demographic differences in the pain descriptors used. The study reported here identified the words children most frequently selected to describe pain and examined the intensity values assigned to these words and the demographic influences on children's choices of words. The goal was to develop a list of words children could use to report the quality of their pain.

METHOD

The investigators compiled a list of 129 words that children had reported using to describe pain in two previous studies (Savedra et al., 1982; Tesler et al., 1983; Savedra et al., 1988) and from M. E. Jeans (personal communication, October, 1985). These words were printed on individual cards and randomly presented to 958 students in grades 3–12 in five urban and suburban high schools (grades 9–12; 14–17 yrs.), seven middle schools (grades 6–8; 11–13 yrs.), and five primary schools (grades 1–5; 8–10 yrs.). The children were asked to sort the words into three categories: "words they knew and used" to describe pain, "words they did not know," and "words they knew but did not use" to describe pain. The children were also asked to assign an intensity value to the words they used to describe pain, by sorting them into categories denoting small, medium, large, and worst pain.

RESULTS

The multiethnic sample of 958 students reflected the diverse population in the greater San Francisco Bay Area. Fifty-three percent were girls, 47% boys. A fourth of the sample (26%) were in grades 3–4, 24% were in grades 5–6, 20% in grades 7–8, 17% in grades 9–10 and the remaining 12% in grades 11–12. Thus the sample was fairly evenly distributed over the age range 8–17. Twenty-six percent of the children reported that English was not their first language.

Seventy-five percent of the sample knew at least 115 of the 129 words. Only 3 words (remorse, inhibiting, pulsating) were not known by more than half of the children. However, only 67 of the 115 "known" words were selected by 50% or more of the sample as words they used to describe pain. Six words or similes—hurting, sore, burning, stinging, aching, and like a sharp knife—were selected by more than 75% of the sample as words known and used to describe pain. Other words chosen by well over a majority included sharp, like a sting, pinching, cramping, swollen, uncomfortable, pounding, and awful (see Table 7.1).

The children assigned widely differing intensity values to the 67 words they knew and used. For example, words like pinching, scratching, and like a pin were assigned small pain values, reflecting the common cuts and scrapes of childhood. Medium intensity pain values were assigned to words like aching, swollen, cramping, and pounding, while large intensity values were assigned to words like sharp, awful, throbbing, and terrible. The worst pain intensities were assigned to violent, intrusive procedures such as shooting, stabbing, like a sharp knife, and for affective responses such as killing, deadly, torturing, and terrifying. Overall (using the modal intensity), 9 words were designated small, 27 medium, 15 large, and 17 worst pain intensities.

Girls selected 8 words significantly more frequently ($p < .001$) than boys (crying, frightening, frustrating, hurting, like a hurt, miserable, sickening, and scary). Children for whom English was not the first language selected 9 words significantly less frequently ($p < .001$) than native English speakers (annoying, cramping, numb, pricking, sharp, stabbing, suffocating, throbbing, and unbearable). Whites and Filipinos tended to select all the words more frequently than did Chinese, blacks, Hispanics, or others. Children in grades 3–6 (ages 8–11) selected fewer words than other children. Eleven words (aching, cramping, uncomfortable, hot, throbbing, annoying, unbearable, pricking, sharp, torturing, and piercing) were selected more and more often as the children's ages increased ($p < .001$ in each case). There were no significant differences in word selection between children previously hospitalized and those with no previous hospitalization.

Thirty-one (46%) of the 67 words identified by at least half the children as words they used to describe pain are words that appear on the McGill Pain Questionnaire; 5 additional words selected by at least half of the children appear on the McGill scale in a slightly different form ("itching" vs. "itchy"). Thus, while 36 words were related to the McGill, there were 31 additional different words that were useful for this population. When the 67 words used by the children were classified according to the McGill Pain Questionnaire into sensory, affective, and evaluative categories, 39 (58%) were considered sensory, 13 (19%) affective, and 9 (13%) evaluative, while 7 (10%) were miscellaneous.

TABLE 7.1 Words Selected by 50% or More of the Sample ($n = 958$)

Word	%	Modal[a] Intensity
Hurting	88.4	Med
Sore	83.9	Med
Burning	83.7	Wst
Stinging	80.1	Med
Aching	79.1	Med
Like a sharp knife	76.0	Wst
Sharp	74.0	Lg
Like a sting	73.5	Med
Pinching	73.4	Sml
Cramping	72.9	Med
Swollen	72.3	Med
Uncomfortable	71.6	Med
Pounding	71.0	Med, Lg
Awful	70.5	Lg
Stabbing	69.6	Wst
Cutting	69.2	Lg
Killing	68.6	Wst
Beating	67.3	Med
Terrible	67.2	Lg
Horrible	65.5	Lg
Like a pinch	65.4	Sml
Dizzy	65.4	Med
Like an ache	65.1	Med
Punching	65.1	Med
Miserable	64.9	Lg
Crushing	64.8	Lg
Itching	64.7	Sml
Biting	64.0	Med
Hot	63.8	Lg
Pressure	63.5	Med
Like a hurt	63.4	Med
Never go away	63.2	Wst
Shocking	62.6	Lg
Scratching	62.1	Sml
Numb	60.7	Med
Splitting	60.7	Lg
Hitting	60.4	Med
Blistering	59.2	Med
Throbbing	59.2	Lg
Like a pin	59.0	Sml
Crying	58.7	Sml
Sickening	58.2	Med

(continued)

TABLE 7.1 *(continued)*

Word	%	Modal[a] Intensity
Like a scratch	57.4	Sml
Dying	56.9	Wst
Bad	56.8	Med
Frightening	56.4	Lg
Tight	56.2	Med
Pin like	55.7	Sml
Screaming	55.7	Wst
Suffocating	55.5	Wst
Deadly	55.2	Wst
Annoying	54.3	Med
Uncontrollable	54.0	Wst
Stiff	54.0	Med
Tearing	53.7	Lg
Unbearable	53.0	Wst
Like a bullet	52.8	Wst
Shooting	52.7	Wst
Paralyzing	52.6	Wst
Piercing	52.5	Lg
Frustrating	51.8	Med
Pricking	51.4	Sml
Terrifying	51.3	Wst
Dreadful	51.2	Wst
Scary	51.1	Med
Torturing	50.3	Wst
Fear	49.7	Med

[a]Modal intensity: Sml = small, Med = medium, Lg = large, Wst = worst.

DISCUSSION

The number of words these children selected increased with age, reflecting cognitive development. This raises questions about the usefulness of a single tool for children across a broad age range. The intensity values assigned to the words appear to accurately reflect children's experiences with pain and the qualities of the pain. Most words assigned to the "worst" pain intensities were affective words reflecting feelings associated with pain. Only 13% of the words from the list of 67 were assigned a small intensity value. This suggests that children view pain as having a moderate to high intensity.

Words are the most discriminating tool to describe private, subjective experiences such as pain. Most children and adults, however, do not have ready pain vocabularies to use when in pain, though they can readily pick out words in a list that are useful. Having such a list is most helpful in clinical settings during stressful situations when the ability to think clearly is affected. The choice of words clearly reflects the course of the pain experience: words reflecting higher intensity values and more intrusive qualities can be expected at the time of the injury or painful procedure, and as the time from injury increases, words should reflect decreased intensity.

[8]

The Oucher: A Pain Intensity Scale for Children

Judith E. Beyer

Joann Eland, who was the first researcher to suggest that postoperative children were being seriously undermedicated, found that adults received 16 times the number of doses of analgesics that children with similar surgical conditions received (Eland & Anderson, 1977). Eland questioned not only management practices but also many of the assumptions held about children's pain.

This study was conducted while Dr. Beyer was a Fellow of the Robert Wood Johnson Clinical Nurse Scholar Program at the University of Rochester.

Eland's work was extended in our study of analgesics ordered and administered to both adults and children after open heart surgery (Beyer, DeGood, Ashley, & Russell, 1983). A review of randomly selected charts of 50 children and 50 adults showed that adults received almost two and a half times the doses of analgesics that children received; a fourth of the sample of children did not receive any analgesics after open heart surgery. In another study, researchers examined the administration of narcotics to adults and children with burns and orthopedic and abdominal surgery (Schechter, Allen, & Hanson, 1986) and found that adults received one and a half to three times the number of doses that children received.

Of key importance in the management of pediatric pain is the determination of whether or not the analgesics given to children result in adequate pain relief. Counting the doses of medications given, as in the above studies, does not provide sufficient information to determine the adequacy of analgesia. If we are to decide whether the fewer medications given to children are sufficient, too little, or too much for their individual needs, it is also necessary to know how children perceive their pain experiences.

Several self-report instruments have been developed to quantify the intensity of pediatric pain. However, while the self-report instruments have been used in research (Abu-Saad, 1984; Eland, 1981; Hester, 1979; LeBaron & Zeltzer, 1984; McGrath et al., 1985; Varni, Thompson, & Hanson, 1987), few have been tested thoroughly for validity. Self-report instruments can enhance the accuracy of subjective data collected by nurses during the assessment of pain experiences, but until they are improved, there will be uncertainty in the clinical management of pediatric pain.

THE OUCHER

To facilitate assessment and management of pediatric pain, the author developed the Oucher (Figure 8.1), a self-report tool for quantifying pain intensity in 3–12 year old children. The Oucher consists of two scales: a 0–100 numerical scale for older children who can use numbers, and a six-picture photographic scale for younger children. If children are unable to count to 100 by ones, they use the photographic scale. The photographs show the face of a child at what appear to be increasing levels of discomfort: the child's facial expression is neutral to begin with and becomes increasingly intense.

When using the Oucher to measure pain, nurses must orient children to the instrument by giving them the opportunity to remember

FIGURE 8.1.   The Oucher. (Copyright©1983, by The University of Virginia).

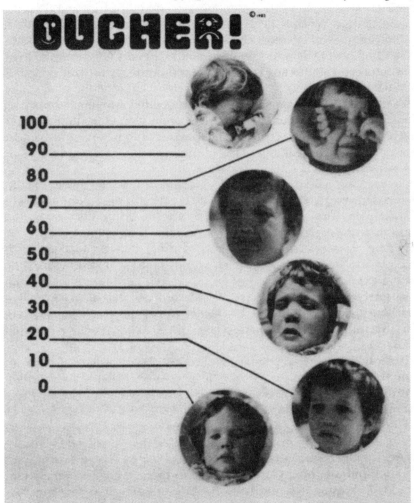

and rate past pain experiences on the instrument. This both enables the nurse to judge if the child is able to understand the Oucher and shows the child graphically that he or she has experienced varying levels of pain intensity. Although it is not always possible, teaching the child to use pain intensity instruments is best accomplished in a quiet environment at a time when the child is not experiencing pain. For example, in surgical situations, it would be best to teach the child to use the Oucher during preoperative teaching. The nurse explains that the bottom picture means no hurt and the top picture means the "biggest hurt you could ever have." The crucial question for obtaining scores is

"How much hurt do you have right now?" The photographic scale is scored from 0–5, with 0 representing the bottom picture and 5 representing the top picture. It is essential that the person collecting data not be judgmental of the child's score since children know quickly what adults want them to say or do and will generally comply. There is an important difference between clarifying the score with the child and being critical of it.

A series of methodological studies designed to examine the construct validity of this instrument have been conducted. One hundred and twelve 3–12-year-old, primarily Caucasian children were involved in one or more of these studies. The children were mentally and developmentally normal and English-speaking.

Convergent validity was tested by administering the Oucher to children concurrently with two other self-report tools to rate the intensity of their pain. The scores were highly correlated; in other words, the three instruments seemed to measure the same phenomenon. The other two measures used were Hester's Poker Chip Tool (Hester, 1979) and a visual analogue scale, which was simply a 100 mm vertical line with anchor points on each end to represent "no hurt" and the "biggest hurt you could ever have." Children were instructed to make a mark on the line to indicate the intensity of their pain, and the score was the number of millimeters from the 0 point (Beyer & Aradine, 1988).

To test the ability of the Oucher to discriminate between fear and pain, two instruments to measure fear were administered concurrently with the Oucher; the two fear measures used were the Hospital Fears Rating Scale (HFRS) (Melamed & Siegel, 1975) and the Scare Scale. The HFRS is administered by asking children how afraid (or scared) they are of 25 different items, 16 of which are related to hospital fears. The Scare Scale is a single-item measure designed by the author in which children indicate how scared they are of their particular situation; circles of increasing size are used to indicate increasing levels of fear. Each child is asked, "How scared are you of being in the hospital right now, two days after you had your heart fixed?" The Oucher scores were not correlated with scores on the fear instruments, suggesting that the Oucher is able to discriminate fear from pain (Beyer & Aradine, 1988).

Additional evidence of construct validity was obtained by a study in which patterns of pain scores were found to vary in expected directions before and after surgery and before and after analgesic administration. The presurgical pain score was 0 for 90% of the children in this study ($n = 102$). Only 10 of the children reported pain, and all but one could identify a reason for the hurt. A group of children with more extensive surgical procedures reported more pain after surgery than children with less extensive procedures. Pain scores were highest immediately after major surgery, gradually decreasing almost to baseline by the fifth postoperative day. Pain scores were also high before analgesics were given; they decreased the hour after administration and then gradually began to increase three hours later (Aradine, Beyer, & Tompkins, 1988; Beyer & Aradine, 1987).

A major study of the Oucher examined the content validity of the photographic scale (Beyer & Aradine, 1986). Essentially, the researchers wanted to know if the pictures were in the right order according to children; the children themselves served as expert judges.

The following research questions were explored in this study:

1. Are 3–7 year old children able to discriminate the facial expressions shown in the photographs of the Oucher?
2. Do children agree in sequencing the photographs of the Oucher?
3. Are there differences in the ways that children sequence the photographs?
4. What percentage of children agree with the original placement of the photographs of the Oucher?
5. How consistent is the sequencing by the children with the sequencing of the Oucher?

METHOD

To answer these questions, 26 3–7-year-old children were obtained from each of three sites: a day care center, a hospital, and a presurgical orientation program. The parents of the hospitalized and presurgical children were approached for permission directly. Consent forms were mailed to the parents of the day care children.

The subjects were asked if they would help the researcher make a poster and were then shown the six photographs of the Oucher. They were asked to sequence them according to their perceptions of the amount of "hurt" shown.

Specific instructions to the children were these:

Will you help me make a poster? Let me show you what we have to do. The poster is about hurting. Do you know what I mean by hurt? [The child explains and the researcher confirms and/or clarifies.] All of these pictures are about hurting. There is one picture there that shows no hurt at all. Can you pick it out? Now, there is just one picture that shows the biggest hurt you could ever have. Can you pick that one? Now of these four pictures that are left, can you show me the biggest hurt that's left? [This is done until all pictures have been chosen.]

RESULTS

The 78 subjects ranged in age from 3.1 to 7.9 years (mean = 4.8). The majority were below the age of five (62%). The hospitalized group consisted primarily of children who had had surgery. All of the children in the presurgical group were scheduled for surgery within a week of their orientation programs. The day care children were essentially healthy children engaged in day care activities.

Although some variation was found in the way children sequenced the photographs, overall, 77% of the sample sequenced five or six of the six photographs in the order they appear on the Oucher, with 41% correctly sequencing all six of the photographs and 36% correctly sequencing five. Seventeen percent correctly placed four out of the six photographs, and only 6% placed three or fewer in the same order as displayed on the Oucher. Not only did the entire sample show this degree of accuracy, but so did age, sex, and site subsamples, with one exception: 3-year-olds had a bit more difficulty with the task; only 52% of these children correctly sequenced five or six of the photographs.

Mean ranks were calculated for each photograph based on the average number of times children placed it first, second, third, etc., in the sequence. These mean ranks were found to correspond closely to the order of the pictures on the Oucher, again lending support for the validity of the ordering of the photographs.

DISCUSSION

The results of the series of studies of the Oucher indicate that it is possible to get children to quantify pain through the use of an appropriate self-report scale. A valid scale to measure pain intensity in children 3–12 years old has important implications for practice.

First, the Oucher provides a means to more closely monitor the pain experiences of children. This is important not only for pain assessment but also for pain management. If pain can be measured precisely and systematically, nurses will be able to better test interventions to relieve pain. These interventions may include medications, relaxation techniques, position changes, distraction, or other techniques. All of these methods need to be tested for their efficacy. In addition, with a valid assessment tool painful situations can be examined more closely so that health providers can be more sure about what children are experiencing.

In order to use the Oucher, a nurse needs to have rapport with the child. If it is used in conjunction with decisions on how much medication to give, injections must be avoided. That is because children will quickly tie their self-reports to getting "shots"; it will only take one injection before they report "no hurt" on any pain scale. As far as they are concerned, getting a shot is punishment for being honest.

The photographic scale has both advantages and disadvantages. First, the photographs serve as relevant cues for pain when presented to most 3–7-year-old children. They are attracted to the photographs, which are colorful, real, and rich with information. There are, however, some 3 year olds who cannot use the Oucher, particularly those who have just turned three. Because of their cognitive immaturity, they may not understand the idea of describing how they feel by pointing to a picture. It is readily apparent when they do not understand. A prime example was the little 3-year-old boy who said to the research assistant, "No, the hurt is on my arm, not on the board [Oucher]." Until more testing is done, it would be best to use caution when administering the Oucher to 3-year-olds.

The photographs of the Oucher are also culturally specific; they are of a white child. It is uncertain at this time whether that is a problem. Additional research to test the content validity and acceptability of the photographic scale of the Oucher with large groups of black and Hispanic children is being done by a nurse administrator/clinical specialist at the Children's Hospital of Michigan and a professor at Wayne State University School of Nursing (Denyes & Villarruel, 1988; Villarruel & Denyes, 1988). It is essential to determine whether all ethnic groups can use the Oucher as it currently exists, or whether it is necessary to construct other models of the instrument to accommodate children of different cultural backgrounds.

Data are beginning to accumulate to suggest that the Oucher is a valid and useful tool for assessment and management of pediatric pain. The patient's subjective report of pain intensity should count heavily in the nurse's diagnosis and treatment decisions. As Margo McCaffery points out, "Pain is whatever the experiencing person says it is, occurring whenever he or she says it does" (McCaffery, 1977, p. 12).

[9]

The Relationship Between Assessment and Pharmacologic Intervention for Pain in Children

Roxie L. Foster and Nancy Olson Hester

The nurse handed me the rating sheet on which she had recorded her assessment of 5-year-old Tanya's pain. She had rated her 6.5 on a scale of 10, and had noted that her assessment was based upon the child's irritability and sleepiness and the fact that she was being repositioned in bed at the time of the measure (see Figure 9.1). This was Tanya's first postoperative day following bilateral tibial osteotomies. Two hours earlier Tanya had received 10 ml of Tylenol with codeine elixir.

The next step in the pain assessment was to obtain the child's own rating of her pain. As I entered the room, Tanya lay quietly sucking her thumb. Her eyes closed intermittently but she was not asleep. I showed her a ladder picture and explained that at the bottom of the ladder there was no hurt, but with each step up the hurt got worse and worse until, at the top, the hurt was as bad as it could be. Tanya was then asked to mark on the ladder or point to the place that was like the way she felt. She pointed to the bottom. "Do you feel just fine—no hurt?" I asked. "It hurts," she said irritably, "but I want to go to sleep."

Tanya was not medicated during the hour and a half between the first and second assessments of her pain. At the second assessment, the nurse again rated the child's pain at 6.5 on the 10-point pain ladder. She recorded that Tanya had complained of pain and asked for pain medication. When Tanya was asked to indicate the place on the ladder that was like her pain at that moment, she pointed to the top. Upon questioning she confirmed that the pain was much worse than before. She was whining and fretful, sucking her thumb, and lying very still in the bed. Despite the nurse's assessment of Tanya's pain at 6.5, the child still received no medication until one and a half hours later, two hours after she was eligible for a dose.

This case illustrates the clinical problem that is the focus of the research reported here: the undertreatment of pain in children. The pioneering work of Eland (Eland & Anderson, 1977) alerted the nursing profession to this problem. Since then researchers have developed a number of instruments and techniques for assessing children's pain (Abu-Saad & Holzemer, 1981; Beyer, 1984; Craig, McMahon, Morison, & Zaskow, 1984; Hester, 1979; Jeans, 1984; Katz, Kellerman, & Siegel, 1980; LeBaron & Zeltzer, 1984; McGrath et al., 1985; Molsberry, 1979; Savedra, Gibbons, Tesler, Ward, & Wegner, 1982; Scott, 1978; Szyfelbein, Osgood, & Carr, 1985; Taylor, 1983), have studied the assessment criteria nurses use to assess pain (Bradshaw & Zeanah, 1986; Burokas, 1985; Lukens, 1982; Varchol, 1983) and have questioned children about their experience of pain (Hester & Barcus, 1986; Ross & Ross, 1984b). Sadly, the problem remains. In 1986 the NIH Consensus Development Conference on the Integrated Approach to the Management of Pain noted that, "Even when pain is reported and assessed, it may not necessarily be attended, monitored, treated, and satisfactorily managed" (p. 6).

FIGURE 9.1. Nurse's rating of Tanya's pain on the pain ladder.

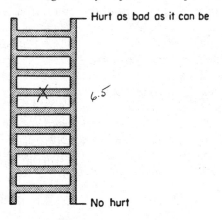

Hurt os bod os it con be

6.5

No hurt

METHOD

This research explored the relationship among nurses' ratings of pain in children, the cues upon which nurses based those judgments, and the medications administered for pain. Data were gathered from pain ratings, nurses' assessment cues, and medication records.

The research was part of a larger study (Hester, 1986–88) of the generalizability of two instruments designed to assess children's pain—the Hester poker chip tool and the pain ladder (Hay, 1984). Findings are presented here for 120 cases, representing 60 children who were assessed with the poker chip tool and 60 children who were in the pain ladder group. The boys and girls ranged in age from 4 to 13 years, and were either postoperative or determined to be experiencing pain by virtue of their medical diagnosis and prior assessments by nursing staff. The children were largely Caucasian and from middle-class families. The study was conducted at a large regional children's hospital with an all-RN staff.

Children in the study were randomly assigned to one of two pain assessment groups—the Hester poker chip group or the pain ladder group. The pain ladder instrument is shown in Figure 9.1. The poker chip tool consists of four red poker chips. Children in that group were told that each chip represented one piece of hurt. They were then asked to indicate how many "pieces of hurt" they were experiencing at the time. Pain ratings (up to four in an eight-hour period) were made by both the nurse and the child. The ratings were independent of one another, with neither the nurse nor the child knowing the level of pain indicated by the other. Nurses also wrote on their assessment sheet the cues they used to determine the child's level of pain.

Data on medications were also collected. Medications were recorded that were given (1) within four hours preceding the first pain measure, (2) between measures, and (3) within one hour after the final measure. Using this information, profiles were developed to describe each child's analgesia during the hours when pain measures were obtained. Tanya's profile, cited earlier, is an example.

The percentage of possible medications administered to each child was determined based on the actual number of medications given divided by the number of times when it would have been possible to medicate the child. Medication was considered a potential nursing action if (1) at least one analgesic was ordered, (2) sufficient time had elapsed since the last medication, and (3) the nurse rated the child's pain greater than zero on the assigned scale.

RESULTS

Overall, children were medicated approximately 48% of the time when medication was an alternative. Children who were rated on the poker chip tool were given medications more often (52%) than those who were rated on the pain ladder (42%). The reason for this difference may be related to the fact that children rated on the pain ladder were, on average, three days postoperative while those rated on the poker chip averaged two days postoperative. Except for this difference, however, the groups were similar. Children in both groups had similar rating patterns for pain across the measures, as did the nurses who rated them. The groups were evenly distributed among diagnoses, clinical units, age, and sex.

This study was concerned not only about whether the children received or did not receive medication for pain, but also about the relative dosage of the medications ordered and administered. It was necessary, therefore, to calculate the maximum recommended therapeutic dose for each analgesic ordered. These calculations were based upon nationally recognized standards (see Table 9.1).

The percent of maximum therapeutic dose was computed as the dosage ordered divided by the maximum dose recommended. First the maximum therapeutic dose was computed by multiplying the maximum recommended dosage by the child's body weight (see Table 9.2). For example, if the child weighed 24 kg, this weight times the maximum recommended dose for morphine (0.1 mg) would yield a maximum dose of 2.4 mg of morphine. The minimum and maximum doses ordered were then divided by the maximum therapeutic dose. If the order, in this case, was for 2 to 3 mg of morphine, 2 mg would represent 83% of the dose that could be safely administered, whereas 3 mg would be 125% of the maximum amount recommended.

The three most commonly ordered analgesics were morphine, Tyle-

TABLE 9.1 Standards Used to Calculate Maximum Recommended Therapeutic Dose

Drug	Recommended Therapeutic Range[a]
Morphine Sulfate IV	0.05 - 0.1 mg/kg of body weight
Tylenol with Codeine #3	0.5 - 1.0 mg/kg of body weight
Tylenol	10 - 15 mg/kg of body weight

[a]Biller & Yeager, 1987; U.S. Pharmacopeial Convention, 1987.

TABLE 9.2   Calculation of Maximum Therapeutic Dose

	Formula
Step 1	Compute the maximum therapeutic dose for the child. Multiply the high end of the maximum recommended range times the child's weight in kilograms. e.g., 0.1 mg morphine $\times$ 24 kg = 2.4 mg maximum dose
Step 2	Compute the percent of maximum therapeutic dose represented by the dose (or dosage range) ordered. Divide the minimum and maximum doses ordered by the maximum therapeutic dose. e.g., If the order reads 2–3 mg morphine IV: 2/2.4 = 83% of recommended maximum 3/2.4 = 125% of recommended maximum

nol with codeine #3 and plain Tylenol. Means and ranges for the doses ordered by physicians for the 120 children are presented in Table 9.3. Although the average orders ranged from 47% to 114% of the maximum recommended dose, the range of individual orders among these three analgesics was remarkable—from 7 to 224%. The findings emphasize the need for nurses to calculate recommended therapeutic doses based upon each child's body weight, to calculate the percentage of therapeutic maximum that is represented by the ordered dose or dosage range, and to include that information in judgments about medication administration.

Data from this study indicate that nurses tend to give higher doses of Tylenol and Tylenol with codeine #3 (with respect to therapeutic maximum) than of morphine (see Table 9.4). Additional research is needed to determine why nurses are more reluctant to administer maximum therapeutic doses of morphine. It would be interesting, for example, to see whether administration patterns would change if nurses based dosage judgment on knowledge of the maximum amount of the drug that could safely be administered.

TABLE 9.3   Medications Ordered by Physician

Medication	Means	Range
Morphine Sulfate (% of 0.1 mg/kg)	47% to 99%	7% to 200%
Tylenol with Codeine #3 (% of 1.0 mg/kg)	64% to 114%	31% to 224%
Tylenol (% of 15 mg/kg)	52% to 96%	39% to 180%

TABLE 9.4 Analgesics Administered by Nurses: Percent of Maximum Therapeutic Dose

Name of drug administered	Minimum dose administered	Maximum dose administered	Mean of doses administered
Morphine Sulfate (% of 0.1 mg/kg)	38%	131%	68%
Tylenol with Codeine (% of 1.0 mg/kg)	31%	209%	88%
Tylenol (% of 15 mg/kg)	41%	180%	92%

Surprisingly, the nurses' self-reported assessment cues often provided little rationale for their interventions for pain and sometimes seemed inconsistent with their pain ratings. The following profiles help to illustrate these findings. In the first example medication was given despite low pain ratings; in the second example, medication was withheld despite identified pain.

Profile 1. Sherry, age 10, was three days postoperative following removal of a dermoid tumor and adhesions on her spinal cord. She had received a Tylenol suppository 650 mg (118% of therapeutic maximum) at 6 A.M. At 9:40, the time of the first pain measure, the nurse rated Sherry's pain as 1 on the 4-point poker chip tool. She indicated that this judgment was based upon the child's expression and verbal comments. Sherry rated her pain as a 2 at this time, but she was not medicated. At 11:15 she was medicated with Tylenol with codeine #3, one tablet (82% of therapeutic maximum for her weight). Ten minutes later, before the Tylenol with codeine #3 had time to absorb, both Sherry and her nurse rated the pain as 1. The nurse wrote that Sherry had told her, "It hurts less than last time." The nurse offered no further cues to explain why medication was given when the child's pain was apparently less severe than at the first rating, when she received nothing for pain.

Profile 2. Roger, age 6, participated in the study on the first day after surgery on both feet to correct a congenital flexion deformity. The analgesics ordered postoperatively were morphine, Tylenol with codeine #3, and plain Tylenol. Tylenol with codeine #3 was ordered 5 to 10 ml every 3 to 4 hours. Roger received 5 ml at 8:30. This was 64% of the maximum recommended dose.

At 10:15 Roger's nurse gave him a rating of 2 on the 4-point poker chip scale. She noted that he was "fussy when his toes were lightly touched" and that "he refused to wiggle his toes." She indicated that he was "playing a game with Mom." Following this measure the nurse remarked that the mother and child seemed extremely anxious about pain. When I approached Roger for his rating of pain he was crying. He said the pain was "bad" and rated his pain as a 4.

At 11:25 the nurse rated Roger's pain as 1 and recorded that he was "asleep with easy respirations." When I entered the room moments later, however, Roger was awake and I wondered if he had only pretended to be sleeping. He told me the hurt was as bad as before, indicated a rating of 4, and said that the pain was in his legs.

At 12:50 the nurse again rated Roger's pain as 1 and recorded that the child had told her he didn't hurt. She repeated that he seemed very anxious. Clearly, Roger was giving different signals to the nurse and the researcher, because when asked to rate his pain he indicated four poker chips, tearfully pointed to his legs, and said that the pain was no better. Once again, I confirmed with him that he meant the pain was as bad as it could be. At this time, on his first postoperative day, it had been more than five hours since his last medication for pain and that had been only 64% of what might safely have been administered.

The last measure was at 2:05 P.M. This time the nurse's rating matched Roger's: both indicated 4 on the 4-point scale. The nurse said that her judgment was based on Roger's "crying, short attention span, and rejecting questions." Yet Roger received no medication within four hours after that measure.

DISCUSSION

These examples illustrate the perplexing findings from this study: high pain ratings by either the nurse or the child were only moderately associated with administration of analgesia; physicians' orders for analgesics deviated widely from the recommended maximum dosages; pain ratings by nurses were sometimes inconsistent with their self-reported assessment cues; and nurses' assessment cues often provided little rationale for their interventions. Further, the study demonstrates some of the complexities of pain assessment in children: the difficulty of obtaining an accurate assessment when the child chooses not to participate in evaluating pain (as in the case of Tanya, who just wanted to sleep), the difficulty of knowing when anxiety is related to pain and when it is associated with fears of hospitalization in general, and the possibility that the child may deliberately mislead the nurse to avoid "that nasty medicine" or because of fear of other interventions.

The study of the relationships between nurses' ratings of children's pain, nurses' assessment cues related to pain, and the medications administered for pain raises many questions:

- What, besides pain rating, goes into the nurse's decision to administer analgesia?
- Is there an allowable level of pain? If so, what is that level?
- Are some nurses still concerned about the safety of administering analgesics to children?
- Are some nurses overzealous in their attempts to discriminate between anxiety and pain? Does pain increase anxiety? Does anxiety increase pain?
- Can a child be in significant pain and still fall asleep?
- Are decisions about pain medication based upon professional knowledge and research?
- How do personal values affect clinical decision making?
- Are dosage decisions related to knowledge of the drug's recommended therapeutic range?
- Are recommendations for therapeutic dosages unnecessarily conservative? Is it safe to give more than 100% of the recommended therapeutic maximum?
- Is pain relief routinely evaluated following administration of analgesia to children?
- What comfort measures might be used in addition to or in place of analgesia?
- At what level of pain are nonpharmacologic measures indicated?

This research offers no clear answers to the questions. Those answers will come when the body of knowledge concerning pain in children is sufficient for use as a base for practice. In the meantime, every nurse has the responsibility to critically analyze clinical decision making in concert with the currently available research and theoretical knowledge about pain in children.

[10]

Use of Patient-Controlled Analgesia by Children

Catherine J. Webb, Debra A. Stergios, and Bradley M. Rodgers

Current research on pediatric pain shows that we are not adequately administering postoperative analgesics (Beyer, DeGood, Ashley & Russell, 1983; Eland & Anderson, 1977; Mather & Mackie, 1983; Schechter, Allen, & Hanson, 1986; Strauss, Fagerhaugh, & Glaser, 1974; Swafford & Allen, 1968). There are many factors that contribute to this. Typical medical orders for analgesics allow great variation in their administration because the orders usually specify a range in dosage and frequency. The time when medication is given and the dosage are both determined by the nurse. Therefore, the same patient may receive different dosages for the same level of pain depending on the nurse who administers the medication. Factors affecting the nurse's ability to discern a child's need for pain medication include the busyness of the clinical setting and the nurse's previous experiences with children in pain, experiences with his or her own pain, values and beliefs about administering narcotics, and knowledge of children's developmental stages.

Some children verbalize their need for pain medication more quickly than others, and there are children who cannot communicate their experience of pain at all. Variables that can affect the child's ability to

Funding for this study was provided by the University of Virginia School of Nursing. Patient-controlled analgesia infuser pumps were provided by Abbott Laboratories, Chicago, Illinois 60064. We gratefully acknowledge the technical assistance of Don Delk.

communicate pain include speech impediments, shyness, fear, inability to speak, cultural values regarding medicines, and the parents' absence or presence. In an unfamiliar environment without a parent present, the child will often try to hide pain.

School-age and adolescent surgical patients sometimes experience considerable difficulty with pain management. Various drugs, including antianxiety agents, dosages, and schedules have been tried without much success. Some of these children express the fear that they will not get pain medication when they ask for it or will have to wait for it to be administered. The situation is frustrating for children, their parents, nursing and medical staff.

Self-administration of intravenous narcotics or patient-controlled analgesia (PCA) is well documented as an effective method of pain treatment for adults (Atwell et al., 1984; Bennett, Batenhorst, Bivins et al., 1982; Bennett, Batenhorst, Graves et al., 1982; Check, 1982; Citron et al., 1986). Children aged 11–18 have adequate cognitive ability to manage PCA, with the added security that PCA devices' safety features will prevent inadvertent overmedication. Therefore, PCA should be an effective method of pain control for these children.

METHOD

The purpose of this study was to determine if 11–18-year-olds could use PCA for relief of postoperative pain. In particular, we wanted to ascertain whether children can manage PCA, whether they assess PCA as an effective method for the relief of postoperative pain, whether parents of these children assess PCA as an effective method for relief of pain, and whether 11–18-year-old children use less analgesia with PCA than with traditional methods of pain medication.

SUBJECTS

The study was conducted at the University of Virginia Children's Medical Center in the pediatric intensive care unit and the school-age medical-surgical unit. The experimental group consisted of 15 pediatric surgery patients who had undergone elective surgery, were mentally alert without head injury, were able to understand and comply with instruction, had no known allergy to morphine sulfate, and had no history of narcotic abuse or addiction.

The control group was made up of 15 children who met the same criteria as the experimental group and who received intravenous morphine by the traditional bolus method. The control group children had received treatment prior to this study and the amount of medication administered was assessed by chart review.

Intervention

Children were taught by the researchers how to use the PCA device at least 6 hours prior to surgery. The basic concept of PCA was explained in simple terms: the child was to push the button when feeling pain and thus receive medication. The researchers pointed out to the children the differences between PCA and asking nurses for pain medication.

The safety of PCA was reviewed, and the children were told they would receive exactly the amount of medicine their doctors had ordered because the infuser was very accurate. The researchers also explained that the nurse would check on the child and the infusers every 2–4 hours, the child could not give himself too much medicine, and he had to press the button to make the infuser work, thereby preventing an accidental dose of medicine. The child was told that when he started to feel pain he should push the button (unless he was extremely sleepy). If the child experienced pain despite having pushed the button, he was to call his nurse.

The researchers demonstrated use of the PCA infuser with a syringe and tubing containing water by pressing the button so the child could see the fluid infusing from the open end of the tubing. The child was encouraged to practice using the machine during the evening.

A verbal pain rating scale ranging from 0 to 10 was explained to each child, who was told to expect his nurse to ask him to rate his pain every two hours during the day and evening shifts and every four hours at night. He was assured that the nurse would not wake him if he was sleeping, however. The Visual Analogue Scale (VAS) was also explained, and the child practiced using the VAS by rating his present pain. He was told that the nurse researcher would ask him to rate his pain on the VAS twice a day. The child was then given an opportunity to ask questions about PCA and the pain rating scales.

All of the children learned to successfully manage the PCA infuser during the teaching session though three children required reinforcement. In those cases, one of the researchers returned later to review the basic concepts and answer questions.

For the experimental group, PCA was begun two hours after the child returned from the recovery room. If the analgesics administered in the recovery room did not provide sufficient pain relief, IV analgesics were administered by a nurse prior to the initiation of PCA. All of the PCA orders were written by the attending physician or chief surgical resident. These orders included (1) dose of morphine sulfate (usual range = 0.05 mg–0.1 mg/kg); (2) lockout time interval, the period during which the PCA cannot be activated (usual range = 10–15 minutes); and (3) 4–hour limit setting, the maximum amount of morphine a patient can receive in 4 hours (preset maximum = 30, range = 5–30 mg in 5 mg increments). PCA was discontinued when the child was ready for oral medication.

Data Collection

The following information was obtained from all of the children: date of birth, sex, race, admission height and weight, admission vital signs, type of surgery, any existing chronic illness, current medications, previous hospitalizations, and level of education. We also recorded how well the experimental group children understood PCA and the infuser device after a teaching session.

Using the verbal report scale ranging from "no pain" at 0 to "the worst pain possible" at 10, each child in the experimental group was asked by the nurse at the bedside to rate his pain every 2 hours during the day and evening shifts and every 4 hours at night.

The nurse recorded the amount of morphine sulfate administered by the child on a bedside flow sheet and in the medication Kardex. The nurse also recorded the child's pain rating, and his or her assessment of the child's pain on the flow sheet. The sheet also provided space for vital signs and comments.

Twice a day the researchers asked the children to rate their pain using this same verbal report scale and a 10 cm visual analogue scale (VAS), one end of which indicated no pain and the other extreme pain. This information was recorded on a separate flow sheet. If a parent was staying at the bedside, he or she was asked to also rate the child's pain. A simple questionnaire was given to the child and parent 24 hours after PCA was discontinued to obtain general comments and to discern whether the child and parent felt PCA was effective for postoperative pain.

RESULTS

The two groups in the study were similar in type of surgery, age, gender, race, hospital experience and education ($p > .01$). All of the children in the study had been admitted for major abdominal or chest surgery.

FIGURE 10.1. The average amount of morphine sulfate administrated by each group.

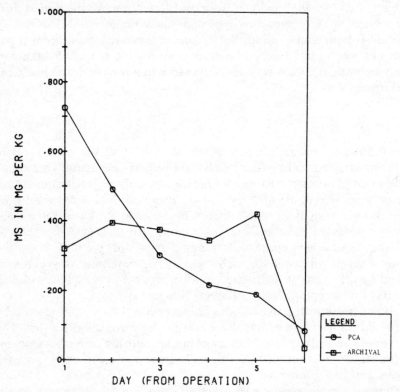

When we compared the amount of morphine (mg/kg/24-hour period) administered to each group, we found that during the first 24 hours the experimental group (the PCA group) used 2.3 times as much morphine (.73 versus .32) as the control group (the chart audit group). The overall number of patients using IV morphine declined each day, which made it hard to accurately interpret the data after day three or four. However, on the third day the PCA group had tapered its use of morphine to less than the control group (0.30 versus 0.37) and continued to use less (Figure 10.1).

The PCA children received adequate and even pain relief throughout each day; the mean self-report of pain was 4.01 on the 10-point verbal scale. Nurse ratings were slightly lower. Of the few parents who stayed with their children 24 hours a day, only two assessed their children's pain. The other parents felt their child could better assess his pain and therefore declined to do so themselves.

The questionnaires documented a high degree of satisfaction with PCA. Eleven children and 10 parents (only 11 of the 15 parents answered the questionnaire) said that they would like to use PCA again. The majority of children and parents indicated that PCA was a better method of administering pain medication than the methods they had previously experienced.

Children and parents felt the advantages of PCA use included (1) not having to wait to receive pain medication, (2) longer and more effective pain relief, (3) not having to call the nurse, (4) giving their own medication, and (5) ease of operating the PCA device. The disadvantages they saw with PCA were related to medication side effects: nausea, dosage adjustment, and burning sensation at infusion site; and restriction of activity from short intravenous tubing and the size of the pump.

Informally the nursing staff expressed satisfaction with the pump, noting that PCA provided their patients with good pain control. They also felt that the nursing time saved by self-medication could be used to provide better nursing care. The nurses reported that the self-care and control aspects of PCA were valuable for their patients.

Parent and nurse comfort with PCA, the satisfactory pain relief, and the lack of harmful incidents all indicate that, overall, the children were able to manage the PCA device. However, two 11-year-olds had some minor difficulty using the PCA infuser post-operatively. At times they were reluctant to self-administer their pain medication. When prompted by parents or nursing staff, however, they sometimes did trigger the device.

Some problems arose during the study: the fact that the 4-hour limits could be set in 5 mg increments was problematic; often physicians would have preferred more precise dosages. Also, at times it was difficult to assess the patient's pain management and regulate medication because of inability to discern how long the patient needed to wait when the 4-hour dose limit had been reached. Several children complained of burning at the IV site when the morphine was infusing, which may have been caused in part by the rate of infusion (1 mg/14 sec; nurses usually give 1 mg/min). All of these problems, however, have been solved by the recent design of a new PCA device.

One patient accidentally received a dose of morphine when his push button fell on the floor and landed with the button down. Following this incident it became policy to pin the push button to the child's bed linen.

DISCUSSION

This study indicates that PCA is an effective method of postoperative pain treatment for children 11–18 years of age. These children obtained good pain relief and expressed satisfaction with the treatment, and parents and nurses were enthusiastic about this method of administering pain medication. PCA also gave the children some control over their care. In many postsurgical situations, this may be one of the few areas of control open to the child. This was seen as a positive aspect of PCA by the children, their parents, and the nursing staff.

Following this study, the use of PCA has become a common method of pain relief for children in this age group at our medical center. PCA has been used effectively by children with these medical and surgical conditions: orthopedic surgery, sickle cell crisis, cancer, cystic fibrosis and multiple trauma (where no head injury occurred). For some children it has been found that PCA is a good adjunct to an initial loading dose and/or continuous infusion of morphine sulfate.

PCA can be used on any nursing care unit that already practices intravenous administration of narcotics. PCA is safe and does not require additional patient assessment; the patient is assessed for pain and the amount of medicine administered every 2–4 hours. The use of PCA is attractive because it increases nursing productivity by eliminating the time required for narcotic administration.

The nursing staff can learn quickly how to program and operate PCA devices. The children in this study demonstrated that patient teaching is easily accomplished and requires minimal nursing time. Preoperative instruction can provide the nurse with a good opportunity for patient assessment as well.

The initial cost of equipment can be significant; however, the positive patient outcomes and nursing productivity should be considered as a balance for this expense. Nurses should therefore consider the use of PCA as an intervention for the treatment of 11–18 year olds who are experiencing pain requiring intravenous analgesics.

[11]

The Effectiveness of Transcutaneous Electrical Nerve Stimulation (TENS) with Children Experiencing Cancer Pain

Joann M. Eland

When I was a new staff nurse in 1970, a seven-year-old boy, Scott, was dying from a metastatic brain tumor on the unit where I was working. Scott and his family had been favorites of the nursing staff since his diagnosis nine months previously and in spite of the seriousness of his illness, he maintained his sense of humor and always looked on the bright side of his situation. Things did not go well for Scott, and his condition had worsened to the point that he was admitted to the hospital at his parents' request. It was not difficult to understand that request, because whenever anyone came into contact with his body or even bumped the bed slightly, he screamed in pain. Whenever a member of the staff entered his room he said with terror in his voice, "What are you going to do to me?" and began to cry. An evaluation revealed that there was nothing more that could be done for Scott to stop the advancing disease. The nursing staff repeatedly requested analgesics from the physicians caring for him, but they refused to order even a single acetaminophen (Tylenol) for him and he remained in intense, uncontrolled, 24-hour-a-day pain. As his condition deteriorated it was highly likely that Scott was going to have a respiratory arrest and his parents were asked if they wanted his life maintained on life support systems. The very morning this issue was raised, Scott had a respiratory and cardiac arrest. An aggressive physician and three *obedient* nurses including me resuscitated Scott for over an hour. The result of this "heroic" effort was 72 more hours of agony for Scott until his parents could make the decision to stop the vasopressor that was maintaining his blood pressure. *Never* have I felt less like a nurse than on that occasion when we maintained a life with no hope of cure and no relief of symptoms, when living only meant a "living hell" for Scott and those who loved him. The one thing (in addition to requesting a resuscitation status from the family earlier) the health care team could have done for Scott in his final weeks was to relieve his pain and that was not done.

Fortunately pain control in pediatrics has come a very long way, and it is highly unlikely that this situation would repeat itself today. However, Scott and many other children have left me with memories that provide a challenge for me to continue working on behalf of children in pain. I believe that if we keep the interests of the children first, the knowledge on which to base our practice will continue to develop as rapidly as time will allow.

This study was designed to determine whether transcutaneous electrical nerve stimulation (TENS) can be used in children ages four and older experiencing pain associated with cancer. The earliest reported use of electrical stimulation for pain relief is believed to have been among the ancient Egyptians, who in 600 B.C. used the electricity of the lung fish (related to the eel) in basins of water to rid themselves of the pain of gout. Since the early 1970s, the beginning of the modern TENS era in the United States, TENS technology and its application to the clinical setting have been changing rapidly. To compare the technical specifications of a device manufactured in 1973 to one of the new models of TENS would be like comparing the engine of a Model T Ford to a modern race car. In the early 1970s the devices were large, heavy (because they required four D cell batteries), noisy, and had two controls (amplitude and rate). A TENS unit in 1988 is a small silent device with capabilities far beyond the earlier versions. The controls and functions of the newest models are summarized in Tables 11.1, 11.2, and 11.3.

Research reporting the effectiveness of TENS has varied depending on the focus of the research. Various health care providers have explored (1) which types of pain could be relieved by TENS, (2) stimulation parameters, (3) electrode placement, and (4) the applications of the evolving technological improvements. When critiquing TENS research, a reader must recognize the impact these four approaches have had and how they have affected the success or failure of a given project. Nurses' contributions to TENS research have been infrequent, but TENS is a powerful intervention with expansive applications that are

TABLE 11.1   TENS Parameters

Control	Adjustments	Function
Amplitude	0-60	Determines amount of energy to skin
Rate	2-125 pps	Indicates the number of times per second the nerve is stimulated
Pulse Width	30-250 u sec	Controls depth of stimulation

TABLE 11.2   Stimulation Variations

Normal
Modulate Rate
Modulate Pulse Width
Modulate Rate and Pulse Width
Burst
Modulate Pulse Width and Amplitude

TABLE 11.3   Stimulation Modalities of TENS

	Rate	Pulse Width	Amplitude
Conventional	75-100 pps	>250 u sec	No Contraction
Low Rate			
Acupuncture Like	1-4 pps	200-300 u sec	Visible muscle twitches
Brief Intense	150 pps	150+ u sec	Early muscle twitches

not yet recognized by our colleagues in physical therapy, who have been responsible for most of the clinical knowledge about TENS. Nurses, by virtue of their role, are exposed to a greater variety of patient situations and have contact with hospitalized patients 24 hours a day; also, they are often the most frequent resource for community clients.

This study was designed to answer the following questions: (1) Is TENS effective in reducing cancer-associated pain in children aged four and older? (2) Is TENS an acceptable pain relief alternative to children who have undergone a large number of painful episodes associated with cancer? (3) Can TENS be used for some nontraditional types of pains that children with cancer experience, such as painful intravenous infusions, bone metastasis, or phantom limb pain?

The research was intended to be a preliminary project that would provide a basis for a larger, more comprehensive project.

METHOD

Subjects

Subjects between the ages of 4 and 17 years with pain related to cancer or its treatment that was unrelieved by conventional methods were referred to the investigator by the pediatric oncologists at a 1,100 bed Midwestern university teaching hospital. The physicians were aware of the investigator's expertise in pain management and knew that the investigator had a clinical base in the use of TENS with adults experiencing pain and was interested in examining its effectiveness with children.

Because so little is known about the use of TENS with children or its use with cancer pathology, the investigator decided to use a case study approach with several children as subjects. No attempt was made to control the subjects' various pathologies, previous pain experiences, current pain producing processes, use of analgesics, stage of the disease process, sex, or any other extraneous variables.

Procedure

After appropriate introductions were made, it was explained to the child and family that the oncologist and researcher were unsure whether the device might benefit them but that the device would certainly not hurt the child in any way. The use of TENS was the sole decision of the child and parents. If the child and family consented to participate, the protocol in Table 11.4 was followed.

Conventional TENS (see Table 11.1) was used for the study because it is the most comfortable type of stimulation and is well tolerated by most people (Mannheimer & Lampe, 1984). The single principle guiding electrode placement is that the electrode must be placed so that the stimulus is directed at the central nervous system. Optimal electrode placement can best be accomplished at the spinal column, at superficial aspects of peripheral nerves and at acupuncture, motor, and trigger points (Mannheimer & Lampe, 1984). In this study the specific location of pain was determined from descriptions by the children and elec-

TABLE 11.4 Pediatric Protocol for TENS

---

1. Place two electrodes on one of the parents and stimulate a superficial nerve such as the radial and the base of a finger using conventional TENS settings.
2. Have the parent adjust the amplitude control to produce a strong comfortable sensation.
3. After a few minutes have the parent readjust the amplitude to produce a strong comfortable sensation.
4. Allow the child to touch the parent and the electrodes while they are still attached to the parent.
5. Ask the parent if this hurts or causes pain in any way.
6. After about 15 minutes have the parent compare sensation in the stimulated finger and the same finger (nonstimulated) on the opposite hand.
7. Ask the child if he would like to try the TENS Unit on his hand (provided the hand is not the current source of pain).
8. Give the child the TENS unit to hold and tell him the unit is "off" and he will be in control of it.
9. Place the electrodes on the same finger/hand as the parent had stimulated.
10. Allow the child to adjust the amplitude to comfort and assess sensation.
11. Ask the child if he would like to try the TENS on _____ (the painful body part).
12. Apply the TENS very carefully to the painful body part and once again allow the child to adjust the amplitude.

---

trode placement was based on the suggestions of Mannheimer and Lampe (1984), Stux and Pomeranz (1987), Travel and Simons (1983), and Yu and Carroll (1982).

Initially one electrode was placed at the distal extent of pain and one proximal in an attempt to send energy through the painful area. Relief using this method was usually apparent in 10 to 20 minutes. If relief was not obtained in this period, the TENS unit was turned off and the electrodes were rearranged.

Assessment

Pain was assessed using either the Eland Color Tool (Eland, 1981) or a 0–10 numerical scale. The Eland Color Tool was developed to assess pain in the 4- to 10-year-old age group but has been used with younger children and some developmentally disabled adults. It is inexpensive, requires little equipment (eight colored markers or crayons and front and back body outlines) and can be used with little difficulty. Children select pain colors from red, orange, yellow, brown, blue, black, purple, and green crayons or markers. Having children show the nurse on a

TABLE 11.5   Eland Color Tool Protocol

1. Present eight markers to the child in a random order.
2. Ask the child, "Of these colors, which color is like _____?" (the event identified by the child as having hurt the most).
3. Place the marker away from the other markers (represents severe pain).
4. Ask the child, "Which color is like a hurt, but not quite as much _____?" (the event identified by the child as having hurt the most).
5. Place the marker with the marker chosen to represent severe pain.
6. Ask the child, "Which color is like something that hurts just a little?"
7. Place the marker with the others.
8. Ask the child, "Which color is like no hurt at all?"
9. Show the four marker choices to the child in order from the worst to the no hurt color.
10. Ask the child to show on the body outlines where he hurts using the markers he has chosen.
11. After the child has colored the hurts, ask if they are current hurts or hurts from the past.
12. Ask if he knows why the area hurts (if it is not clear to you why it does).

body outline where they hurt as well as their pain intensity can be useful as a diagnostic tool. The protocol for using the Eland Color Tool is in Table 11.5. The Eland Color Tool has been widely and successfully used to measure pain in children (Clinton, 1983; Gordon, 1981; Hester, 1979; Hester, Davis, Hanson, Hassanein, 1978; Lee, 1986; Loebach, 1979; Lukens, 1982; Schroeder, 1983; Varchol, 1983; Zavah, 1986) and is currently being used in numerous studies conducted both here and abroad.

If the child did not want to color his pain, he was asked to give it a number from 0–10, with zero representing no pain and 10 representing "as bad as pain could possibly be." The children who used numerical ratings of pain were asked to specify the exact location of their pain. (The child's coloring from the Eland Color Tool was used to provide a basis for electrode placement.)

RESULTS

Chad. Chad was four years old and suffering from an end-stage Ewings sarcoma with rib metastasis pain. He had been taking ibuprophen (Motrin) and small amounts of slow release morphine sulfate (MS Contin) for his pain, but they had not been successful in relieving the pain. The usually talkative Chad was quiet, withdrawn, motionless, and had

FIGURE 11.1.   Electrode placement used for Chad #1, who suffered from rib metastasis.

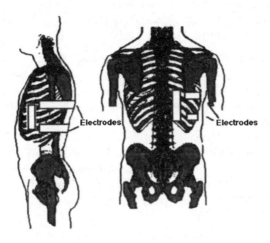

not been out of bed for three days. He colored his rib pain using the Eland Color Tool with the "worst" pain color.

Two six-inch long and two four-inch long electrodes were applied in the shape of a rectangle around the area of hurt (see Figure 11.1). After 15 minutes of conventional TENS stimulation he colored his pain with his "little" hurt color. Chad used his TENS unit almost constantly although he probably would have received the same amount of relief with stimulation for 30 minutes three times a day. It is possible that he was fearful that the pain might return or that he preferred being in control of the situation and the TENS unit itself was exerting a significant placebo effect.

The following day the investigator found Chad skipping down the hall. When asked about his pain, he colored using his "no hurt" color and said it didn't hurt anymore "because of the magic box." The TENS unit was the only parameter of his care that had changed in the previous 24 hours. Chad continued to use his TENS unit, ibuprophen (Motrin), and slow release morphine sulfate (MS Contin) until his death three months later.

Dave. Dave was a 17-year-old leukemic with two pain problems: a systemic fungal infection requiring amphotericin B (Fungizone) and perineal herpes zoster. He had been receiving acetaminophen (Tylenol) and codeine sulfate for his pain. The herpes zoster covered his scrotum and penis so the two 2 × 2 inch electrodes were placed on intact skin near the dorsal penile and inguinal nerve where they become superficial. Almost immediately his pain went from a "9" on a 10-point scale to a "1" using conventional TENS settings. Dave used his TENS unit on a prn basis whenever pain returned or when he needed to void or move around in bed.

At Dave's suggestion two electrodes from a second TENS unit were placed above and below the IV insertion site on his arm where he was receiving amphotericin B (Fungizone) (see Figure 11.2). Prior to use of the TENS unit he would lie silently in bed with tears streaming down his cheeks from the pain of this infusion and he rated his pain a "7"; after institution of the TENS unit this pain was reduced to a "0." Dave wanted the TENS unit on only for the duration of the daily amphotericin B (Fungizone) infusion.

Tracy & Stacy. Tracy, age 18, and Stacy, age 16, both had phantom limb pain from above-the-knee amputations associated with osteogenic sarcoma. Their electrodes were placed on the opposite side of their bodies at the location of their pain on the amputated limb (contralaterally), based on previous research (Gvory & Caine, 1977; Miles & Lipton, 1978). Both were stimulated using conventional TENS settings for 30 minutes twice a day but were told if pain returned they could use the TENS unit as needed.

Tracy had tried other pain relief alternatives that were unsuccessful; she was currently undergoing no treatment for her phantom pain because "none of them work!" Her phantom pain was at the base of her toes so two electrodes were placed over the traditional acupuncture points of Kidney 1 and Stomach 44 (see Figures 11.3 & 11.4). The points were stimulated twice a day for 30 minutes using four 1 × 2

FIGURE 11.2. Electrode placement used for Dave's IV amphotericin B and the traditional acupuncture points Lung 7 and Intestine 11 used for Zach's boney metastasis to the radius.

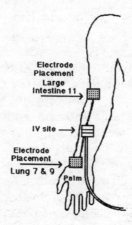

FIGURE 11.3. Electrode placement for the traditional acupuncture point Kidney 1 used for Tracy's phantom limb pain and for Matt's buring paresthesias of the feet.

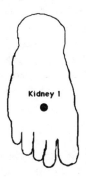

inch electrodes. Prior to stimulation, Tracy's pain was an "8" when it was at its worst and a "4" occasionally. Stimulation using conventional settings resulted in pain ratings of "0" and "1." For the next eighteen months Tracy's phantom pain had numerous peaks and valleys. When her pain recurred, she successfully used the TENS unit to relieve it.

Stacy's *nightmare* began one month prior to the investigator's contact with her. Over the course of 30 days, she was diagnosed with an osteogenic sarcoma, received toxic chemotherapy, lost all of her hair, had her leg amputated, required an appendectomy for appendicitis, and developed phantom limb pain. At the time of the investigator's first visit Stacy was in bed in her darkened hospital room with the drapes pulled shut and the sheets pulled over her head. When the investigator introduced herself, there was no response from Stacy. Ten minutes later the investigator said, "Stacy, if I had a magic wand, which I don't, what would you like for me to do for you?"

FIGURE 11.4. Electrode placement for the traditional acupuncture point Stomach 44 used for Tracy's phantom limb pain.

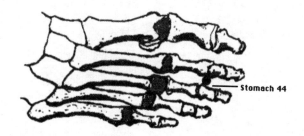

Slowly the sheets were pulled back to reveal a thin, emaciated, bald "birdlike creature" with two piercing eyes who said, "Take away the pain in the leg I don't have!" After several minutes Stacy identified the location of her worst pain, which was across the top of her amputated foot, and said that it "feels like my foot is in a vice." She had been receiving intermittent slow release morphine sulfate (MS Contin) for bone pain unrelated to her phantom pain but felt the morphine was ineffective for her phantom pain. The acupuncture points of Kidney 6 and Bladder 60 (see Figure 11.5) were used with conventional settings, which reduced her pain from an "8" "most of the time" to a "1" or "2." After that initial bout with phantom pain, which she used TENS to control, Stacy had no recurrence of her phantom pain.

Zach. Zach was an eight-year-old suffering from a widely metastasized neuroblastoma. Upon admission, Zach denied all pain in spite of his pathology, would remain in his bed staring at the television, and was not the person the staff had known previously. Pharmacologic intervention including slow release morphine sulfate (MS Contin), dexamethasone (Decadron) and ibuprophen (Motrin) was instituted based on his pathology and lack of affect and activity. After a few days a TENS unit was requested in the hope of providing additional pain relief and increasing his activity. At the time the TENS unit was ordered Zach would admit to many pains, but the worst pain was from bone destruction of the right radius and right tibia. He refused to rate or color pains and would only say they were the "worst."

The pain in the radius was stimulated using the traditional acupuncture points of Lung 7 and Large Intestine 11 (see Figure 11.2) while the tibia was stimulated using Stomach 36 and Stomach 41 (see Figure 11.6). All points were stimulated with conventional settings. Although there was no baseline pain rating from Zach, the addition of TENS

FIGURE 11.5. Electrode placement for the traditional acupuncture points Kidney 6 and Bladder 60 used for Stacy's phantom limb pain and for Matt's burning paresthesias of the feet.

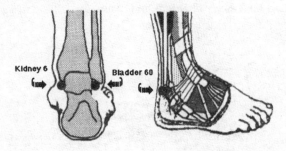

FIGURE 11.6. Electrode placement for the traditional acupuncture points Stomach 36 and 41 used for Zach's boney metastasis to the tibia and for Matt's burning paresthesias of the feet.

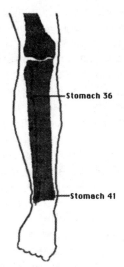

changed his activity and his affect. He was up spontaneously in the hall, requested to go out on pass for dinner and to go fishing with his dad, and later in the week asked to be discharged from the hospital. Relief with the pharmacology and TENS continued even after he herniated his spinal cord as a result of boney destruction. In the final week of his life he went fishing with his dad on two occasions and left his home to go "out for junk food" on one occasion.

Matt. Matt is probably the most complex adolescent in severe cancer-induced pain that the investigator has ever encountered. Matt was diagnosed with a multifocal osteogenic sarcoma that included 12 primary sites. His worst pain was a "12" on a 10-point scale and was the result of spinal cord herniation at T_8 that resulted in complete paralysis below that level and created burning paresthesias in both feet. His pain was being aggressively treated pharmacologically with intravenous morphine sulfate, dexamethasone (Decadron), and ibuprophen (Motrin), but the burning paresthesias persisted. The sign in his own handwriting at the head of his bed stated: "Don't Bump My Bed and Don't Touch My Feet!"

A total of eight one-inch square electrodes from two TENS units were placed on Kidney 6, Bladder 60, Kidney 1, and Stomach 41 (see Figures 11.3, 11.5, and 11.6) using conventional settings. After several adjustments of the amplitude and pulse width controls over a 24-hour period, Matt reported that his feet were numb! Matt insisted that his TENS units remain on 24-hours a day, which was done because less frequent use resulted in a return to pain. Matt continued to use the TENS unit for his foot pain up until his death eight weeks later.

Chad #2. Chad, age seven, had a Stage IV Wilm's Tumor and was suffering from herpes zoster along an intercostal nerve. He had been placed on codeine sulfate and diphenhydramine hydrochloride (Benadryl) for the associated pain, but they did not relieve the pain and often made him fall asleep in school. He was very fearful of the investigator but finally colored his skin pain with the "worst" hurt color. Chad was skeptical of having the electrodes placed over an area that was so very painful so the investigator suggested that he return to the playroom with the electrodes stimulating his arm and return to the exam room when/if he wanted to. Approximately 30 minutes later he returned and requested that the electrodes "fix" the pain on his side.

Four electrodes were placed on intact skin so that they boxed in the affected area (see Figure 11.7). Within two minutes of stimulation, Chad grabbed the markers and colored his side with the "little" hurt color. Chad and his mom were instructed to stimulate twice a day for 30 minutes or whenever the pain returned. When Chad returned to clinic the following week, he reported that "the box was magic!" He no longer required pain medicine, was not falling asleep in school, and his classmates were convinced that he had a pager.

Jacque. Jacque, age four, had leukemia. The treatment for his disease required that he receive 30 subcutaneous injections of cytarabine (Ara-c) five days a week for six weeks. He had received four injections before

FIGURE 11.7. Electrode placement used for Chad #2, who suffered from herpes zoster involving the intercostal nerve.

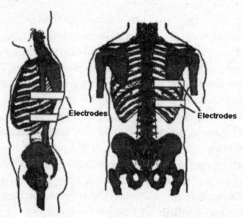

the investigator came in contact with him. His response to these injections was continual crying and tears for approximately 30 minutes after receiving the injection, and he colored the pain from his injections with his "worst" hurt color. One electrode was placed above the patella while the other was placed along the inguinal crease. After stimulation for 15 minutes with conventional TENS he received his injection, cried for 30 seconds and used his "little" hurt color to represent his pain. Jacque went from a crying, fearful child who was physically fighting his parents as they attempted to bring him to the outpatient clinic, to a child who would come skipping into the clinic holding his TENS unit. When the author asked him why he was skipping, he replied, "My magic box makes the hurt go away!"

DISCUSSION

Based on the study results, the *only* thing the investigator can say about the use of TENS with children experiencing pain associated with cancer is that it significantly reduced the pain these eight children were experiencing. Four children continued to use TENS, which contributed significantly to their pain relief and overall quality of life. For Chad, Dave, Zach, and Matt, TENS provided a powerful adjuvant to other pain relief measures and allowed them to be "themselves" until their deaths. Relief was obtained using conventional TENS settings with electrodes applied in most instances to areas proximal and distal to the area of pain. Most of the children's pain was relieved when they were stimulated two or three times a day for 30 minutes, although some insisted that the TENS units remain "on" 24 hours a day. None of the children experienced any negative side effects from the TENS units.

Every child and his parents in this study liked the TENS units and had little difficulty adjusting the controls, reapplying the electrodes, or recharging the batteries. It is certainly possible that the children enjoyed the control they had over their pain, and this may have exerted a significant placebo effect. The nontraditional types of pain experienced by the children in this study, including painful intravenous infusions and phantom limb pain, were relieved.

Clinicians must recognize that this is an extremely small number of children to study and represents a *preliminary* effort to ascertain the effectiveness and acceptability of TENS with children suffering cancer pain. They must not assume that TENS will be of benefit to all children suffering from the pain of cancer because the study itself had no experimental control. There are also problems with saying that a TENS unit would work over time, though TENS continued to be effective for the children who remained alive. Of the children in this study who have died, all were using TENS at the time of their deaths and continued to receive pain relief. Clinicians should view TENS as a device that (1) may well benefit children in pain, (2) will not be harmful to them, (3) is worth the effort. They can consult physical therapists and others knowledgeable about TENS and consult the references at the conclusion of this section of the book for additional information.

Researchers are encouraged to undertake controlled studies to provide specific guidelines for the use of TENS and to discover which applications are most appropriate for ill children, including those with cancer. Children suffering from the advanced pain of cancer are certainly worthy of our study, but studying them is complicated by the extent of their pathology and by the myriad of physical and psychological problems associated with their illness. They also pose the additional problem that long-term study with many of them is impossible, which has a disastrous effect on evaluation of the reliability of an intervention.

There seems to be something very wrong in the fact that many children have cancer and many will die from their disease. The health care team has to make a conscious decision on how many of these children will live and die in pain. The investigator believes the only thing worse than seeing a child die is seeing one die in agony from unrelieved pain. TENS appears to represent a piece of the puzzle of children's pain, but it needs much more research before its specific uses are known and it can be used to the fullest. The vivid memories of the parents and children with cancer must serve as a stimulus for all of our continuing efforts on behalf of children in pain.

[12]

The Effect of Musical Distraction on Pain in Hospitalized School-aged Children

Eileen A. Ryan

Helping children cope with pain is demanding and difficult. It is especially difficult when the procedures that nurses perform on hospitalized children cause pain. In a study of pain in prekindergarten children, for example, Eland (1981) found that 49% of these young children said that needles and injections were the worst hurts they had ever experienced. Nurses responsible for inserting intravenous catheters know the risks of nerve damage due to improper restraint of an extremity (Guhlow & Kolb, 1979). Unfortunately, the risk is increased by the behaviors children exhibit when confronted with painful stimuli like venipunctures. The tensed muscles, jerking away from the painful stimulus, refusal to change position, and twisting and arching body have been described by numerous authors (Abu-Saad, 1981; Baer, Davitz, & Lieb, 1970; Beyer & Levin, 1987; Hester, 1979). These manifestations of pain make venipuncture difficult for even the most skilled nurse; thus, minimizing the pain experience would help the nurse as well as the child. This study, therefore, was designed to determine the effects of musical distraction on hospitalized children's perception of pain during venipuncture. The long-term goal was to find a method of reducing the acute pain associated with many of the procedures to which hospitalized children are subjected.

METHOD

The study was conducted at St. Christopher's Hospital for Children, a 140-bed pediatric referral center in Philadelphia. Data were collected over a three-week period on inpatient units and the emergency room.

The sample included children between the ages of 9 and 12 who were hospitalized and required venipuncture as part of their diagnosis and treatment. Children of this age group were selected because they have been shown to be able to evaluate pain intensity and identify approaches they use to cope with pain (Tesler, Wegner, Savedra, Gibbons, & Ward, 1981). When a potentially eligible patient was found, the staff nurse would page the nurse investigator, who would evaluate the patient. Patients judged eligible were approached by the investigator, who gave a brief explanation of the study and then answered any questions the child or parent might have. All the children who were approached agreed to participate in the study. The accessible sample, however, was limited because often venipunctures were done before staff remembered to page the investigator or two venipunctures were happening at once.

The children were assigned nonrandomly to either a comparison or experimental group with some attempt to equally distribute participants by age and sex in each group. The experimental group listened to music during the procedure; the comparison group received routine care.

Music was selected for distraction because older school-aged children and adults have identified musical and visual distraction as approaches they use to cope with pain. Further, several authors (Beales, 1982; McCaffery, 1977; McGrath & Vair, 1984) have indicated that auditory distraction using headphones is effective with brief episodes of painful stimuli like needle sticks. This type of intervention has the additional advantage of giving the child some control over one aspect of the hospital experience through participating in the selection of music. Stereo headphones are also widely accepted, relatively inexpensive, and easy to convince children to use.

Headphones were placed on the child several minutes prior to the actual venipuncture to enhance the effectiveness of the distraction by minimizing external stimuli related to the procedure. The children chose from several popular musical tapes and put on their own headphones to maximize their involvement and sense of control. All venipunctures took place in a treatment room or cubicle to minimize external variables or distractions from TV, roommates, or hospital activity.

The venipunctures were performed by registered nurses or resident pediatricians; therefore, techniques and skill level varied. Thus, pain produced by catheter insertion was a potential variable that was not controlled.

After venipuncture the children were asked to complete a pain assessment scale. A visual analogue scale was used since this has been found valid for the age group used in this study (Abu-Saad, 1984; Beyer & Byers, 1985). The scale is a simple line, measured in centimeters, that represents a continuum from 0 (no pain) to 10 (pain as bad as it can be). This scale is simple, it is easy for nurses and patients to learn to work with, and it requires no special equipment. The scale can give children a sense of control as they mark their perceptions on it. Demographic data obtained included diagnosis, rationale for venipuncture, age, sex, and whether the child had previously experienced venipuncture.

RESULTS

The sample consisted of 14 children: 7 male and 7 female. The experimental and comparison groups were similar in sex and age distribution; 71.5% had previously had a venipuncture, and the most common reason was intravenous fluids or antibiotics.

Results of the pain scale ratings for comparison and experimental subjects are reported in Table 12.1. Scores for children in the comparison group ranged from 0, for one child who reported no pain, to a maximum of 9. The mean pain level for these children was 6.14. Children in the group who listened to music reported lower pain levels, with the scores ranging from 0 to 7, and a mean of 4.14. While this difference was not statistically significant ($U = 29$, $p > .05$), perhaps due to the small sample size, we believe pain scores that average two points lower on an 11-point scale have clinical significance. No relationship between level of pain and either age or sex of the child was noted.

An interesting finding was that pain scale ratings frequently did not correlate with the investigator's *subjective* assessment of behavioral cues exhibited by the children. Those exhibiting the most facial and motor behaviors often rated the experience low on the pain scale, and those who were nonvocal about their pain sometimes gave it high ratings. This finding supports the need to replace unscientific, intuitive assessment strategies frequently used by nurses with reliable and valid pain indicators.

Both the children and nursing staff reacted positively to the use of stereo headphones. Given their minimal cost and wide availability, this is an intervention that is practical and feasible in the clinical setting. Staff showed a high level of interest in the study; they were interested

TABLE 12.1 Pain Scale Ratings and Age and Sex Distributions for Experimental and Comparison Groups

	Comparison Group n = 7				Experimental Group n = 7		
Patient	Age	Sex	Pain Scale Rating	Patient	Age	Sex	Pain Scale Rating
A	9	M	7	H	9	F	2
B	10	M	0	I	9	M	6
C	12	F	6	J	9	M	6
D	9	F	7	K	12	M	3
E	9	F	6	L	9	F	7
F	9	F	9	M	9	F	5
G	10	M	8	N	10	M	0
Mean			6.14				4.14

in discussing pain and many asked for copies of the articles used in planning the study. Moreover, they indicated interest in becoming involved in research themselves.

DISCUSSION

Small investigations like this should be replicated in clinical settings to expand the knowledge base of pediatric nurses and encourage interventions based on empirical findings. The investigator was excited by the enthusiasm generated by this study; staff nurses should be involved in more clinical research.

The results of this study have relevance for nurses concerned about minimizing the pain experienced by hospitalized children undergoing procedures like venipuncture. Given the relative ease and minimal cost of musical distraction and its potential ability to help children in pain, this intervention should be tried more broadly. Nursing administrators should be receptive to such strategies as they seek to enhance patient and family satisfaction within federally mandated cost restrictions.

This type of intervention has two additional advantages: it can enhance staff nurse autonomy in planning care and instituting non-pharmacologic pain control techniques (music, breathing, focused imagery) as an adjunct to analgesics for hospitalized children, and it can give the child some control over one aspect of the hospital experience.

[13]

Approaches to Pain
in Infants and Children:
A Discussion

Margaret Shandor Miles and Virginia J. Neelon

One of the hardest parts of being a pediatric nurse is having to see children suffer pain. What is even harder, nurses themselves often must impose pain on children as part of routine care. Providing pain relief, then, is an important aspect of nursing care. Managing pain in infants and children requires adequate knowledge of their pain responses. The chapters in this section provide useful information about the uniqueness of the pain response in children of various ages, the complexity of assessing and measuring children's pain responses, and the various approaches to intervening with children experiencing pain. The clinical implications of these chapters are both simple and complex.

THE PAIN RESPONSE IN CHILDREN

All of the chapters on pain in children reemphasize the accumulating scientific and clinical evidence that children, even small prematures, experience pain. The chapters also underscore the fact that pain responses differ greatly in children at various developmental ages. When working with children in pain, health care providers must be alert to how developmental age may affect both the response to pain and the ability and willingness to share that response. The infant may spontaneously cry or moan when in pain, whereas the older child may suppress his response for a variety of reasons. The small child may blame pain on caregivers, whereas an older child may perceive pain as punishment for wrongdoing.

These chapters underscore the fact that the pain response involves behavioral, physiological, cognitive, and psychological components. Thus, clinicians must be skilled in assessment in each of these fields and use multiple means of assessing the pain response of a child.

The responses of children experiencing pain are dependent on a number of other variables that must be considered within the context of the illness and related treatments. A child whose autonomic responsiveness is suppressed may not show the increased activity of that system that is usually considered an indicator of acute pain. Anesthesia or other drugs may influence the response of a child to painful stimuli. Stresses associated with illness and hospitalization such as fear, anxiety, loss of control, and lack of understanding about treatment may influence the pain response. Frequently, the child who is drowsy or who denies pain because of anxiety is thought by others not to have pain. Foster and Hester suggest that children may underreport pain for fear of getting an injection. Awareness of the extraneous variables that may affect a child's pain response is important in understanding the pain of children.

To date, much of the focus on pain in children has been on its short-term impact. However, the consequences of severe pain can extend beyond the immediate manifestations. For example, relief of acute behavioral responses does not necessarily indicate that the physiological or psychological responses have been controlled. Thus, the management of pain in children should include an awareness of potential long-term physiological and psychological consequences of pain, including psychological stress, cardiovascular changes, sleep disturbances, and muscular damage. The management of pain in children requires understanding of prolonged and chronic pain, as well.

ASSESSING AND MEASURING PAIN IN CHILDREN

The assessment of pain in children is the first step toward planning interventions. Assessment is also extremely important (though often ignored) in the evaluation of the effectiveness of interventions.

Behavioral responses are important in assessing pain in children, especially the premature, infant, and toddler. It is essential to become familiar with the behaviors of children of various ages that indicate pain. Davis and Calhoon provide clues to behaviors in the preterm infant that are associated with painful stimuli, particularly negative facial expressions and large body movements. Fuller and colleagues have examined subtle differences in the crying behavior of infants experiencing pain. Mills has carefully documented behaviors in infants and toddlers that indicate pain and has shown that even within this age group, behavioral responses differ.

Dependence on behavioral cues has risk. Their predictability, pattern, and character depend on the coping patterns of the individual child and the specific pain situation. Thus, the behavioral, physiological, and psychological responses of an infant or child under our care need to be identified, documented, and used in our assessment of the child. The Fuller et al. study, for example, suggests that nurses may be able to identify the pitch and tenseness of an infant's crying that indicate pain and distinguish this from other types of arousal.

Nurses need to increase the repertoire of words used to discuss pain with children. The ability of even young children to verbalize their pain is suggested in the study by Mills. Tesler et al. have shown that children have a rich vocabulary to describe pain and that the number and complexity of words they use increases with age. It is especially important to be sensitive to the particular words that an individual child understands and uses to describe pain. Parents can be an important resource in learning about the child's words for pain. These words should be recorded in the child's record or care plan.

Self-report tools can be used as adjuncts in the assessment of pain in children starting with preschoolers. Beyer has demonstrated that young children can visually rate the amount of pain experienced using a six-picture photographic scale, and older children can use a 0–100 numerical scale. Foster and Hester have successfully used a poker chip method with young children and a pain ladder tool with older children.

However, the use of self-report measures requires an understanding of the concept of pain and the ability to visually rate the level of the pain. This is a complex task for a child, especially in the preschool years. Tools are best used in conjunction with behavioral and physiological assessment. Ryan's study indicates that the self-reports of children do not always correlate with the observations of nurses. What is not clear is which assessment is more valid.

Assessment tools and self-report measures, if used in clinical assessment, should be recorded in the child's medical record and used to guide treatment and continued evaluation of the child's pain. Foster and Hester found that nurses' assessments of children's pain were not used to intervene with the children in pain; high pain ratings were only moderately associated with the administration of analgesia.

INTERVENTIONS WITH CHILDREN

The main concern for children in pain is pain relief, particularly for children experiencing pain associated with acute or chronic illness. However, it is also important to plan interventions to reduce the pain caused by treatment itself—such as invasive medical procedures. Davis and Calhoon, for example, point to the need to use analgesia and anesthesia to reduce or prevent pain in preterm infants experiencing procedures, unless these drugs would cause life-threatening complications.

One of the most important means of reducing pain in children as well as in adults is analgesia. However, studies are increasingly showing that pharmacologic pain relief in children is often inadequate. There is continued underestimation of the dosages children need and can tolerate for pain relief. As patient advocates, nurses need to anticipate the pain that illness, care, or treatment may cause, and they need to evaluate the orders written by physicians to be certain that the amount ordered will be sufficient to relieve the child's pain. Further, pain medications that are ordered should be given to the child in pain in a timely fashion.

Webb et al. have demostrated the efficacy of patient-controlled analgesia (PCA) to ease pain in some children. A significant factor in the use of PCA may be the psychologic aspect of control, which may reduce the anxiety that is closely related to the pain response. Thus, allowing the child control over the method of giving a pain medication (oral, suppository, intramuscular injection, or intravenous) may make the medication more effective.

Transcutaneous electrical nerve stimulation (TENS) has a psychophysiological basis for relieving pain through nonpainful nerve stimulation and through altering pain perception and increasing pain tolerance. Based on her clinical work with children with terminal cancer, Eland suggests that TENS may be highly effective in reducing pain in children, particularly when the painful area can be localized. Although the effective use of TENS requires demonstration and instruction by a professional experienced in its use, it allows the child a measure of control over the pain through adjustment of the frequency, intensity, and placement of the stimulation. This intervention may ultimately be a powerful tool for pain reduction in children experiencing prolonged and chronic pain, and it should be further explored as an adjunct therapy with these children.

While management of pain primarily involves reducing the painful stimuli, interventions that relieve the distress associated with pain and refocus attention away from the painful stimuli can be used as an adjunct to pharmacologic and other interventions with children. Thus, distraction and other associated interventions such as relaxation, guided imagery, and visualization, discussed in other sections of this book, may be effective in reducing the emotional response to pain and to painful procedures such as injections, bone marrow aspirations, and lumbar punctures. Ryan's study, for example, demonstrates the efficacy of music as a distractor for children undergoing intravenous insertion. Musical distraction has also been used with children undergoing cardiac catheterization. Other research has shown success in using guided imagery and relaxation with children undergoing bone marrow examinations and with burned children undergoing painful dressing changes. These methods are noninvasive, they are low in cost, and they do not take a large amount of time. Furthermore, parents can be taught to coach their child in using these methods and children can eventually learn to use them as a self-care measure. Distraction measures need to be based on what the child perceives as helpful and not on staff interpretations. Overuse and prolonged use of distraction may cause more problems than it solves.

Nurses need to explore carefully how comfort measures might be used to relieve pain in infants and children. Davis and Calhoon point to the importance of comfort measures as the only method available to help small, sick, premature infants with pain caused by procedures. Yet the nurses in their study did not often provide comfort to infants following the painful procedures.

SUMMARY

The clinical implications of these chapters are both simple and complex: (1) yes, infants and children of all ages do experience pain; (2) although complicated by developmental issues, it is possible to assess the pain of children using behavioral and physiological cues, self-report, and verbal description; (3) there are many nonpharmacologic means for intervening with children in pain and they need to be used more often; (4) pharmacologic interventions remain important in pain relief for children but are often used inadequately; and (5) interventions that allow the child control, such as PCA or TENS, may be especially helpful.

Nursing research, with increasing basic science support, has made great advances toward understanding the pain responses of children. The research is still in its infancy, however, and much more is needed to truly understand the complexities of the pain experienced by children. Certainly we need to know more about what the pathways of pain are in children and about how children of various ages experience pain. There is a need to develop more valid and reliable assessment tools and research instruments to measure the pain response of children, especially very young children. Clinical research is urgently needed to identify comfort measures that reduce pain and enhance recovery from painful procedures. Other nonpharmacologic means of pain control need to be studied. Finally, a great deal more information is needed on the efficacy of various pain medications with children, including dosages, timing, self-administration, and side effects. Continued advancements will require the integration of knowledge into clinical practice and feedback from this clinical experience to guide future research.

References on Pain in Children

Abu-Saad, H. (1981). The assessment of pain in children. *Issues in Comprehensive Pediatric Nursing,* 5(5–6), 327–335.

Abu-Saad, H. (1984). Assessing children's responses to pain. *Pain, 19,* 163–171.

Abu-Saad, H. (1984). Cultural components of pain: The Asian-American Child. *Children's Health Care,* 13(1), 11–14.

Abu-Saad, H., & Holzemer, W. (1981). Measuring children's self-assessment of pain. *Issues in Comprehensive Pediatric Nursing, 5,* 337–349.

American Academy of Pediatrics (1987). Neonatal anesthesia. *Pediatrics, 80,* 446.

Anand, K. J. S., & Hickey, P. R. (1987). Pain and its effects in the human neonate and fetus. *The New England Journal of Medicine, 317,* 1321–1329.

Anders, T. F., & Chalemian, R. J. (1974). Effect of circumcision on sleep-wake states in human neonates. *Psychosomatic Medicine, 36,* 174–179.

Aradine, C., Beyer, J., & Tompkins, J. (1988). Children's perceptions before and after analgesia: A study of instrument construct validity. *Journal of Pediatric Nursing, 3,* 11–23.

Atwell, J. R., Flanigan, R. C., Bennett, R. L., Allen, D. C., Lucas, B. A., & McRoberts, J. W. (1984). The efficacy of patient-controlled analgesia in patients recovering from flank incisions. *Journal of Urology, 132,* 701–703.

Baer, E., Davits, L. J., & Lieb, R. (1970). Inferences of physical pain and psychological distress in relation to verbal and nonverbal patient communication. *Nursing Research, 19,* 388–392.

Bailey, C. A., & Davidson, P. O. (1976). The language of pain: Intensity. *Pain, 2,* 319–324.

Beales, J. (1982). The assessment and management of pain in children. In P. Karoly, J. J. Steffen, & D. J. O'Grady (Eds.), *Child health psychology: Concepts and issues.* Toronto: Pergamon.

Beaver, P. K. (1987). Premature infants' response to touch and pain: Can nurses make a difference? *Neonatal Network,* 6(3), 13–17.

Bennett, R., Batenhorst, R. L., Bivins, B., Bell, R. M., Graves, D. A., Foster, T. S., Wright, B. D., & Griffen, W. O. (1982). Patient-controlled analgesia: A new concept of postoperative pain relief. *Annals of Surgery, 195,* 700–705.

Bennett, R. M., Batenhorst, R., Graves, D., Foster, T. S., Baumann, T., Griffen, W. O., & Wright, B. D. (1982). Morphine titration in postoperative laparotomy patients using patient-controlled analgesia. *Current Therapeutic Research,* 32(1), 45–52.

Beyer, J. (1984). *The Oucher: A user's manual and technical report.* Evanston, Illinois: The Hospital Play Equipment Company (1122 Judson Avenue, Evanston, Illinois 60202).

Beyer, J., & Aradine, C. (1986). Content validity of an instrument to measure young children's perceptions of the intensity of their pain. *Journal of Pediatric Nursing, 1,* 386–395.

Beyer, J., & Aradine, C. (1987). Patterns of pediatric pain intensity: A methodological investigation of a self-report scale. *Clinical Journal of Pain, 3*, 130–141.

Beyer, J., & Aradine, C. (1988). The convergent and discriminant validity of a self-report measure of pain intensity for children. *Children's Health Care, 16*, 274–282.

Beyer, J., & Byers, M. L. (1985). Knowledge of pediatric pain: The state of the art. *Children's Health Care, 13*, 150–159.

Beyer, J. E., DeGood, D. E., Ashley, L. C., & Russell, G. (1983). Pattern of post-operative analgesia with adults and children following cardiac surgery. *Pain, 17*, 71–81.

Beyer, J. E., & Levin, C. R. (1987). Issues and advances in pain control in children. *Nursing Clinics of North America, 22*(3), 661–675.

Biller, J. A., & Yeager, A. M. (Eds.). (1987). *The Harriet Lane handbook*. Chicago: Year Book Medical Publishers, Inc.

Bosma, J. F., Truby, H. M., & Lind, J. (1965). Cry motions of the newborn infant. *Acta Paediatrica Scandinavica Supplement, 163*, 61–92.

Bradshaw, C., & Zeanah, P. D. (1986). Pediatric nurses' assessments of pain in children. *Journal of Pediatric Nursing, 1*(5), 314–322.

Brenner, M., Shipp, T., & Doherty, E. T. (1983). *Voice measures of psychological stress—laboratory and field data*. Paper presented at the Iowa Conference on Physiology and Biophysics of Voice.

Burokas, L. (1985). Factors affecting nurses' decisions to medicate pediatric patients after surgery. *Heart and Lung, 14*(4), 373–379.

Check, W. A. (1982). Results are better when patients control their own analgesia. *Journal of American Medical Association, 247*, 945–947.

Citron, M. L., Johnston-Early, A., Boyer, M., Kransnow, S. H., Hood, M., & Cohen, M. H. (1986). Patient-controlled analgesia for severe cancer pain. *Archives of Internal Medicine, 146*, 734–736.

Clinton, P. K. (1983). *Music as a nursing intervention for children during painful procedures*. Unpublished master's thesis, University of Iowa, Iowa City.

Craig, K. D. (1980). Ontogenetic and cultural influences on the expression of pain in man. In H. W. Kosterlitz and L. Y. Terenius (Eds.), *Pain and society* (pp. 37–52). Weinheim: Dahlem Konferenzen, Verlag Chemie Gmbh.

Craig, K., McMahon, R., Morison, J., & Zaskow, C. (1984). Development changes in infant pain expression during immunization injections. *Social Science and Medicine, 19*, 1331–1337.

D'Apolito, K. (1984). The neonate's response to pain. *Maternal-Child Nursing Journal, 9*, 256–258.

Davis, D. H., & Thoman, E. B. (1987). Behavioral states of premature infants: Implications for neural and behavioral development. *Developmental Psychobiology, 20*, 25–38.

Denyes, M., & Villarruel, A. (1988). *Content validity of a self-report pain intensity instrument with young black children*. Unpublished manuscript, Wayne State University, Detroit.

Eland, J. E. (1981). Minimizing pain associated with prekindergarten intramuscular injections. *Issues in Comprehensive Pediatric Nursing, 5*, 361–372.

Eland, J. M. & Anderson, J. E. (1977). The experience of pain in children. In A. Jacox (Ed.), *Pain: A source book for nurses and other health professionals* (pp. 453–473). Boston: Little, Brown and Company.

Emde, R. N., Harmon, R. J., Metcalf, D., Koenig, K. L., & Wagonfeld, S. (1971). Stress and neonatal sleep. *Psychosomatic Medicine, 33*, 491–496.

Fabrega, H., Jr., & Tyma, S. (1976). Language and cultural influences in the description of pain. *British Journal of Medical Psychology, 49*, 349–371.

Field, T., & Goldson, E. (1984). Pacifying effects of nonnutritive sucking on term and preterm neonates during heelstick procedures. *Pediatrics, 74,* 1012–1015.

Fischer, A. (1987, October). Babies in pain. *Redbook.*

Franck, L. S. (1986). A new method to quantitatively describe pain behavior in infants. *Nursing Research, 35,* 28–31.

Franck, L. S. (1987). A national survey of the assessment and treatment of pain and agitation in the neonatal intensive care unit. *JOGN Nursing, 16,* 387–393.

Fuller, B. F., & Horii, Y. (*in press*-a). Differences in fundamental frequency, jitter and shimmer among four types of infant vocalizations. *Journal of Communications Disorders.*

Fuller, B. F., & Horii, Y. (*in press*-b). Spectral energy distribution among four types of infant vocalizations. *Journal of Communications Disorders.*

Gaston-Johansson, F. (1984). Pain assessment: Differences in quality and intensity of the words pain, ache and hurt. *Pain, 20,* 69–76.

Gordon, D. J. (1981). *The developmental characteristics of pain in children.* Unpublished master's thesis, McGill University, Montreal, Canada.

Gorski, P. A., Hole, W. T., Leonard, C. H., & Martin, J. A. (1983). Direct computer recording of premature infants and nursery care: Distress following two interventions. *Pediatrics, 72,* 198–202.

Gottfried, A. W. (1985). Environment of newborn infants in special care units. In A. W. Gottfried & J. L. Gaiter (Eds.), *Infant stress under intensive care: Environmental neonatology* (pp. 23–54). Baltimore: University Park Press.

Guhlow, L., & Kolb, J. (1979). Pediatric IV's: Special measures you must take. *RN, (12),* 40–51.

Gvory, A. N., & Caine, D. C. (1977). Electric pain control of a painful forearm amputation stump. *Medical Journal of Australia, 2,* 156–158.

Hammond, N. I. (1982). *Nitrous oxide analgesia and children's perception of pain.* Unpublished master's thesis, University of Washington, Seattle.

Hay, H. (1984). *The measurement of pain intensity in children and adults—A methodological approach.* Unpublished raw data in unpublished master's research report, School of Nursing, McGill University, Montreal, Canada.

Hester, N. (1979). The preoperational child's reaction to immunization. *Nursing Research, 28,* 250–254.

Hester, N. (1986–1988). *Generalizability of procedures assessing pain in children* (NIH Grant No. NR23 1382 01). Bethesda, MD: National Institutes of Health.

Hester, N., & Barcus, C. (1986). Assessment and management of pain in children. *Pediatrics: Nursing Update, 1*(14), 1–7.

Hester, N., Davis, R., Hanson, S. H., & Hassanein, R. S. (1978). *The hospitalized child's subjective rating of painful experiences.* Unpublished manuscript, University of Kansas, Kansas City.

Hollien, H., Michel, J., & Doherty, E. (1973). A method for analyzing vocal jitter in sustained phonation. *Journal of Phonetics, 1,* 85–91.

Horii, Y., & Hughes, G. W. (1972). Speech analysis by computer. *Proceedings of the National Electron Conference, 27,* 74–79.

Horii, Y. (1979). Fundamental frequency perturbation observed in sustained phonation. *Journal of Speech and Hearing Research, 22,* 5–19.

Izard, C. E., & Dougherty, L. M. (1982). Two complementary systems for measuring facial expressions in infants and children. In C. E. Izard (Ed.), *Measuring emotions in infants and children* (pp. 97–126). Cambridge: Cambridge University Press.

Jeans, M. E. (1984). *The experience of pain in children*. Paper presented at the National Conference on Pediatric Nursing: Challenges in Health Care for Children, San Francisco, California.

Katz, E., Kellerman, J., & Siegel, S. (1980). Behavioral distress in children with cancer undergoing medical procedures: Developmental considerations. *Journal of Consulting and Clinical Psychology, 48,* 356–365.

Koivisto, M., Michelsson, K., Sirvio, P., & Wasz-Hockert, O. (1974). Spectrographic analysis of pain cry of hypoglycemic newborn infants. *Proceedings of the Fourteenth International Congress of Pediatrics* (p. 250). Buenos Aires, Argentina.

Koivisto, M. (1987). Cry analysis in infants with Rh haemolytic disease. *Acta Paediatrica Scandinavica Supplement, 335,* 1–73.

Laver, J. (1980). *The Phonetic Description of Voice Quality*. Cambridge: Cambridge University Press.

LeBaron, S., & Zeltzer, L. (1984). Assessment of acute pain and anxiety in children and adolescents by self-reports, observer reports, and a behavior checklist. *Journal of Consulting and Clinical Psychology, 52,* 729–738.

Lee, C. (1986). *Korean children's reactions to painful experiences*. Unpublished master's thesis, University of Iowa, Iowa City.

Levi, L. (1975). *Emotions—Their parameters and measurement*. New York: Raven Press.

Levine, J. D., & Gordon, N. C. (1982). Pain in prelingual children and its evaluation by pain-induced vocalization. *Pain, 14,* 85–93.

Loebach, S. (1979). *The use of color to facilitate communication of pain in children*. Unpublished master's thesis, University of Washington, Seattle.

Lukens, M. (1982). *The identification of criteria used by nurses in the assessment of pain in children*. Unpublished master's thesis, University of Cincinnati.

Mannheimer, J. S., & Lampe, G. N. (1984). *Clinical transcutaneous electrical nerve stimulation*. Philadelphia: F. A. Davis.

Mather, L., & Mackie, J. (1983). The incidence of post-operative pain in children. *Pain, 15,* 271–282.

McCaffery, M. (1977). Pain relief for the child. *Pediatric Nursing, 3*(4), 11–16.

McGrath, P., Johnson, G., Goodman, J., Schillenger, J., Dunn, J., & Chapman, J. (1985). The Children's Hospital of Eastern Ontario Pain Scale (CHEOPS): A behavioral scale for rating post-operative pain in children. In H. L. Fields, R. Dubner, & F. Cervero (Eds.), *Advances in pain research and therapy, 9,* (pp. 395–402). New York: Raven Press.

McGrath, P., & Vair, C. (1984). Psychological aspects of pain management of the burned child. *Children's Health Care, 13*(1), 15–19.

McGraw, M. B. (1941). Neural maturation as exemplified in the changing reactions of the infant to pin prick. *Child Development, 12,* 31–41.

Melamed, B., & Siegel, L. (1975). Reduction of anxiety in children facing hospitalization and surgery by use of filmed modeling. *Journal of Consulting and Clinical Psychology, 43,* 511–521.

Melzack, R., & Torgerson, W. S. (1971). On the language of pain. *Anesthesiology, 34,* 50–59.

Melzack, R., & Wall, P.D. (1972). *The puzzle of pain*. New York: Basic Books.

Michelsson, K. (1971). Cry analysis of symptomless low birth weight neonates and of asphyxiated newborn infants. *Acta Paediatrica Scandinavica Supplement, 216,* 10–45.

Michelsson, K., Sirvio, P., & Wasz-Hockert, O. (1977). Pain cry in full-term asphyxiated newborn infants correlated with late findings. *Acta Paediatrica Scandinavica, 66,* 611–616.

Miles, J., & Lipton, S. (1978). Phantom limb treated by electrical stimulation. *Pain, 5,* 373–382.

Molsberry, D. (1979). *Young children's subjective quantifications of pain following surgery.* Unpublished master's thesis, University of Iowa, Iowa City.

National Institutes of Health. (1986). *Consensus development conference statement. The integrated approach to the management of pain.* USHHS, 6(3) (document number 491–292: 41148).

Nelson, K. (1973). Learning to talk: A process model, Section 6. *Monograph of Society for Research in Child Development, 34*(149), 95–136.

Norris, S., Campbell, L. A., & Brenkert, S. (1982). Nursing procedures and alterations in transcutaneous oxygen tension in premature infants. *Nursing Research, 31,* 330–336.

Owens, M. E. (1984). Pain in infancy: Conceptual and methodological issues. *Pain, 20,* 213–230.

Owens, M. E., & Todt, E. H. (1984). Pain in infancy: Neonatal reaction to heel lance. *Pain, 20,* 77–86.

Peiper, A. (1963). *Cerebral function in infancy and childhood.* New York: Consultants Bureau.

Porter, F. L., Miller, R. H., & Marshall, R. E. (1986). Neonatal pain cries: Effect of circumcision on acoustic features and perceived urgency. *Child Development, 57,* 790–802.

Porter, F., Miller, J. P., & Marshall, R. (1987, April). *Local anesthesia for painful medical procedures in sick newborns.* Poster presented at the biennial meeting of the Society for Research in Child Development, Baltimore, MD.

Price, D. D., & Dubner, R. (1977). Neurons that subserve the sensory-discriminative aspects of pain. *Pain, 3,* 57–68.

Ross, D.M., & Ross, S.A. (1984a). Childhood pain: The school-aged child's viewpoint. *Pain, 20,* 179–191.

Ross, D.M., & Ross, S.A. (1984b). The importance of type of question, psychological climate and subject set in interviewing children about pain. *Pain, 19,* 71–79.

Savedra, M., Gibbons, P., Tesler, M., Ward, J., & Wegner, C. (1982). How do children describe pain? A tentative assessment. *Pain, 14,* 95–104.

Savedra, M., Tesler, M., Ward, J., & Wegner, C. (1988). How do adolescents describe pain? *Journal of Adolescent Health Care, 9,* 315–320.

Schechter, N., Allen, D., & Hanson, K. (1986). Status of pediatric pain control: A comparison of hospital analgesic usage in children and adults. *Pediatrics, 77,* 11–15.

Scherer, K. R. (1981). Vocal indicators of stress. In J. K. Darby (Ed.), *Speech evaluation in psychiatry* (pp. 66–71). New York: Grune and Stratton.

Schroeder, P. (1983). *A descriptive study of pain associated with therapeutic procedures in the burned school age child.* Unpublished master's thesis, University of Cincinnati.

Scott, R. (1978). It hurts red: A preliminary study of children's perception of pain. *Perceptual and Motor Skills, 47,* 787–791.

Shearer, M. H. (1986). Editorial: Surgery on the paralyzed, unanesthetized newborn. *Birth, 13,* 79.

Stevens, B., Hunsberger, M., & Browne, G. (1987). Pain in children: Theoretical, research, and practice dilemmas. *Journal of Pediatric Nursing, 2,* 154–166.

Strauss, A., Fagerhaugh, S., & Glaser, B. (1974). Pain: An organizational-work-interactive perspective. *Nursing Outlook, 22,* 560–566.

Stux, G., & Pomeranz, B. (1987). *Acupuncture: Textbook and atlas.* New York: Springer-Verlag.

Swafford, L. I., & Allen, D. (1968). Pain relief in the pediatric patient. *Medical Clinics of North America, 52*(1), 131–135.

Szyfelbein, S., Osgood, P., & Carr, D. (1985). The assessment of pain and plasma β-endorphin immunoactivity in burned children. *Pain, 22,* 173–182.

Taylor, P. (1983). Postoperative pain in toddler and pre-school age children. *Maternal-Child Nursing Journal, 12,* 35–50.

Tesler, M., Wegner, C., Savedra, M., Gibbons, P., & Ward, J. (1981). Coping strategies of children in pain. *Issues in Comprehensive Pediatric Nursing, 5,* 351–359.

Tesler, M., Ward, J., Savedra, M., Wegner, C., & Gibbons, P. (1983). Developing an instrument for eliciting children's description of pain. *Perceptual and Motor Skills, 56,* 315–321.

Thoman, E. B. (1985). *Sleep and waking states of the neonate* (rev. ed.). Unpublished manuscript, University of Connecticut, Storrs.

Thoman, E. B., Davis, D. H., & Denenberg, V. H. (1987). The sleeping and waking states of infants: Correlations across time and person. *Physiology and Behavior, 41,* 531–537.

Travel, J., & Simons, D. G. (1983). *Myofascial pain and dysfunction of the trigger point manual.* Baltimore: Williams & Wilkins.

U.S. Pharmacopeial Convention (1987). *Drug information handbook: Vol. 1.* Easton, Pennsylvania: Mack Publishing Company.

Varchol, D. (1983). *The relationship between nurses' and children's perceptions of pain in the acute and chronic pain experiences of children.* Unpublished master's thesis, University of Cincinnati.

Varni, J., Thompson, K., & Hanson, V. (1987). The Varni/Thompson Pediatric Pain Questionnaire. I. Chronic musculoskeletal pain in juvenile rheumatoid arthritis. *Pain, 28,* 27–38.

Villarruel, A., & Denyes, M. (1988). *Content validity of a self-report pain intensity instrument for young black children.* Unpublished manuscript, Wayne State University, Detroit.

Volpe, J. J. (1987). *Neurology of the newborn* (2nd ed.). Philadelphia: W.B. Saunders.

Wasz-Hockert, O., Lind, J., Vuorenkoski, V., Partanen, T., & Valanne, E. (1968). The infant cry: A spectrographic and auditory analysis. *Clinics in Developmental Medicine, 29.* Lavenham, Suffolk: Spastics International Medical Publications.

Williams, C., & Stevens, K. (1972). Emotions and speech: Some acoustic correlates. *Journal of the Acoustical Society of America, 52,* 1238–1250.

Yaster, M. (1987). Analgesia and anesthesia in neonates. *The Journal of Pediatrics, 111,* 394–395.

Yu, J., & Carroll, W. (1982). *Electrode placement manual for TENS.* Minneapolis: Medtronic, Inc.

Zavah, M. F. (1986). *Ice as a pain relief measure after subcutaneous injection.* Unpublished master's thesis, State University of New York, Buffalo.

Zeskind, P. S., & Lester, B. M. (1978). Acoustic features and auditory perceptions of the cries of newborns with prenatal and perinatal complications. *Child Development, 49,* 580–589.

Zeskind, P.S., & Lester, B.M. (1981). Cry features of newborns with differential fetal growth. *Child Development, 52,* 207–212.

Section B

PAIN IN ADULTS

[14]

Pain Control Behaviors of Patients with Cancer

Diana J. Wilkie, Nancy Lovejoy,
Marylin J. Dodd, and Mary D. Tesler

Cancer pain, like other pain, is best understood as multidimensional, with affective, cognitive, behavioral, and physiological-sensory dimensions (Ahles, Blanchard, & Ruckdeschel, 1983; Chapman et al., 1985; McGuire, 1987; Melzack, 1983). The behavioral dimension is particularly important for clinicians, who rely upon verbal and nonverbal behaviors when assessing pain (Chapman et al., 1985). However, nonverbal behaviors related to cancer pain have not been well described, particularly as they relate to the magnitude of pain.

The amount of pain a patient perceives is determined by the neurochemical events that occur within a complicated neural network (Basbaum & Fields, 1984). Pain signals can be modulated or altered by endogenous opiates and other neurotransmitters located throughout the nervous system (Fields & Levine, 1984). Because of the physiological circuitry of pain perception, pain intensity may be regulated by behaviors that alter ascending pain input to the central nervous system and/

The authors gratefully acknowledge the American Cancer Society for supporting this research through an Oncology Nursing Master's Program grant and the University of California, San Francisco, for an Instructional Use of Computers grant. Manuscript prepartion was supported by PHS grant number 42 USC 288 42 CRF 66, awarded by the National Cancer Institute, DHHS. Appreciation is expressed for statistical consultation provided by Don Chambers and Mark Hudes.
Reprinted in part from: Cancer Pain Control Behaviors: Description and Correlation with Pain Intensity. *Oncology Nursing Forum*, 15(6), 1988.

or stimulate descending pain modulating mechanisms (Yaksh & Hammond, 1982). Theoretically, the more intense the pain, the more likely it is that pain control behaviors will be used.

However, researchers have found that not all patients who use pain control behaviors find them completely or even partially effective (Barbour, McGuire, & Kirchhoff, 1986; Bressler, Hange, & McGuire, 1986; Donovan & Dillon, 1987; Rosenstiel & Keefe, 1983). Most behaviors have been found to provide inconsistent pain relief and in some cases to increase pain intensity.

Findings from these studies are difficult to interpret because pain etiology varied among subjects, and for studies using cancer populations, stage of disease was not held constant. Furthermore, most studies lacked valid and reliable instruments for pain behavior measurement, and, finally, they failed to examine the relationship between pain control behaviors and pain intensity. The present study addressed these deficits by using semistructured interviews and direct observation to validate use of pain control behaviors by patients with advanced stage cancer and to correlate pain control behaviors with pain intensity.

METHOD

Subjects

The convenience sample included 17 adults hospitalized in a 560-bed, acute care teaching hospital who met the following eligibility criteria: the patient was (a) an adult reporting pain; (b) diagnosed with Stage III or Stage IV solid tumor malignancy; (c) hospitalized for at least 24 hours and expected to be hospitalized for at least four days; (d) recommended by his/her nurse for inclusion in the study; (e) mentally competent and able to speak English; and (f) willing to consent. Eligible patients were approached on the second day of hospitalization, informed of study procedures, and invited to sign the consent form.

Data Collection Procedure and Instrumentation

Data were collected by one researcher on three consecutive days. On Study Day 1 the patient verbally answered interview questions using a Demographic-Pain Data Form (D-PDF), a modified version of the McGuire Pain Assessment Tool (McGuire, 1981), and the McGill Pain Questionnaire (Melzack, 1983). The D-PDF was designed to collect data on variables that could influence the perception of pain intensity, such as sex, age, education, ethnicity, disease process, character and location of pain, and analgesic therapy. During the interview, patients were also asked, "What makes your pain better?" and "What makes your pain worse?" After the D-PDF was completed, patients were instructed in the use of a 100-mm visual analogue scale (VAS) to report pain intensity. The patient reported pain intensity by drawing a vertical mark at the appropriate interval on the horizontal VAS line with "no pain" at the extreme left and "pain as bad as it could be" on the extreme right. The pain intensity score was determined by measuring the number of millimeters from the left side of the line to the place marked by the patient.

In order to prevent patient participation from affecting analgesic intake, the data collection schedule was not revealed to the patients or the nurses. However, the following schedule was observed: On Study Day 2 at 8 A.M. (Time 1), the researcher asked the patient to report present pain intensity using the VAS. The patient then was instructed to resume activities and disregard the researcher's presence. Body position and all subsequent actions and verbalizations for 15 minutes were observed and recorded by the researcher using a Behavioral Observation-Validation Form (BO-VF). The BO-VF was designed to allow verbal and nonverbal behaviors to be recorded and subsequently validated or denied by the patient as pain control behaviors. If the patient directed questions to the researcher, a brief answer was given, but conversation was not encouraged.

The procedure was repeated on Study Day 2 at 4 P.M. (Time 2), and on Study Day 3 at 8 A.M. (Time 3) and 4 P.M. (Time 4). After the final observation on Study Day 3, a final, unstructured interview was conducted in which the patient either confirmed or denied whether each behavior recorded on the BO-VF was used to control pain, by responding to the question, "Do you do this to control or reduce your pain?" Analgesic consumption was documented from review of the patient's medical record.

RESULTS

The 13 patients who completed all study measures consisted of predominantly white females with a mean age of 49 years. Patients had multiple solid tumor malignancies that had been diagnosed a mean of 67 months prior to the study. Most had no metastatic disease but had experienced pain for a mean of 18 months. Up to 14 anatomically distinct sites of pain were reported by a single patient and pain intensity scores ranged from 0 to 102 on the 100 mm VAS (one patient marked the VAS 2 millimeters beyond the upper limit of the scale). Most of the pain was constant, yet all patients but one were on an as needed (prn) analgesic schedule. Most of the patients received a combination of narcotic and nonnarcotic analgesic medications, such as morphine ($n = 6$), meperidine ($n = 3$), acetaminophen and codeine ($n = 5$), hydromorphone ($n = 2$), levodromoran ($n = 1$), steroids ($n = 3$), and nonsteroid anti-inflammatory drugs ($n = 3$). The largest dosage received was of continuous intravenous morphine, 30 milligrams (mg) per hour. The average intramuscular morphine equianalgesic dose was 5.5 mg every three to four hours prn. Many of the patients (38–46%) had not received an analgesic within four hours at each of the *four* measurement periods. However, there was no significant relationship between pain intensity and the length of time since the last analgesic dose.

In the initial interview, patients reported one to six behaviors known to them that "made the pain better." Use of medications was the behavior that patients most frequently reported to reduce their pain ($n = 11$) (see Table 14.1.).

The behavior observation revealed that patients used a total of 37 different behaviors during the 52 15-minute observation periods. Of these, 30 behaviors were validated by at least one patient as a behavior that controlled pain. Behaviors were classified into six categories by three researchers who independently reached 93% agreement on the categorization with the first investigator.

Eight patients used behaviors associated with analgesics to control pain and reported these to be directly or indirectly effective. These behaviors included consuming analgesics, discussing analgesic effectiveness, complaining of pain to request analgesics, and monitoring the medication schedule. Frequently, patients commented that analgesics were only partially effective in controlling pain despite their attempts to help monitor the medication schedule. This is important considering that nearly all of the patients were on prn analgesic schedules. Only 39% of all observed analgesic-use behaviors were identified by subjects as pain control behaviors.

All patients confirmed that positioning behaviors (assuming a special or favorite position, repositioning, or stretching) helped to reduce pain. One patient, for example, experienced severe pain each time he turned his head left of midline, and his hospital bed was positioned such that he had to turn to the left to interact with people entering the room. So whenever possible, this patient shifted his entire body rather than turning his head. Only 32% of the observed positioning behaviors were reported as pain control behaviors. These behaviors were specific to each individual and varied greatly from one individual to another. It is therefore important to establish that the patient's use of a particular positioning behavior is actually for pain control.

TABLE 14.1 Pain Control Behaviors Reported by Each of Two Methods—Interview and Validation of Observed Behaviors (n = 13)

Type of Behavior Reported to Control Pain	Method of Reporting Pain Control Behaviors[a]		Comparison of D-PDF Interview & Validated-Behaviors		
	D-PDF Interview (I) (n)	Validated Observed Behaviors (OB) (n)	Behaviors Identified by		
			I & OB (n)	I only (n)	OB only (n)
Analgesic Use Behaviors	11	8	7	4	1
Positioning Behaviors	6	13	6	0	7
Distractive Behaviors	4	12	4	0	8
Pressure Manipulative Behaviors	2	8	2	0	6
Immobilizing/Guarding Behaviors	2	5	2	0	3
Apply Heat	2	0	0	2	0
Alter Attitude	1	0	0	1	0
Other Behaviors:					
Sleep	0	7	0	0	7
Food/Drink	0	2	0	0	2
Moaning	0	1	0	0	1
	Col 1*	Col 2**	Col 3	Col 4	Col 5

D-PDF = Demographic Pain Data Form
* Col 3 + Col 4 = Col 1
** Col 3 + Col 5 = Col 2
[a]n = number of patients

Distractive behaviors were used as pain control behaviors by 12 patients, the most common means being watching or listening to television. Reading, socializing, and slow breathing were also reported as effective behaviors to control pain "because it takes my mind off of the pain." As with positioning behaviors, only 34% of all observed distractive behaviors were reported by patients to be pain control behaviors.

Pressure manipulative behaviors were used to control pain by 8 patients. Rubbing, massaging, applying pressure to a body area, or removing pressure from a body part are examples of this type of pain control behavior. A woman with liver metastases applied pressure to the liver region with her hand or a folded blanket. Another patient used a pillow folded around the edge of the over-bed table and leaned over the table to apply pressure to his upper abdomen. Although these behaviors were infrequently observed, 67% of those observed were confirmed by patients to be pain control behaviors. Hence, observation of a patient using a pressure manipulative behavior may be a good indicator that he or she is trying to control pain.

Five patients validated that immobilizing/guarding behaviors were effective in reducing pain. These behaviors included having one's eyes open and maintaining one body position during the observation period, or keeping the body or a body part rigid while walking. Again, few of these behaviors were observed, but 54% were confirmed by patients as pain control behaviors.

Seven patients validated other behaviors of pain control. Sleep reduced pain for all of these patients. Eating, drinking, and moaning were also observed as behaviors to control pain. However, only 13% of behaviors observed in this category were identified by patients as pain control behaviors.

Pain control behaviors observed and validated by patients were compared with patients' responses to the D-PDF interview question: What do you do that makes the pain better? Only two patients reported and were observed using the same types of behaviors for pain control. Eleven patients used up to four types of behaviors that they did not report during the interview.

The relationship between the summed number of validated pain control behaviors and pain intensity was examined at each of the four data collection points (see Table 14.2). There were moderate, signifi-

TABLE 14.2   Mean Number of Summed Pain Control Behaviors Correlated with Pain Intensity Ratings on Visual Analogue Scale at Four Measurement Times ($n = 13$)

Measurement Time	Number of Validated Pain Control Behaviors				Pain Intensity Ratings on Visual Analogue Scale (VAS)		
	Range	Grand Mean	SD	Correlation[a]	Mean	SD	Range
One (8 a.m.)	1–23	1.38	.31	.54**	30.7	26.4	0-81
Two (4 p.m.)	1–17	1.39	.22	.08	27.7	35.6	0-97
Three (8 a.m.)	2–22	2.03	.73	.64**	39.5	36.6	2-102
Four (4 p.m.)	0–20	1.73	.32	.46**	45.1	25.1	0-94

[a]Kendall Correlation Coefficient for summed pain control behaviors and VAS
**$p < .02$

cant correlations at Times 1, 3, and 4, which indicates that with higher pain intensity patients used more behaviors to help control pain. At Time 2, mean pain intensity was slightly lower and patients were involved in more daily activities while still using some pain control behaviors. No significant correlation was found between the number of behaviors *observed* and pain intensity, indicating that the association between pain control behaviors and pain intensity was not an artifact of the number of behaviors observed by the investigator.

DISCUSSION

Cautious interpretation of these study findings is warranted because of the small, nonrandom sample. Yet the findings suggest that observation may be more effective in identifying some pain control behaviors than an open-ended interview. Although patients were observed using pressure manipulative, positioning, and distractive behaviors and confirmed the use of these behaviors to reduce pain, they often did not report using them when asked a common pain assessment question. On the other hand, two patients reported heat as helpful for pain at home, but no patient was observed using heat in the hospital. Therefore, pain control choices may vary by setting (hospital versus home), and a combination of verbal and observational assessment methods may be necessary to thoroughly assess and manage cancer pain.

These findings suggest that nurses should recognize that pain is reduced by a variety of behaviors, particularly positioning and distraction, and should encourage the use of these behaviors. When nurses observe a favored position, it should be documented in the care plan and patients should be asked to move from favored positions *only when necessary*. Further, they can be helped to maintain favored positions with pillows or other supports. For example, the patient who experienced pain when turning his head to the left could have been reassigned to a room where the door was located to the patient's right.

Nurses can encourage distractive behaviors by assigning patients with pain to rooms with operating television sets, keeping the television control apparatus near the patient, and ensuring that the television screen can be seen by the patient. In this study, it was observed that doctors and nurses frequently moved televisions and control devices when caring for patients but did not return them before leaving the room. Patients often had to endure additional pain in reaching for the television controls.

Additionally, these results suggest that nurses should be cognizant of how much time has passed since an analgesic was administered to the patient with cancer pain. Offering analgesics to patients engaged in purposeful distraction, positioning, or pressure manipulation may augment pain control. Nurses should encourage pain control behaviors before pain intensity becomes critical and prohibits activity.

This research clearly indicates that patients with cancer pain use particular behaviors to help relieve their pain. Some of these behaviors, such as watching television or chatting with family and friends, may be misinterpreted by health professionals as indicating lack of pain. Then clinicians may not recognize the need to offer analgesic interventions to patients engaged in distractive behaviors. Similarly, positioning behaviors may be interpreted as pain expression behaviors rather than pain control behaviors. Furthermore, analgesic-use behaviors may be misinterpreted as drug-seeking behavior and the need for pain control ignored. Clinicians need to recognize the effective pain control behaviors, as well as the behaviors such as excessive immobilization, guarding, or restrictive positioning, that may actually produce tissue damage and more pain, such as from decubitus ulcers and contractures. Further research in this area may improve initial and follow-up assessment of cancer pain, especially if adaptive and maladaptive behaviors are well described in particular pain populations. Assessing and promoting usual pain control behaviors or teaching new ones may be effective nursing interventions for cancer pain management.

[15]

The Accuracy of Nurses' and Doctors' Perceptions of Patient Pain

Nancy J. Krokosky and Richard C. Reardon

A group of clinical nurse specialists in our acute care hospital felt the staff could do more for patients with pain. We began sharing articles and books. *Pain: A Source Book for Nurses and Other Health Professionals* by Ada Jacox (1977) covers a broad range of topics, and McCaffery's books (1979; Meinhart & McCaffery, 1983) offer practical suggestions for relieving pain and discuss comparable medications and strengths. Turk and Meichenbaum (1983) focus on assessing and treating chronic pain. Fagerhaugh and Strauss (1977) make the point that often within institutions, pain relief is everyone's and no one's responsibility. As a consequence patients may learn to ask for relief before they need it, or they may play staff one against the other. Staff may retaliate by labeling patients complainers and/or by delaying pain medication.

METHOD

Before proposing a way to improve the management of pain in our hospital, we decided that we should establish the existence of a problem. Realizing that if we did find deficiencies in pain relief, we would need help to remedy them, we asked the Hospital Quality Assurance Committee to appoint a multidisciplinary task force on pain to survey inpatients about their pain experiences and to compare their replies with the perceptions of their doctors and nurses.

To collect data, we designed a shortened version of the McGill Pain Questionnaire. We made two forms, one for patients that used the pronoun "you," and one for physicians and nurses with the same questions, but using "the patient" rather than "you" where appropriate. The patient's name appeared on both forms so they could be compared, but staff did not see the patient's answers.

Our general, acute care hospital has 10 units with an average of 37 beds apiece. We randomly sampled 7 patients from each unit. Our 10 interviewers consisted primarily of nurses, but included one psychologist and one physician. All received instruction sheets along with the data collection forms. After explaining the survey to the charge nurse and selecting the sample, they approached the patients. Each interviewer asked if the patient had had any pain during his hospitalization, and if so, asked for permission to ask questions or to leave the questionnaire.

The last step for each interviewer was to review patients' charts for pain medication ordered. Some surveyors noted what medications were actually given, but that was not uniformly done.

Our interviewers surveyed 50 patients. We had nurse responses for most of these and physician responses for 43. Not all patients answered all questions, nor did all nurses and physicians complete the questionnaires, so the actual number of respondents varied from question to question.

RESULTS

The diagnoses of patients were both medical and surgical. Patients reported pain of lower extremities most often, followed by chest pain, and upper extremity or neck pain.

This study found that 64% of the patients were having pain at the time of the interview. Interestingly, sometimes patients talked about pain in one part of their body, while their doctors or nurses talked of pain in another part. This was more often true when the patient had chronic pain in addition to an acute problem. Such discrepancies highlight the importance of questioning a patient about pain location, rather than making assumptions based upon diagnosis.

Ten percent of patients classified their duration of pain as brief (less than 15 minutes), 36% as intermittent (comes and goes), and 54% as persistent (never free of pain). Patients', doctors', and nurses' assessments of pain duration are illustrated in Figure 15.1.

Two different methods were used to assess the extent of agreement between patient–nurse and patient–doctor ratings of pain duration.

FIGURE 15.1 Responses to the question "How long does the pain last?"

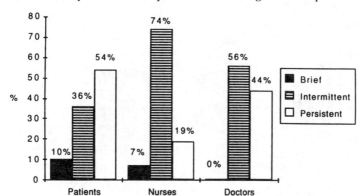

First, percentage of agreement scores were calculated on a case by case basis. Patients and nurses agreed in 47.5% of cases (19/40) and patients and doctors agreed in 34% (11/32). Second, correlations were computed for the same sets of pain duration ratings; the coefficients were these: patient–nurse $r = .29$, nonsignificant *(ns)*; patient–doctor $r = .07$, *ns*. These results indicate that doctors and nurses have difficulty in accurately gauging the duration of the pain experienced by their patients.

Sixty-two percent of the patients described their pain as acute and 38% reported it as chronic (present for six months or more) (see Figure 15.2). Case-by-case comparisons showed 70% agreement between the patients' and nurses' ratings (28/40) and 84% agreement (27/32) between the patients' and doctors' ratings. Doctors and nurses assumed more acute and less chronic pain than patients reported.

Eight percent of the patients rated their pain as mild, 20% as discomforting, 36% as distressing, 24% as horrible, and 12% as excruciating. As Figure 15.3 shows, professionals tended to significantly underestimate the amount of severe pain and to overestimate the amount of moderate pain. This underestimation of pain also was reflected in mean pain intensity ratings given by patients, nurses, and doctors (means = 3.12, 2.64, and 2.48, respectively, on a 5-point scale ranging from 1 = mild to 5 = excruciating pain). These differences were significant [one-way ANOVA, $F(2, 122) = 5.49$, $p < .01$]; further, post hoc Scheffé comparisons revealed that patients' pain intensity ratings differed significantly from those of the nurses and doctors ($p < .05$) while there was no significant difference between nurses' and doctors' rat-

FIGURE 15.2   Responses to the question "How long have you (or has the patient) had this pain?"

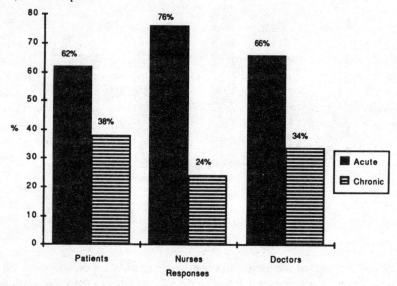

FIGURE 15.3   Responses to the question "How would you rate the amount or degree of your (or the patient's) pain?"

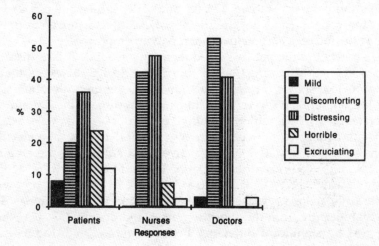

ings. Correlations between pain intensity ratings again showed little relationship between patient and nurse ratings ($r = -.01$, *ns*) and between patient and doctor ratings ($r = .30$, *ns*).

Responses to the question, "How pleased are you with the way your pain is being managed?" are shown in Figure 15.4. While the modal rating for patients, nurses, and doctors was "satisfactory," nurses and doctors tended to underestimate the number of patients who reported minimal or no relief—which was one fourth of the sample. The mean satisfaction ratings given by patients, nurses, and doctors were, respectively, 3.46, 3.63, and 3.60 (5 = total satisfaction, 1 = not at all satisfied) [one-way ANOVA, $F(2, 138) = .479$, *ns*]. Correlations between pairs of satisfaction ratings were patient–nurse $r = .23$, *ns*; patient–doctor $r = -.04$, *ns*. As with the pain intensity ratings, it appears that it is difficult for doctors and nurses to gauge the extent to which patients are satisfied with pain management attempts.

Pain intensity and satisfaction scores showed only a modest negative correlation ($r = -.31$, $p < .05$). That is, some patients with relatively mild pain were quite dissatisfied with the management of their pain, while others with severe pain were pleased with their pain control. Type of pain, however, did affect satisfaction: chronic pain patients expressed significantly less satisfaction than acute pain patients [chronic mean = 2.7, acute mean = 3.9; $t(48) = 3.907$, $p < .0005$].

FIGURE 15.4 Responses to the question "How pleased are you with the way your (or the patient's) pain is being managed?"

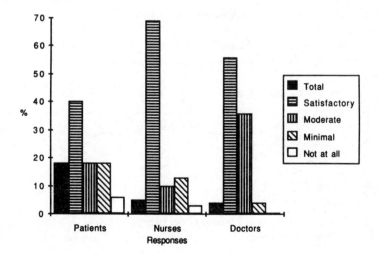

FIGURE 15.5 Responses to the question "Aside from medication, what relieves your pain?"

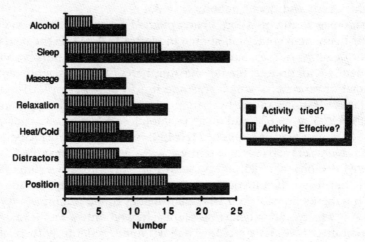

Pain medication was rated as effective by 87% of the patients. The duration of relief from medication ranged from .08 to 12 hours, with a mean of 3.79 hours. While this mean corresponds well with the frequency for which most prn orders are written, the range indicates that some patients waited a very long time from the end of their medication's effectiveness until they could have it again.

Other measures that patients reported using are shown in Figure 15.5. In all, 39 of the 50 patients were able to find some pain relief from at least one of these. Sleep helped the largest number of patients, lasting an average of 5 hours. Other measures were helpful for only 1 to 2 hours. Many patients, however, reported using several measures. It was not noted whether staff encouraged patients to try any of these methods.

Sixteen patients said walking and fatigue exacerbated their pain. Eleven mentioned dressing changes, 9 said visitors, 4 cited physical therapy and movement, 3 noted weather, and 2 said noise and sitting exacerbated pain.

DISCUSSION

We found that pain was a common occurrence, with two-thirds of patients surveyed experiencing acute pain and one-third experiencing chronic pain. While doctors and nurses generally recognized the presence of pain, they underestimated its severity and duration, and overestimated patients' satisfaction with pain management. Though one might expect those patients with greatest pain to be least satisfied, there was only a modest degree of association between patients' ratings of pain and their satisfaction with its management. There was, however, a high degree of association between pain chronicity and dissatisfaction.

Medication appeared to be most effective in relieving patients' pain, but more than three-quarters of the sample had also tried other means of pain relief. Most pain medication was ordered on a prn basis, usually every 4 hours, even though for many patients it did not remain effective for that long. Forty percent of the patients in pain were also receiving psychoactive medications, primarily Valium and Restoril.

Following analysis of our findings, our task force recommended that the hospital form a Pain Consultation Group composed of a physician, nurse, pharmacist, and psychologist, with a physical therapist and social worker if possible. We urged that the group be established as a staff resource when the usual methods were not effective in relieving patients' pain. Members would see patients on a consult basis, making suggestions to the primary physician and helping to implement these when desired. In addition, the group would help coordinate staff education on the subject of pain and collaborate in evaluating new technology such as fentanyl patches or patient controlled analgesia pumps for introduction into our hospital. Finally, the group would design and conduct further research on pain management.

While we did not have "pain experts" on staff, we recognized that we did have a core of people willing to devote the time and energy to develop expertise and to share it with others. We anticipated that by rotating duties, the Pain Consultation Group would require four to eight hours per month per member. We argued that such a group could improve patient care without raising costs to the hospital. The Hospital Quality Assurance Committee sent our proposal to the Clinical Executive Committee, which approved it with the proviso that we begin by concentrating on oncology patients. We therefore added an Oncology Clinical Nurse Specialist to the group.

Our group met first to familiarize ourselves with the contributions each could make and to share resources. We decided on an assessment format and a procedure (see Table 15.1). We then wrote a memorandum describing our functions for the Hospital Director, and a more detailed description to share with the oncology staff. We are currently reviewing cases with the oncology CNS preparatory to announcing that we are ready to receive consults.

TABLE 15.1 Proposed Pain Consultation Group Procedure

Physician Consult
Clerk routes to member "on call" that week
  During regular duty hours only
  If member unable to take case,
  must find another member to do so.
Member does assessment
  Reviews chart
  Assesses patient
  Talks with staff
Confers with other group members as needed
Makes recommendations orally and on consult
Reevaluates within 24–48 hours
  Patient's pain status and satisfaction with interventions
  Staff's opinion of situation
  If recommendations implemented, were they successful?
  If not, reassess, confer, make new plan
Periodically (more frequently at first), whole group to meet and review cases

---

Those of us who worked on this study feel that through it we were able to resensitize many professionals to the problems of patients with pain. Without the study, the idea for a Pain Consultation Group would probably never have arisen, or if it had, the chances for its acceptance would have been much smaller. We are hopeful that the Pain Consultation Group can provide patient service and staff education, and conduct future research. We think that a group similar to ours would work wherever a core of interested professionals are willing to collaborate to reach the goal of pain relief.

[16]

The Use of Patient-Controlled Analgesia for Burn Pain

Marlene A. Moyer

Problems associated with pain are the foremost difficulties faced by the health care team managing burn trauma victims. Burn pain is intense and it lasts a long time. While hospitalized, the burned patient is subjected to numerous treatments, including hydrotherapy (tubbing/debridement), surgical procedures, application of topical agents, and physical therapy; the treatments themselves cause pain, especially in the acute phase of the injury. Wagner's survey of 87 patients found that dressing changes, tubbing or debridement, active exercises, and procedures related to grafting all caused pain (Wagner, 1977). Patients' reactions to the pain of dressing changes and debridement in the tub vary from stoicism to complete loss of control. This is clearly the most frustrating and grueling experience for both patient and staff. Therefore, any measure that may be used to make this situation more tolerable for the patient is worth investigating.

Treatment-inflicted pain poses problems because, short of complete anesthesia, drugs alone cannot adequately relieve that pain; this is particularly true of the debridement procedure. Nevertheless, management is primarily directed toward reducing the pain through narcotics.

Many psychological processes also can influence the reaction to pain (Sternbach, 1968). Control has been shown to be a mediating variable in both acute and chronic pain. There is substantial evidence for the view that there is a relationship between perceived control, anxiety, and perceived pain. Mandler and Watson (1966) reviewed the evidence for a link between control and anxiety and concluded that "if the organism has some control over the onset and offset of potentially stressful stimuli, or even if it simply expects to have such control, there is likely to be less anxiety or arousal" (p. 271). Many laboratory studies (Averill, 1973; Bowers, 1968; Geer, Davison, & Gatchel, 1970; Glass, Singer, Skipton, & Krantz, 1973; Staub, Tursky, & Schwartz, 1971) have shown that if subjects do not believe they can control or terminate an aversive event, they perceive the event as more aversive or painful. Taylor (1982) suggested that many hospitalized patients might be in a state of "anxious helplessness"; the hospital environment engenders loss of control, which may actually increase the experience of aversive symptoms.

If there is a relationship between control and pain tolerance, then the most therapeutic approach to the burn patient should include increasing his control over such unpleasant events as the tubbing/debridement procedure. Control over this procedure has been shown to be associated with significantly less depression and anxiety in young patients who were in pilot studies at the Shriners' Burn Institute in Boston and the University of Wisconsin Center for Health Sciences (Kavanaugh, 1984).

The concept of patient-controlled analgesia (PCA) is currently gaining acceptance as an alternative to the traditional method of administering narcotic analgesics to patients in pain. With this technique, patients activate an electronic syringe pump connected to their intravenous line when they feel the need for analgesia. The frequency of administration is controlled by an adjustable lockout mechanism that prevents the patient from receiving the drug for a predetermined period following each dose.

Demand analgesia techniques such as PCA, which give the patients some measure of control over their pain medication, have been explored recently in several acute pain settings. However, while a number of clinical trials have used PCA with various patient populations, very little documentation exists in regard to the use of PCA with burn patients. The two studies recently reported (Sandidge, Marvin, & Heinbach, 1987; Wolman, Lasecki, Alexander, & Luterman, 1987) give conflicting results. Wolman and associates concluded that PCA was not successful in providing adequate analgesia based on its use in the acute phase of burn therapy for 52 patients. Sandidge and associates concluded that PCA was equivalent to the standard prn system in terms of pain relief and amount of medication required over a period of seven days.

This study explored the efficacy of PCA with a small sample of burned patients, looking specifically at its benefit for the patient during the debridement procedure. The provision of some control to burn patients over the pain they experience during this procedure could, theoretically, enhance pain tolerance or decrease the amount of pain perceived.

METHOD

In this experimental, two-group, posttest-only study, burn patients were requested to indicate on a pain-color scale what their perceived pain level was during the tubbing procedure on two consecutive days, one using PCA and one the routine administration of analgesia by the nurse researcher. Each patient's sets of responses were compared to each other to determine whether PCA influenced the perception of pain.

Subjects

The setting for the study was a 14-bed burn unit in a large, private, university-affiliated hospital in a metropolitan area. The first 15 acutely injured burn patients who were admitted to the unit, met the study criteria, and agreed to participate were included in the study. Study criteria included having a burn injury that was thermal, chemical, or electrical in nature and of sufficient severity to justify IV therapy and tubbing for at least two days; having the ability to use at least one hand; and being alert, oriented, and English-speaking. It took nine months to acquire subjects for study.

Procedure

The method of narcotic analgesic delivery to be used first was randomly assigned, so that some patients received the nurse-administered medication during the tubbing procedure on the first day while others received the PCA system initially. On the next day, the alternate method of medication delivery was used for each patient. The medication administration protocol for both methods of delivery is illustrated in Figure 16.1. Every effort was made to ensure that the tubbing procedure was performed by the same personnel on both days and the duration of the procedure was similar on both occasions. The investigator monitored the procedure to ensure that extraneous variables did not interfere.

The instrument used for this study was the Stewart Pain-Color Scale (Stewart, 1977), which consists of a color continuum of yellow-orange-red-black arranged from left to right. The instrument was selected because it indicates perception of pain, is easy to administer and requires

FIGURE 16.1 Morphine administration protocol.

Minutes:	-10 (prescrub)	0 (scrub begins)	5	10	15	20
PCA	Morphine in mg : 5.0 (loading dose)	1.0	1.0	1.0	1.0	1.0
		-------------patient choice--------------------				
Nurse-administered injections	5.0 (bolus)	1.0	1.0	1.0	1.0	1.0
		-------------nurse-administered-------------- (not patient choice)				

very little time or effort on the part of the subject. On both days, the investigator requested subjects to point to the color on the scale that best represented what they perceived their pain level to be at two distinct times: (a) while at rest, before being premedicated for the tubbing procedure and (b) near the end of the tubbing or approximately 20 minutes after commencement of the procedure. The subjects were apprised of the color scale continuum before each measurement. To facilitate data analysis, each color on the instrument was assigned a numerical value ranging from 0 to 10, with 0 at the extreme left representing no pain and 10 on the extreme right representing severe pain.

RESULTS

The study subjects had from 14% to 60% of total body surface area burned. The majority of patients ($n = 12$; 80%) had flame burns. While many of the patients had a mixture of partial thickness (second degree) and full thickness (third degree) burns, 80% had primarily partial thickness burns; the remaining 20% had predominantly full thickness burns. The age of patients ranged from 24 to 55; 80% (12) were between the ages of 24 and 36. All but one were male.

Each patient's sets of responses on the Stewart Pain-Color Scale were compared to each other; thus, the patients served as their own controls. One set of pain scores was obtained when the patient was medicated using the PCA pump and another set of scores was obtained on an alternate day when the medication was administered by the nurse researcher.

A paired *t*-test was done to determine whether the two pain perception scores obtained during tubbing differed significantly. There was no significant difference in the pain perception of burn patients when analgesia was delivered via the PCA pump and when analgesia was administered by the nurse [$t(14) = .64$, $p > .05$]. In fact, the mean pain perception scores for the PCA procedure (6.60) and the nurse-administered analgesia procedure (6.93) were surprisingly similar. Thus, these burn patients did not perceive a lower level of pain when allowed to administer their own pain medication using the PCA pump. In fact they perceived comparable levels of pain during the two treatments.

It is important to note that all of the patients self-administered a minimum of 8 mg of narcotic (morphine) during the tubbing procedure; the mean received dose of narcotic was 8.93 mg via PCA. When medicated by the nurse researcher, the patients received 10 mg of morphine. An independent *t*-test indicated that there was no significant difference between the two doses at the .05 level.

DISCUSSION

The equivocal results of the study may be associated with differences between patients in locus of control. Patients who are more sensitive to loss of control may benefit more from demand analgesia, while other patients may actually prefer to have the nurse or physician in control (Peck, 1986). Perhaps locus of control should be examined in further studies of PCA.

Gal and Lazarus (1975) found that engaging in activity is preferable to being passive when one is in a stressful situation. In addition to providing a sense of control, PCA may be distracting. And indeed, one patient in this study noted that the PCA pushbutton served as a desirable distractor. However, other patients said that PCA was simply an extra thing to deal with and preferred the nurse to administer the pain medication. Thus, being able to take action during stressful periods was of positive value for some individuals, but it seemed a negative for others. PCA is clearly not for every patient.

While a few of the patients expressed a preference for PCA, the data do not indicate that it significantly reduced patients' pain. PCA may not be appropriate for the kind of acute episodic pain suffered during debridement, especially when a caregiver is readily available to administer medication. This implies that other strategies should be explored to try to help burn patients better tolerate the dreadfully painful tubbing procedure. Maybe the provision of control in some other aspect of the tubbing procedure should be considered. Another suggestion for research would be to examine the effects of various relaxation techniques (e.g., music therapy, imagery, Lamaze-type breathing) during tubbing. There are innumerable strategies to explore as adjuncts to administration of analgesia. Research should focus on finding which of these are better ways to manage pain.

[17]

The Effects of Transcutaneous Electrical Nerve Stimulation (TENS) on Postoperative Patients' Pain and Narcotic Use

Terry S. Nelson and Norann Y. Planchock

Transcutaneous electrical nerve stimulation, TENS, was introduced in 1970 as a pain relief method. TENS is a battery-powered generator that transmits electrical impulses through electrodes placed on the skin, and it appears to present few unwanted side effects. Hymes, Raab, Yonehiro, Nelson, and Printy (1973, 1974) found that TENS users reported 60–80% less pain after using TENS. No incidence of ileus was observed in TENS users, and they had a significantly lower incidence of postoperative atelectasis.

Bussey and Jackson (1981), who compared the frequency of intramuscular injections of meperidine in TENS and non-TENS users, found that among cholecystectomy patients, the frequency of narcotic use was 70% less for TENS users than for non-TENS users. For herniorraphy patients, frequency of narcotic use was 65% less among TENS users. Some patients in each TENS group required no postoperative narcotics, and many herniorraphy TENS users were discharged from the hospital one to two days before non-TENS users.

Rosenberg, Curtis, and Bourke (1978) and Schuster and Infante (1980) reported that TENS users in their study had significantly lower mean narcotic dosages than non-TENS users. Rosenberg et al. (1978) contended that TENS could increase ambulation, respiratory activity, awareness, and appetite, and decrease the potential for drug addiction. Likewise, Schomburg and Carter-Baker (1983) found that among post-laparotomy patients, the frequency of meperidine and other analgesic use was significantly lower for TENS users than for non-TENS users.

The possibility of a placebo effect with TENS use was investigated by Ali, Yaffe, and Serrette (1981) using the frequency of analgesic requests as a dependent variable and by Taylor, West, Simon, Skelton, and Rowlingson (1983) using milligram equivalents of morphine taken by patients. Both investigations found that TENS users took fewer narcotics than placebo users. VanderArk and McGrath (cited in Tyler, Caldwell, & Ghia, 1982) also concluded that patients who used functioning TENS took fewer narcotics than those with placebo TENS.

However, despite positive findings about TENS, many users have not reported complete pain reduction. In a study by Hymes et al. (1974), 97% of TENS users reported at least mild pain. VanderArk and McGrath (cited in Tyler, Caldwell, & Ghia, 1982) found that 23% of TENS users still reported pain. Likewise, Schomburg and Carter-Baker (1983) found that TENS was not completely effective for 17% of their subjects.

Since reports of the effectiveness of TENS are inconsistent, this investigation studied the effects of TENS upon perceived pain and narcotic use. It was expected that TENS users would experience less pain than non-TENS users, though for both TENS and non-TENS groups, pain was expected to decrease over time. It was also expected that TENS users would use fewer narcotics than non-TENS users, though narcotic use was expected to decrease over time for both groups.

METHOD

The study was conducted in a 175-bed acute care medical center in a south-central state. A deliberate sample of 40 subjects was selected from the list of scheduled surgical cases. Twenty subjects were TENS users and 20 were non-TENS users. Potential subjects had to meet the following criteria: (1) 18 years of age or older, (2) oriented to person, place, and time as judged by a researcher and an R.N. who worked on the unit with the subject, (3) scheduled for an abdominal surgery case (excluding caesarean sections), (4) able to see well enough to read the Visual Analogue Scale used by the researchers, (5) not preselected by the physician to be postoperatively admitted to the intensive care unit, (6) no narcotic usage exceeding two weeks during the previous six months, and (7) willing to participate in the study and signify agreement by signing a consent form.

All TENS units were of the brand name Neuromod by Medtronic, Incorporated. According to medical center policy, on the first postoperative day, a physical therapist instructed each TENS user how to adjust stimulation intensity according to individual pain relief needs.

Instruments used in the investigation were a visual analogue scale (VAS) and a medication data collection instrument. For the medication collection sheet, developed by the researchers, interrater reliability was 100% as determined by chart review by a researcher and two other registered nurses. Face and content validity were determined by a panel of experts.

Subjects were asked to complete the VAS for perceived pain at 8:00 A.M., 2:00 P.M., and 8:00 P.M. of their first, second, third, and fourth postoperative days. Each day, narcotic usage of each subject was recorded from the medication chart record. Narcotic usage was calculated using equianalgesic doses compared to intramuscular morphine. Medications taken on a prn basis were noted for frequency.

RESULTS

The sample consisted of 20 TENS users and 20 non-TENS users. There were few demographic differences between the groups. Most of the sample consisted of women who were in their 30s, white, married, and experiencing recovery from an abdominal hysterectomy with nonmalignant findings.

VAS scores indicated that there was no significant difference in pain perception between the TENS and non-TENS groups [F $(1,35) = .29$, $p > .05$], although TENS users had less pain on all but the first postoperative day (see Figure 17.1). As expected, both groups indicated a decrease in pain over time, except for a slight increase among TENS users on the third postoperative day. Most patients attributed their pain increase on the third day to "gas pain." Seventy percent of TENS users had discontinued TENS by the end of the third postoperative day even

FIGURE 17.1   Mean Visual Analogue Scale of TENS and non-TENS users according to postoperative day.

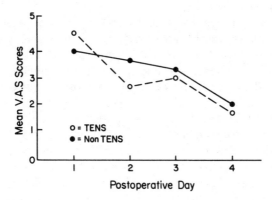

though the mean TENS intensity of the group was highest on this day. If TENS therapy had continued longer, perhaps pain perception in TENS users might have been somewhat less on the third postoperative day.

TENS users used significantly fewer narcotics than non-TENS users [F (1,35) = 9.52, $p < .01$]. As shown in Figure 17.2, this difference held for all four postoperative days; it was significant for days one, two, and three. Likewise, TENS users used fewer prn antiemetics, antihistamines, nonopiate analgesics, hormones, and tranquilizers than non-TENS users, although the only significant difference was in nonopiate

FIGURE 17.2   Mean narcotic usage for TENS and non-TENS users according to postoperative day.

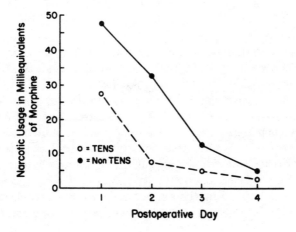

analgesic usage. Non-TENS users used fewer bisacodyl suppositories and suppositories for bladder spasms than TENS users, but this difference was not significant.

As expected, narcotic use in both groups decreased each day after surgery. No significant relationship between pain perception and narcotic usage was evident in either the TENS or non-TENS group. Thus, nurses should not assume that high narcotic use provides total pain relief, nor should they assume that low narcotic use means a patient is not experiencing pain.

TENS users were discharged after a mean 4.7 days postoperatively while non-TENS users' mean hospital stay was significantly longer— 5.8 days [$t(38) = 3.25$, $p < .01$]. The earlier discharge of TENS users, however, may be attributable to physician differences or other differences in the groups.

DISCUSSION

The study findings have a number of implications for nurses dealing with patients in pain. When TENS or any other pain relief method is planned for postoperative use, the patient needs to be taught how to use the method before he or she is confronted with postoperative pain. The standard procedure at the medical center where these data were collected was that the physical therapist explained TENS to the patient during the patient's first postoperative day. Half of the first postoperative day had sometimes passed before the patient fully understood TENS. Fear of TENS and lack of knowledge of how to manipulate the control, and the purpose, safety, and proposed length of use were all concerns expressed by patients to the researchers. Active involvement in pain relief by patients may help lower analgesic use; but only by understanding the pain relief modality can an individual be actively involved in its use.

The nurse must keep in mind that some pain relief modalities may not be well accepted by all individuals. During this study, three TENS users commented that they did not like TENS or found TENS ineffective in providing pain relief. Such patients should clearly not use TENS. Further, nurses should carefully assess the effectiveness of a pain relief measure for each patient because pain is such a subjective response. Narcotic dosages or narcotic frequency intervals may be inadequate for some individuals; individual assessment of pain is crucial to decide this. With ongoing assessments the nurse can provide feedback for the health care team regarding the adequacy of the pain relief approach.

This study indicated that postoperative patients can use techniques such as TENS to supplement narcotics for pain relief. Patients who use TENS may experience great pain relief, use fewer narcotics, and, possibly, have an earlier hospital discharge. In this age of cost containment, increased patient acuity, and decreasing numbers of nursing personnel, time-saving pain relief modalities such as TENS provide promising results for nurses as well as for patients.

[18]

The Effectiveness of Biofeedback in Relieving Childbirth Pain

Pamela Duchene

Pain is an integral component of childbirth. A variety of nonpharmacological pain relief methods have been evaluated for effectiveness in childbirth: transcutaneous electrical nerve stimulation, hypnosis, prepared childbirth training, and relaxation (Brucker, 1984). Another method that has been investigated for efficacy during labor is biofeedback (Basmajian, 1983; Gregg, 1983; St. James-Roberts, Hutchinson, Haran, & Chamberlain, 1983). Biofeedback techniques of relaxation reduce pain associated with childbirth by reducing muscle tension. Decreased muscle tension may reduce stimulation of the pain nerve endings in the uterus, cervix, and peritoneum. Therefore, in keeping with the Gate Control Theory, pain perception may be reduced in two ways by biofeedback: by the woman consciously reducing abdominal muscle tension, thus reducing the risk of childbirth-related perineal trauma;

and by distraction as the woman focuses on relaxing the abdominal muscle (Oriol & Warfield, 1984).

In 1983, St. James-Roberts et al. reported that electromyographic (EMG) biofeedback was helpful during active labor but was discarded during transition in favor of epidural anesthesia. Electromyographic or EMG biofeedback is a method of detecting the amount of electricity generated by a muscle or muscle group. Muscle contraction or tension results in the generation of electricity that can be monitored by an EMG device. The EMG unit translates the electrical impulses produced into audible and/or visible signals. Individuals using EMG biofeedback are informed of subtle changes in muscle tension and can learn to control muscle tension and relaxation. Gregg (1983) studied the use of biofeedback during childbirth for over a decade and found a reduction in the length of labor, reduction in use of medications, and higher Apgar scores when biofeedback was used during labor. However, Gregg did not use any standardized form of pain assessment in the study. In light of the conflicting results reported by St. James-Roberts et al. and Gregg, additional studies of the effects of biofeedback on pain during labor and delivery, using a standard measure of the pain experienced, were needed.

The purpose of this study was to examine the effects of EMG biofeedback on self-reported pain during childbirth. The study compared reports of pain from women using both biofeedback and prepared childbirth training techniques and women using only prepared childbirth training techniques.

METHOD

Subjects

The study was conducted within the labor and delivery unit of a community hospital. Participants were selected who were in their first pregnancy, were not carrying twins, were of 30 weeks or less gestation, attended the full childbirth preparation course, were between 16 and 40 years of age, were married, and were not known to have any major medical or obstetrical complications. Study participants were recruited as they registered for Lamaze classes. After obtaining informed consent, participants were randomly assigned to experimental or control classes.

Training Procedures

All participants attended six weekly prepared childbirth training classes. Participants in the experimental group were also instructed in the use of EMG for the purpose of promoting muscle relaxation according to the following routine:

1. Monitoring of baseline activity   5 minutes
2. Relaxation exercises   35 minutes
3. Training in application and use of biofeedback equipment
                                           20 minutes

The relaxation exercises were integral to the Lamaze classes, and baseline activity was monitored on all participants to ensure that experimental and control groups were comparable. Therefore, adding training in the use of the biofeedback equipment lengthened each session by only 20 minutes.

Biofeedback was taught using an instruction manual and a standardized relaxation tape. Each participant in the experimental group then received a copy of the manual, a relaxation tape, and a biofeedback device for practice at home. Subjects were instructed to practice for 20–30 minutes daily for six weeks and to then continue to practice for 3–5 minutes each day until delivery. They were instructed to bring the biofeedback devices with them when they were admitted to the labor and delivery unit.

Equipment

A J & J portable EMG device, which could be used with an earphone, provided biofeedback through a visual monitor and an audible sound. Three electrodes were placed in close proximity of one another on the abdomen of the participants with the ground electrode in the center. The electrodes were placed to ensure that the device monitored muscle tension rather than fetal or uterine movement. When uterine contractions occurred, the participant focused on relaxing the abdominal muscle. Tension of the abdominal muscle was indicated by clicking sounds, and as EMG activity (muscle tension) increased, there was an increase in the rate of clicks.

Intervention

Biofeedback was initiated upon admission to the labor and delivery unit and was continued throughout labor and delivery. The nursing staff was instructed in the use, purpose, and reading of EMG biofeed-back to increase awareness of and support for the technique.

Pain Assessment

During labor, participants were assessed for pain perception by use of a 10-cm visual analogue scale (VAS) and the present pain intensity portion of the McGill Pain Questionnaire. The instruments were administered during (1) admission to the labor unit (early labor), (2) active labor, (3) transitional labor, and (4) delivery. At each of the assessment times participants were asked between contractions to rate the pain they perceived with contractions, on both scales. An additional 24-hour recall measure was based on the woman's recollection of the overall pain intensity during labor and delivery. Following labor, participants who had used EMG biofeedback were interviewed to determine their perceptions of the technique.

RESULTS

Fifty-five primiparous women began this study; 15 did not complete it because they required caesarean sections. The experimental and control groups were equivalent with regard to age, race, history of miscarriage, and EMG baseline. Twenty subjects in each group completed the study. Characteristics of the infants born to mothers in both groups were similar with regard to birth weight and Apgar scores.

On the present pain intensity scale, women using EMG biofeedback reported lower average pain levels at each of the assessment times than did women in the control group. Using the Mann-Whitney test, statistically significant differences between the groups were found on admission ($z = 1.81$; $p = .035$), at delivery ($z = 2.59$; $p = .005$), and on the recall measurement ($z = 2.25$; $p = .012$) (see Table 18.1).

Average pain ratings with the VAS were also lower for the group using biofeedback at all assessment times except transitional labor. However, analysis of variance indicated that the differences between pain experienced by participants using biofeedback (mean VAS rating = 2.40) and those not using it (mean VAS rating = 4.18) differed significantly only on the admission measurement ($p = .011$).

In the 24-hour postpartum interviews, 85% of patients using biofeedback indicated that it was helpful during labor and delivery, and 80% indicated that they would use biofeedback during future labors.

The use of medications in the control group and experimental group differed significantly. Seventy percent of the women in the control

TABLE 18.1 Means for Present Pain Intensity Index at Four Measurement Times

	Measurement Time				
Study Condition	Admission	Active	Transition	Delivery	Recall
Biofeedback	1.7	3.4	3.2	2.9	2.9
Control	2.2	3.5	3.4	4.0	3.7

group used epidural anesthesia, compared to 40% of the women in the biofeedback group ($p = .023$). Women using biofeedback labored an average of 2 hours less than women in the control group; however this difference was not significant ($p = .25$), perhaps due to the great variation in labor times.

DISCUSSION

Women's experiences of childbirth vary; no two are identical. Additionally, women have different expectations of pain relief; some women want to experience childbirth fully, while others prefer complete anesthesia. Because of these variations, it is appropriate that many alternative pain relief methods be available to the expectant mother. Biofeedback cannot be used spontaneously during childbirth because it requires planning, but EMG biofeedback requires only short practice periods and is suitable for individuals who are motivated to practice the technique. Although in this study less medication was used by women using biofeedback, the technique should be viewed as an adjunct to other pain relief measures and medications. Biofeedback cannot be considered a spontaneous method of pain relief.

Biofeedback, besides being learned easily, is appropriate for instruction in a group format, such as in Lamaze or other childbirth preparation classes. Training in the technique for prospective instructors can be obtained from practitioners or through educational programs. Training for biofeedback requires less time than either hypnosis or prepared childbirth.

The nurse attends the mother throughout labor and delivery and often serves as childbirth coach and support person. EMG biofeedback equipment and techniques provide the nurse with another tool to help reduce the childbearing woman's pain. For childbirth, the most appropriate EMG biofeedback device is a small, portable unit. These devices are relatively inexpensive, $250 to $400, which is substantially less than other types of pain reduction equipment such as transcutaneous electrical nerve stimulation (TENS) units. Once a woman has mastered the relaxation technique, biofeedback may be done without equipment.

EMG biofeedback has been used for several years for chronic pain, and its effectiveness is well documented for reducing muscle tension (Nigl, 1984). However, the use of biofeedback with acute pain, such as childbirth pain, has not been widely reported. The results of this study point to EMG biofeedback's potential for reduction of acute pain.

[19]

The Effectiveness of Relaxation in Relieving Pain of Women with Rheumatoid Arthritis

Theresa P. Dulski and Ann M. Newman

Rheumatoid arthritis is a major health problem for women, affecting them three times more often than it affects men (Pelletier, 1977). Chronic pain is a primary complaint of patients with rheumatoid arthritis and a major problem in managing the disease. The pain can be so disabling that those experiencing it may be unable to participate in normal daily activities.

Pain has been shown to be associated with stress (Clark, 1983; Shearn & Fireman, 1985); therefore, managing stress may be a way to reduce pain. Jacobson and Benson have found that stress management through use of relaxation techniques is a means of self-management of chronic pain (Benson, 1975). These researchers do not suggest that one's pain is eliminated with relaxation techniques, but that the perception of pain decreases because stress is reduced. Building on their work, this study evaluated nurse-taught relaxation as an approach to self-management in reducing the perceived pain of rheumatoid arthritis.

METHOD

The study was conducted at a private rheumatology clinic in a large metropolitan area. Subjects in the study were women receiving treatment for diagnosed rheumatoid arthritis who agreed to participate. They were randomly assigned to either the control or the experimental group. Each group consisted of 30 subjects.

Intervention

Each subject in the experimental group was taught the relaxation technique. This technique combines Jacobson's progressive relaxation and systematic tensing and relaxing of muscles with Benson's breathing awareness and relaxation techniques (Benson, 1975). This script was used to demonstrate the relaxation technique:

1. Sit quietly in a comfortable position.
2. Close your eyes.
3. Deeply relax all your muscles, one at a time, beginning at your feet and progressing up to your face. Keep them relaxed.
4. Breathe through your nose. Become aware of your breathing. As you breathe out, say the word "one" silently to yourself. For example breathe in . . . out, "one"; in . . . out, "one"; etc. Breathe easily and naturally.
5. Continue for 10 to 20 minutes. You may open your eyes to check the time, but do not use an alarm. When you finish, sit quietly for several minutes, at first with your eyes closed and later with your eyes opened. Do not stand up for a few minutes.
6. Do not worry about whether you are successful in achieving a deep level of relaxation. Maintain a passive attitude and permit relaxation to occur at its own pace. When distracting thoughts occur, try to ignore them by not dwelling upon them and return to repeating "one." With practice, the response should come with little effort. Practice the technique twice daily, but not within two hours after any meal, since the digestive processes seem to interfere with elicitation of the relaxation response.

After demonstrating the technique, the researcher asked subjects to demonstrate it. Clients were given copies of the relaxation technique described above and were instructed to perform the activity at least twice a day for four weeks. Subjects also were to keep daily records of the times and length of the relaxation sessions and record any relevant comments.

Data Collection

A three-part questionnaire was used to elicit information about personal and social background (part I), the subject's functional ability (part II), and the subject's perception of pain (part III). Functional ability, which correlates inversely with pain, was measured using the Stanford Arthritis Center Disability and Discomfort Scale. The Disability and Discomfort Scale contains 19 items designed to measure subjects' degree of difficulty in performing daily activities. The higher the score on this scale, the greater the success in performing daily activities. This instrument was chosen since it has been found that disability and pain are highly correlated (Brown et al., 1984).

The 27-item McGill-Melzack Pain Scale measures pain perception (Feldman, 1984). Twenty items describe levels and types of pain that persons may experience, one item asks respondents whether their pain emanates from "deep" or "shallow" levels of the body, and the other six items assess the levels of pain that respondents have experienced.

The three-part questionnaire was administered to all subjects as a pretest and posttest.

Procedure

After the pretest the nurse researcher reviewed an arthritis self-help brochure with all subjects, which is a routine activity at the clinic. Experimental subjects were taught relaxation, while control subjects received only routine care.

All subjects were asked to follow physicians' orders for medications and to keep daily records of their pain medication use for four weeks. Subjects again completed parts II and III of the questionnaire after four weeks based upon pain experience at that time. Subjects mailed completed questionnaires and medication records to the researchers.

RESULTS

Sixty subjects began the study: however, 15 subjects failed to return the posttest, and 2 additional subjects were excluded from the analysis because posttest instructions were inadvertently omitted from their packets. Thus the final sample included 43 subjects.

The groups were roughly equivalent on demographic variables. The sample included 38 white and 5 black women; 34 were presently married, 6 were widowed, 2 were divorced, and 1 was single. Mean age was 55.47 years. Subjects had been diagnosed with arthritis for a mean of 8.70 years; the range of reported years with arthritis was from 1 to 21 years.

Pre- and posttest scores on the Melzack and Stanford scales were compared to evaluate changes in pain perception and functional ability and to determine differences between people who experienced the relaxation technique and those who did not. Two-way repeated-measures analysis of variance was used to analyze differences in scores between pretest and posttest, control and experimental groups. Only the interaction test was significant [$F(1,41) = 7.42$, $p < .01$], indicating that the average change in pain scores between pretest and posttest was different for the experimental and control groups. The control group had a mean Melzack score of 23.80 on the pretest, while the experimental group's mean was 29.65. The control group's mean score on the posttest was almost 4 units higher (27.7) than their pretest group score. The experimental group had a mean Melzack score on the posttest that was 4.65 units lower (25.00) than their pretest score.

The data suggest that the relaxation techniques were responsible for the decrease in pain reported by the experimental group from pretest to posttest. It was interesting that Melzack scores for the control group increased almost 4 units from pretest to posttest. One possible explanation is that when they were at home, subjects perhaps were experiencing more stress than during the initial testing at the clinic and therefore their pain seemed worse.

Because of the large difference in the Melzack pretest scores, experimental and control groups were also compared using regression analysis to control for these differences. The adjusted mean for the posttest experimental group was 23.18 and for the control group it was 30.38. These means differed significantly ($p < .03$), suggesting that even if the groups had been equivalent on the pretest, the relaxation group would have done better on the posttest.

No significant differences were noted between the experimental and control groups in functional ability. Eighteen subjects reported to researchers that the onset and/or increase in symptoms followed stressful events in their lives. Among the stressors were a disabled husband, a family member's involvement in an automobile accident, being post-hysterectomy, unemployment, poor eyesight, death of husband (3 subjects), separation, divorce, and jobs. Patients also reported benefits of the relaxation technique, including improved ability to relax and sleep at night. Some patients reported that they enjoyed using the technique. One woman in the relaxation group reported that she felt her rheumatoid arthritis had resulted from a "complete nervous breakdown" in 1979. The relaxation technique provided her with "a way to just shut off my brain and rest, sleep. This is my way [to] get away from the thoughts going around in my head and the hurt in my body."

DISCUSSION

Use of the relaxation technique reduced perceived pain and thus provides an adjunctive, nonpharmacologic self-help approach to the management of pain in women with rheumatoid arthritis. Whether pain arises from arthritis, a postoperative procedure, cancer, or unknown causes, the relaxation technique used in this study can be offered to patients as a potential means of reducing the anxiety and stress associated with pain, and thus perhaps controlling pain more effectively.

[20]

The Effect of Relaxation Training on Surgical Patients' Anxiety and Pain

Joanne M. Laframboise

Surgery is stressful, painful, and physically dangerous, evoking emotional responses from patients (Scott, Clum, & Peoples, 1983). Thus, surgery provides an ideal situation in which to examine the relationship between anxiety and acute clinical pain and to attempt to alleviate both.

Postoperative pain management is an important part of the care that nurses provide for surgical patients. It includes assessing pain, providing comfort measures, administering prescribed analgesics, and evaluating the effectiveness of these interventions. McCaffery (1979) suggested that patients in pain need care in each of three phases of the pain experience: anticipation of pain, the painful experience, and the period immediately following pain. In light of this, Kim (1980) suggested that nursing should focus as much on the pre- and post-experience phases as on the painful experience phase, because care during the anticipation of pain, for example, can help alleviate the actual experience of pain by reducing state anxiety.

From their review of the literature MacDonald and Kuiper (1983) concluded that the most effective preparations for surgical patients were those that provided patients cognitive and behavioral strategies for coping with the anxiety related to surgery and postoperative pain. One cognitive-behavioral strategy that has been tested with surgical patients is relaxation (Flaherty & Fitzpatrick, 1978; Levin, Malloy, & Hyman, 1987; Wells, 1982; Wilson, 1981). Wells (1982) suggested that relaxation may reduce postoperative pain by decreasing pain from secondary reflex muscle contractions and altering the focus of attention, anxiety, and perceived control.

The purpose of this study was to test the effectiveness of relaxation training in reducing pre- and postoperative state anxiety and postoperative pain in upper abdominal surgical patients. Also, since previous research (Kim, 1980) has shown that sensation information preoperatively increases pain postoperatively in subjects with high physical danger trait anxiety (i.e., likelihood of responding with high state anxiety to a threat such as impending surgery), a secondary purpose was to determine whether these subjects would benefit from relaxation training.

It was reasoned that when surgical patients used a cognitive-behavioral strategy such as relaxation for coping with the surgical situation, their anticipatory coping mechanisms would decrease preoperative state anxiety and their active coping mechanisms would decrease postoperative state anxiety. It was expected that with the reduction of state anxiety, patients would report less pain postoperatively. Figure 20.1 illustrates the predicted relationships among the study variables.

METHOD

A convenience sample of 30 adult patients from two large acute-care teaching hospitals who were scheduled for elective cholecystectomy were randomly assigned to experimental ($n = 15$) and control ($n = 15$) groups. The evening before surgery, state anxiety and physical danger trait anxiety were measured in all subjects.

FIGURE 20.1   Theoretical framework.

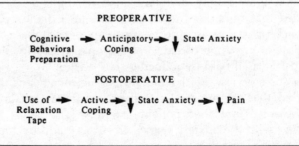

Adapted from: The Pre- and Postoperative Coping Intervention Model, MacDonald & Kuiper, 1983.

Physical danger trait anxiety is defined as the tendency to perceive situations as threatening and to respond to physically threatening situations with elevations in state anxiety (Endler, Edwards, & Vitelli, 1985). Physical danger trait anxiety level was reflected by the score obtained on a 15-item Likert scale—the General Trait Anxiousness–Physical Danger Subscale (Endler et al., 1985). A higher score on the scale indicates more anxiety.

State anxiety is defined as an emotional state characterized by subjective, consciously perceived feelings of tension, apprehension, and nervousness, accompanied by activation of the autonomic nervous system. State anxiety can vary in intensity and fluctuate over time as a function of the stresses that impinge upon the individual (Spielberger, 1972). The subject's level of state anxiety was reflected by the score obtained on a 20-item Likert scale—the State Anxiety Scale (STAI Form Y-1) (Spielberger, Gorsuch, Lushene, Vagg, & Jacobs, 1983). A higher score on this scale indicates greater anxiety.

All subjects were told preoperatively what to expect before and after surgery, and the nature of the pain likely to follow surgery was discussed. They were also given information on physical exercises to aid recovery. Experimental subjects received training in focused relaxation. The relaxation exercise, done with the aid of a 25-minute audiotape, incorporates structured breathing exercises, autogenic muscle group relaxation, and pleasant imagery. Subjects were told that relaxation was one strategy they could use to help relieve postoperative pain by assisting them to relax, physically and mentally. Experimental subjects practiced relaxation once before surgery and as often as they desired after surgery. There was no validation of achievement of the relaxation skill. After preoperative teaching and the relaxation training for the experimental group, all subjects completed the State Anxiety Scale.

On postoperative Days 2 and 3, subjects described and rated their surgical pain using Parts I and II of the McGill Pain Questionnaire (Melzack, 1975) and versions of the Sensation and Distress Scales (Johnson & Rice, 1974). State anxiety was again measured on postoperative Day 2, before pain was measured. The number and types of analgesics received during the first 48 hours postoperatively and from postoperative Day 3 to discharge were recorded, as was the length of postoperative hospital stay.

RESULTS

No significant differences were found between experimental and control groups in state anxiety after preoperative teaching or on Day 2 postoperatively. Pain scores on Day 2 postoperatively also did not differ significantly between the two groups.

However, among subjects who were high in physical danger trait anxiety, those in the experimental group reported significantly less pain intensity [$t(13) = 2.35$, $p < .05$] and less physical sensation of pain [$t(13) = 2.07$, $p < .05$] by Day 3 postoperatively than those in the control group, and they required significantly fewer analgesics for pain relief from Day 3 to the day of discharge [$t(13) = 2.72$, $p < .01$]. These patients also were discharged from the hospital an average of 1.2 days sooner than control subjects with high physical danger trait anxiety [$t(13) = 2.03$, $p < .05$].

Among subjects who were low in physical danger trait anxiety, there were no significant differences between the experimental and control groups in pain scores on postoperative Day 3, analgesic usage, or length of postoperative hospital stay.

For all groups except the low-danger control group, there was a significant decrease in state anxiety after preoperative teaching ($p < .05$ in each case). Also, a moderate, positive correlation was found between physical danger trait anxiety and state anxiety prior to preoperative teaching [$r = .44$, $p < .05$].

DISCUSSION

The lack of significant differences in state anxiety between the overall experimental and control groups after preoperative teaching could be a result of subjects not believing that the relaxation exercise would help to relieve surgical pain. It is also possible that patients expected that using the tape postoperatively when in pain would be an added stressor. In other words, anticipatory coping did not occur possibly because subjects formed negative cognitive appraisals of their situation.

The lack of significant differences between experimental and control groups in state anxiety and pain on postoperative Day 2 could be explained by experimental subjects responding with increased state anxiety when intense pain was not relieved by use of the relaxation tape. It also could be that experimental subjects did not find the exercise helpful in promoting relaxation. It was noted that experimental subjects practiced relaxation infrequently in the early postoperative period, stating either that they felt too ill (groggy from anesthetic, nauseated, or weak) or in too much pain to use the tape. This could explain the lack of significant treatment effect in the early postoperative period.

In future studies, a controlled protocol for relaxation training and use should be carried out so that surgical patients could practice and develop the relaxation skill preoperatively. In addition, attainment of the relaxation skill should be measured. With these changes, it is likely that a stronger treatment effect would be observed. At the same time, it must be remembered that adjunctive therapies like relaxation may not be appropriate for all patients in the early postoperative period.

By Day 3, when experimental subjects had used the relaxation tape, differences in postoperative pain scores emerged for high-danger subjects, though not for low-danger subjects. Low-danger individuals reportedly respond to physically threatening situations with lower state anxiety. Since state anxiety has been shown to relate positively to pain (Chapman & Cox, 1977; Martinez-Urrutia, 1975; Scott, Clum, & Peoples, 1983), an intervention aimed at reducing state anxiety might not show a significant effect with patients who already exhibit low anxiety.

For all groups except the low-danger control group, there was a significant decrease in state anxiety after preoperative teaching. This finding lends support to the idea that preoperative teaching can help alleviate preoperative anxiety in surgical patients, even those who are highly anxious.

The significant effect, in this study, of relaxation training on postoperative pain and recovery in patients high in physical danger trait anxiety supports the idea that this cognitive-behavioral strategy helps such patients cope with the surgical situation. Although a statistically significant effect was not observed for patients low in physical danger trait anxiety, this does not mean that these patients would not benefit from relaxation. Relaxation could be offered to all patients as a strategy to add to their personal repertoires of coping.

Upon admission to the hospital, surgical patients could be offered relaxation instruction. Nurses must be knowledgeable and skilled in the techniques and should encourage patients, especially in the beginning phase of training until they develop the skill. Achievement of the relaxation skill could be assessed by asking patients to rate their relaxation before and after the exercise using a visual analogue scale. Relaxation also could be assessed by measuring pulse, respirations, and systemic blood pressure.

Surgical patients could be encouraged to use relaxation to help cope with anxiety on the day of surgery and postoperatively, when they are experiencing a good deal of pain. The technique could be used after deep breathing and coughing exercises, after moving and turning in bed, after ambulating, at bedtime, or in conjunction with pain medication. However, relaxation should not be used by nurses as a substitute for taking time to sit with patients to discuss their anxieties and concerns or as a substitute for primary analgesic management of acute postoperative pain.

For elective surgical patients, relaxation training could begin in their homes a week or two before admission to the hospital. This would provide patients with the opportunity to practice relaxation and develop the skill. Many subjects in this study acknowledged feeling anxious about their surgery weeks beforehand, and their anxieties might have been alleviated if they had been able to practice relaxation prior to their hospital admissions. Finally, preoperative teaching should be provided for *all* surgical patients, as it was shown to significantly decrease state anxiety.

[21]

The Effects of Self-Guided Imagery and Other-Guided Imagery on Chronic Low Back Pain

Kathleen J. Moran

Chronic pain is a condition that afflicts approximately 65 million Americans, about 50 million of whom are disabled not by underlying pathology, but as a result of the pain itself (Bonica, 1980). To provide care for these individuals is a monumental task and one that requires input from all members of the health care team and, in particular, the nurse, whose work is directed toward relief of human suffering and promotion of wellness. One technique that can be effective in reducing chronic pain is guided imagery (Bresler, 1979; Fezler, 1980; Kroger & Fezler, 1976; McCaffery, 1979; Scott & Barber, 1977a, 1977b; Worthington, 1978; Worthington & Shumate, 1981). Guided imagery is the use of one's mind to form, manipulate, and experience images involving any or all of the five senses for the purpose of achieving pain relief.

Guided imagery is based on the premise that pain is both a psychological and a physiological experience. Recent research on the physiology of pain has revealed the existence of endogenous pain control mechanisms including an analgesia mechanism that descends from the highest levels of the central nervous system. This suggests that pain control is an innate physiologic process that can be triggered by psychogenic methods such as guided imagery (Fields, 1981; Guyton, 1986; Melzak, 1973; Whidden & Fidler, 1977). It also suggests that the key to the effectiveness of imagery lies within the individual (Bresler, 1979; Fields, 1981; Simonton & Simonton, 1974). The individual experiencing pain, therefore, would need only to become aware of and master the methods and techniques for activating these innate processes in order to obtain some relief. Eventually the patient could become independent in using such a technique, enabling him or her to obtain relief when it is most needed. The nurse is the ideal member of the health care team to help patients master such a technique for pain control since the nurse promotes self-care (Orem, 1971).

It appears reasonable to expect that self-guided imagery could be as effective in reducing chronic pain as other-guided imagery, and a chronic pain sufferer could become independent in the use of imagery by learning to initiate his or her own images. The role of the nurse, then, would be to teach the patient to employ self-guided imagery and become independent in using this pain relief technique.

The purpose of this study, therefore, was to determine the relative effectiveness of two imagery techniques in reducing the intensity of chronic pain: self-guided imagery and other-guided imagery. Previous studies have shown that guided imagery can be effective in reducing painful experiences (Blitz & Dinnerstein, 1971; Goldstein & Hilgard, 1978; Olness, Wain, & Ng, 1980; Scott & Barber, 1977a, 1977b; Worthington, 1978; Worthington & Shumate, 1981), but no studies have examined the effect of guided imagery on chronic pain sufferers. The study also examined the influence of selected background and situational variables on the effectiveness of the two approaches to guided imagery.

METHOD

A quasiexperimental design was used to study the effects of other-guided imagery and self-guided imagery on the intensity of pain experienced by adult patients with chronic, myofascial, low back pain. The setting for the study was the outpatient department of a university-based pain control center in Cincinnati, Ohio. Only patients who were 18 years or older, who had the diagnosis of myofascial low back pain, and who had been experiencing pain for six months or longer were included in the study. Patients with multiple pain diagnoses or psychiatric diagnoses were excluded from participation. Each of 40 subjects carried out a technique of imagery using pleasant images involving all of the five senses, guided either by the nurse or self-guided following instruction by the nurse. Each imagery session lasted fifteen minutes and was carried out prior to the patient's other pain relief treatments.

Twenty subjects were randomly assigned to the group using self-guided imagery and were individually instructed to create and experience pleasant mental images. These subjects were taught to use their powers of imagination to recall or invent mental images that were pleasant and were instructed to use images involving all of the senses: sight, sound, taste, smell, and touch. Before the exercise each subject was asked to describe to the researcher the images that he or she planned to include in the exercise. At the completion of the exercise each subject was instructed to describe the images actually used during the exercise. This was done to ensure that each of the subjects carrying out the self-guided imagery technique did so properly.

Twenty subjects were randomly assigned to the group using other-guided imagery and were instructed to listen to the detailed description of a pleasant scene as read aloud by the investigator and to imagine experiencing the scene exactly as it was presented (see Table 21.1). Subjects were instructed to use their imagination to experience the images as fully as possible.

The tool used to measure pain intensity was the Visual Analogue Scale, a 100-millimeter straight line which represents a continuum of pain intensity. "No pain" is the verbal anchor for the extreme left end of the scale, and "Pain as bad as it can be" is the anchor for the right end of the scale. Patients were assisted to a comfortable position, then rated their pain immediately before and after using guided imagery. A numerical value was ascribed to each subject's pain by measuring its distance in millimeters from the left end of the scale.

TABLE 21.1 Text For Other-Guided Imagery

You may close your eyes now. Take a slow, deep breath, breathing slowly and deeply. Feel yourself relax as you breathe out slowly. Concentrate on your breathing, breathing slowly and deeply from your abdomen. . . .

Now, if you wish, you may begin to imagine yourself going for a leisurely stroll. You are walking along the river. It's mid-July . . . and it is very, very hot. The sun is getting low on the horizon line although it has not yet begun to set. . . . The sky is a brilliant blue . . . the sun a blazing yellow. . . . Feel the heat from the sun against your face . . . feel the heat from the sun's rays against your whole body. . . . Now you are barefoot. Feel the damp, cool, plush tickle of the grass on the soles of your feet with each step as you slowly walk along the river's edge. . . . Now you pause and sit on a small ledge on the side of the river. It is shaded from the hot sun by a large willow tree . . . its branches and leaves making a gentle rustling noise as the breeze pushes them to and fro . . . and to . . . and fro. . . . The ledge is made of rock . . . it feels round and smooth as you run your fingers along the surface. . . . Now you dip your hand into the cool water. . . . You can feel the movement of the water as you open your hand against the soft cool flow of the current. Feel the cool water washing over your feet. . . . The water is amazingly clear, clean, and sparkling. . . . Hear the steady soft sounds of the water as it passes by you. . . .

Beside you, by the trunk of the willow tree, you see dozens and dozens of petite wildflowers. Pink ones . . . violet ones . . . yellow ones . . . red ones . . . each one has perfect tiny little petals of every color in the rainbow. . . . As you lean near them you can smell their fragrance. As you inhale deeply . . . you can actually taste the sweetness of the flowers as you breathe in their lovely fresh scent . . . and you feel very relaxed.

The water is like a mirror of silver, reflecting the sun's rays, a mass of pure white light . . . and you are gazing into that light. . . . As you continue to stare at the sun's reflection on the water you begin to see a violet line along the horizon, a purple halo around the skyline . . . everywhere purple and silver. . . .

Now the sun is beginning to set. With each movement, with each motion of the sun into the water you will become more and more relaxed . . . and when the sun has sunk into the river you will be in a profound state of relaxation. . . . The sky is turning crimson . . . and scarlet . . . and gold . . . and amber as the sun finally sets. . . .

You are engulfed in a deep purple twilight, a velvety blue haze. . . . You look up at the night sky . . . it's clear, filled with stars. A brilliant starry night. . . . Listen . . . and you'll hear the sound of the river washing against the rocks. . . . Breathe deeply and you'll taste and smell the sweetness and fresh-ness of the wildflowers. . . . Relax . . . and you'll feel the comforting cool breeze. . . . Look above you and you'll see the beautiful colors of the sky . . . and you feel yourself carried upward and outward into space, at peace . . . and one with the universe. . . .

(continued)

TABLE 21.1   *(continued)*

You may end the guided imagery for yourself when you are ready. . . . Count silently to yourself from one to three. . . . At the count of three inhale fully and deeply, open your eyes, and say to yourself, "I feel relaxed and alert." I will wait now for you to end the imagery when you wish. Take your time. Enjoy the experience.

Adapted from Fezler (1980).

RESULTS

To analyze the effect of each type of imagery on the intensity of pain experienced by chronic low back pain sufferers, a paired t-test was performed on the pre- and posttreatment Visual Analogue Scale scores for each group of subjects, and an analysis of covariance was carried out to examine the difference in effectiveness. The results indicated that either technique could be effective in reducing the intensity of chronic pain. However, other-guided imagery was more effective than self-guided imagery.

The group of subjects using self-guided imagery had an average decrease in pain intensity of 5.4 points on the Visual Analogue Scale. This decrease in pain intensity was statistically significant [$t(19) = 2.9$, $p < .01$], but whether such a small decrease would be clinically significant is questionable. Nevertheless, it is important to note that any reduction in the amount of suffering experienced by a patient is beneficial.

The group of subjects using other-guided imagery had an average decrease in pain intensity of 14.6 points on the Visual Analogue Scale, which was also statistically significant [$t(19) = 3.8$, $p < .01$]. This represents a reduction in pain intensity of approximately 15 points on a 100-point scale. Reducing the intensity of pain from a relatively severe level of 70 (on a scale of 100) to a more moderate level of 55 or from a moderate level of 55 to a milder level of 40 could represent a significant change in the pain experienced by the sufferer.

The mean difference between pre- and post-Visual Analogue Scale scores among those subjects using other-guided imagery was greater than the mean difference in pre- and post-Visual Analogue Scale scores among subjects using self-guided imagery. This difference was statistically significant [$F(1,38) = 4.12$, $p < .05$] and indicated that the effect of other-guided imagery was greater than the effect of self-guided imagery in reducing pain intensity.

The data were analyzed to examine the influence of age, sex, race, pain medications taken within 24 hours of participating in the study, and activity on the effectiveness of each type of imagery in reducing the intensity of chronic pain. None of these variables were significantly associated with effectiveness.

DISCUSSION

A major difference between self- and other-guided imagery is the mode of participation of the subject. Other-guided imagery, in which the subject is provided images and guided through every step of the exercise by the nurse, is a more passive behavior than self-guided imagery, where the subject is required to invent and manipulate mental images without the nurse's guidance. This more active participation on the part of the subject understandably requires more experience for mastery. Subjects may need to repeat the exercise in order to master the new process of an imagery exercise. Possibly on a one-time basis, as in this study, a passive exercise was more easily carried out than an active one; and this may explain why other-guided imagery was more effective than self-guided imagery. This notion is supported by the work of Kroger and Fezler (1976), who reported that a pain-relieving imagery technique became increasingly effective with repeated use.

Another possibility is that other-guided imagery is better suited to patients experiencing moderate and severe levels of pain. The energy required to deal with such suffering is limited, and the patient in pain may have only enough strength to carry out a passive exercise such as other-guided imagery.

Clearly, some relief from chronic pain can be achieved through the use of guided imagery techniques. But the most effective technique for any particular patient is that which is tailored to the individual. In working with a chronic pain patient on guided imagery the nurse should use a trial-and-error approach. Some patients may be able to master self-guided imagery techniques after instruction from the nurse, while other patients may benefit only from imagery techniques in which they can assume a passive role. Some patients may prefer a tape-recorded imagery exercise to use at their convenience such as those available commercially, some of which have soothing background music or nature sounds. Other patients may prefer individualized tape-recorded imagery made by the nurse or significant others. A variety of imagery scenes and techniques should be offered to each patient in order to see what that patient finds most enjoyable and most effective for pain relief.

[22]

The Effect of Music on Adult Postoperative Patients' Pain During a Nursing Procedure

Janet E. Angus and Sandra Faux

One of the ironies of nursing practice is that while nurses work to prevent and relieve pain, they are frequently called upon to perform therapeutic procedures that cause pain (Fagerhaugh & Strauss, 1977; Sandroff, 1983). For example, among postsurgical patients, nursing procedures such as wound packing changes result in episodes of acute pain.

It is encouraging to note that a growing number of nursing interventions are available for the management of pain (McCaffery, 1979; Snyder, 1985). However, many of these interventions have not yet been tested thoroughly in clinical settings (Snyder, 1985).

Music is a pleasant, familiar environmental stimulus that can be used to distract patients from pain during an uncomfortable procedure. Neither the patient nor the nurse requires previous training in this use of cognitive distraction; thus, music is a potential intervention for situations in which pain is acute and episodic.

Music, especially that with a slow tempo and calm or happy overtones, has been associated with lower levels of anxiety and aggression (Fisher & Greenberg, 1972; Peretti, 1975; Shatin, 1970; Stoudenmire, 1975). Locsin (1981) demonstrated that postoperative patients who listened to their preference of music had significantly lower pain scores than did a group who heard music that did not suit their preferences. More recently, anecdotal reports of the successful use of music for pain management have appeared in the nursing literature (Bailey, 1985;

166

Herth, 1978; Jacob & Beyerman, 1986). A tape incorporating music with pleasant guided imagery significantly reduced pain and distress in oncologic patients (Graffam & Johnson, 1987). Music has also been successfully used to distract children from discomfort during immunization (Fowler-Kerry & Lander, 1987).

This study examined the effect of listening to music on the pain perceived by postoperative patients during changes of abdominal wound packing. On the assumption that music can distract patients and that the mood attributes of music may influence the listener's own affective state, it was expected that when the patients listened to music during wound packing changes, they would have less of the sensory component of pain, less negative affect, and less intense pain than when they did not listen to music. Since vital signs tend to rise in response to acute pain, it was also expected that patients would have lower pulse rates and blood pressures when they listened to music.

METHOD

Subjects

Subjects were chosen from one of four surgical nursing units in three large urban teaching hospitals. Patients who had undergone abdominal surgery and were having abdominal wound packing changes were eligible for study if they were free of postoperative complications such as confusion, hypovolemia, or respiratory distress. They also had to be fluent in English, free of aural pathology, and between the ages of 18 and 65.

The Intervention

Each subject had two wound packing changes, once while listening to music and once without music. The two sessions were separated by a 24-hour interval. Patients were randomly assigned to one of two treatment order groups: Group A, which first had treatment without music and then listened to music during their second treatment, and Group B, which listened to music during their first treatment but not during their second. Patients received their routine analgesic at least 30 minutes prior to the start of treatment.

The musical tapes were developed using information from the literature (Cook, 1986; Livingston, 1979; Long & Johnson, 1978; Smith, 1986) and advice from various sources, including a music therapist, a radio station manager, a classical record shop owner, and numerous lay persons. The music was predominantly moderate in tempo and had calm or happy mood attributes. Five lay persons of ages ranging from 26 to 57 assessed the quality of the tapes and assigned them to mood categories. The popular music offered to subjects included sentimental favorites of the 1940s to 1960s, flute renditions of recent movie soundtrack and popular songs, country and western, progressive jazz guitar, ragtime piano, and a semiclassical ballet. Classical selections included a collection of adagios, familiar Baroque pieces, piano classics, and classical guitar music. Music was delivered to subjects using a small tape player with lightweight foam headphones. Subjects selected the tape that best suited their preferences and began listening to music 10 minutes prior to and throughout the wound packing change. All of the wound packing procedures were performed by the investigator. During each of the two procedures, conversation and environmental noise were kept to the minimum level necessary.

Instrumentation

Before their first treatment subjects completed a brief demographic questionnaire. After each procedure, the McGill Pain Questionnaire (MPQ) (Melzack, 1975) was used to measure the intensity of pain as well as the sensory and affective qualities of the pain experienced by subjects during the procedure. Subjects selected adjectives from the 20 subscales of the MPQ that best described their sensations and feelings during the dressing change. The Sensory Pain Rating Index was scored using the first 10 groups of adjectives; the Affective Pain Rating Index was scored using the next five groups of adjectives; and pain intensity was measured by totaling scores on all of the adjectives selected, to obtain the Total Pain Rating Index, and by using the six-point Present Pain Intensity Scale.

The Pain Ladder, a nine-point vertical visual analogue scale (Hay, O'Brien, & Jeans, 1986), was also used to score pain intensity. Subjects were asked to place a mark on the rung of the ladder that corresponded to the amount of hurt they had experienced during the procedures.

Subjects' blood pressure and pulse were measured before and immediately after each procedure. A debriefing questionnaire was completed at the end of the two sessions to obtain subjective descriptions of subjects' experience.

RESULTS

The 26 adult postoperative patients who participated in the study ranged in age from 18 to 65 years, with a mean of 41. Sixty-two percent

($n = 16$) were male, and 65% (17) had midline abdominal incisions. The mean level of education for the sample was Grade 12.

When age, sex, years of education, analgesic intake for 24 hours prior to each treatment, time of day the treatments were done, number of days since surgery and proportions of elective and emergency admissions were compared for the group who had music during the first treatment and the group who listened during the second treatment, no significant differences were found.

Effect of Music on Pain Scores

Individual scores on all of the pain indexes and scales were significantly lower during the wound packing procedures when music was available than when there was no music (see Table 22.1). Thus, the intensity of pain during the procedures was less when patients listened to music than when they did not.

As expected, the sensory quality of pain was also less pronounced when subjects listened to music. For example, those who reported sensations of "tautness," "wrenching," or "stabbing" during the procedure performed without music either reported no such sensations during the procedure in which they listened to music, or reported milder sensations such as "tenderness," "tugging," or "pricking."

The average score for the entire sample on the Affective Pain Rating Index during the procedure performed without music was nearly four times greater than during the procedure performed with music. Those who reported that the pain during the routine wound packing was "frightful" or "exhausting" when they did not listen to music chose no affective terms to describe their pain during the procedure when they had music or described it as merely "tiring."

TABLE 22.1   Mean Pain Scores with Analgesics Only and with Analgesics Plus Music ($n = 26$)

Pain Rating	Possible Range	Analgesic Only Intervention Mean	Analgesic Plus Music Intervention Mean	p^a
Sensory Pain Rating Index	(0-42)	8.19	6.12	.005
Affective Pain Rating Index	(0-19)	.54	.12	.001
Total Pain Rating Index	(0-77)	12.23	8.85	.008
Present Pain Intensity	(0-5)	1.23	.88	.013
Pain Ladder	(0-9)	2.54	1.54	.001

^{a}paired t-tests

However, vital signs were not significantly lower following wound packing changes performed with music as a distractor than following those performed without music.

To eliminate possible effects of order (i.e., whether the individual heard music during the first or second treatment), a second set of analyses (independent t-tests) was performed to compare Groups A and B on data from the first treatment only. Here too, significant differences were found between listening and not listening to music on the Sensory ($p = .015$), Affective ($p = .007$), and Total ($p = .014$) Pain Rating Indexes; differences on Present Pain Intensity and the Pain Ladder were not significant. Again, there were no significant differences in vital signs.

Listening Styles and Size of the Effect

There was a great deal of variation in the ways that subjects received and listened to the music. Some were skeptical or turned the volume down on the tape player to attempt conversation during the treatments. Others were enthusiastic and became immersed in the music, singing along or tapping their fingers in time to the rhythm. Subjects were not instructed to listen to the music in any particular way but were asked at the end of their participation in the study to describe how they had used the music. Three nearly equal groups of listening styles emerged: 9 subjects listened passively or treated the music as background sound; 9 concentrated on lyrics, specific instruments or melodies; and 8 used the music to construct a pleasant, affective milieu by either focusing on the mood attributes of the music or by recalling pleasant images suggested by the music.

To determine the effect of listening style on perception of pain, the difference between each of the pain scores following the two treatment conditions was calculated for each of the three groups. The effect of music was least in the group who listened passively and greatest in those who reported using the music to modify their affective state (see Table 22.2).

Subject Preference

Sixteen (62%) of the subjects reported that they preferred to listen to music during their wound packing changes. The remaining 10 noticed no difference between the treatments and had no preference. Those who used imagery or other forms of distraction as mechanisms to cope with pain found that listening to music was a compatible strategy. Of those who did not find music helpful, 4 explained that they preferred

TABLE 22.2 Changes in Pain Scores for Three Types of Listening Strategies[a]

Pain Score	Passive Listeners ($n = 9$)	Active Listeners ($n = 9$)	Focus on Affect or Imagery ($n = 9$)
	Mean Change	Mean Change	Mean Change
Sensory Pain Rating Index	1.78	1.67	2.88
Affective Pain Rating Index	.11	.56	.62
Total Pain Rating Index	2.00	2.67	5.75
Present Pain Intensity	.22	.22	.63
Pain Ladder	.56	.78	1.75

[a]Change was calculated as the difference between scores for the Analgesic Only Intervention minus scores for the Analgesic Plus Music Intervention; thus, the larger the change score, the greater the effect of music on pain.

to be able to interact with the nurse, and 2 did not enjoy being distracted from watching and directing the wound packing change.

DISCUSSION

In this study, patients who underwent a painful procedure reported significantly fewer sensations, less affective distress, and less intense pain when they listened to the calm or happy music of their choice than when they did not listen to music. These results are sufficient to support the combined use of analgesics and familiar music with calm or happy mood attributes to help patients cope with short-term unpleasant sensory and affective experiences.

Listening to music is economical in time, energy, and funds. Many people have spent their lives developing and enjoying positive associations with music; they do not have to expend energy in developing a new skill, nor do nurses need advanced preparation to successfully use this intervention. Initially, a few moments are required to explain the purpose of the intervention, determine the patient's choice of music, provide instruction on cassette player use, and offer suggestions as to the most effective ways of listening to the music. Additional staff are unnecessary, although if a music therapist is on staff at your facility, his or her input could be solicited. The hospital librarian could assume responsibility for organizing and maintaining a central music collection since music therapy has applications in many of the specialty areas found in a general hospital.

The possibilities are endless; one man who participated in the study suggested that for those who do not enjoy music, recordings of comedy routines or radio dramas would be a good alternative. Several tapes are commercially available that guide the listener in pleasant imagery or relaxation techniques set to music.

Nurses can help their patients use auditory distraction to the best advantage by attending to these details:

1. Have the patients' favorite type of music available. Music is a highly symbolic, personal medium; its meaning varies markedly between individuals.
2. Instruct the patients to concentrate on the music. Encourage them to recall a pleasant scene or event that is connected with or suggested by the music, or to focus on the mood of the song.
3. Allow patients to control the volume of the player so they can "tune out" the rest of their environment or keep in touch with you as they prefer.

Finally, those who benefited most from music during the study were people who also used other forms of distraction to cope with pain. Some patients cope by involving themselves in the painful event in order to somehow control it. For the patient who prefers to watch dressing changes and offer suggestions to the nurse, auditory distraction could be an unwelcome nuisance. Offer the use of music; not everyone will want to use this strategy, but those who accept are predisposed to benefit from it.

[23]

Intervening with Adults in Pain: A Discussion

Mary T. Champagne and Ruth A. Wiese

Pain relief is a prerequisite for optimal recovery following injury or surgery and for maintaining function and quality of life in chronic or terminal conditions. In every instance, pain relief decreases suffering and enhances the patient's ability to cope with other stresses that illness or diagnostic procedures bring. The nine chapters in this section examining interventions for relieving pain in adults not only describe ways that clinicians can improve patient outcomes through relief of pain but also identify issues that warrant clinical exploration and further study.

It is noteworthy that the chapters on pain in adults focus primarily on interventions; this shows that we have made significant progress in developing instruments to reliably and validly measure key aspects of the pain experience in adults, particularly in those who can report their subjective experience to us. Pain is now recognized as a complex experience with at least four main components—nociception, sensation, suffering or distress, and behavior. This clearly refutes the notion that there is a one-to-one relationship between the amount of noxious stimulation and the pain experience.

Although physiological, subjective, and behavioral responses to pain have been identified, the complexity of the pain experience often makes measurement difficult. It is valuable to know that a number of tools are now available to help us assess our patients' pain since this facilitates selecting interventions and evaluating therapeutic efficacy. However, we must chose which tools to use in what context. Such decisions should be based on the type of pain, the characteristics of the patient, and the resources available. If the patient's condition changes or if he is unable to understand the instrument chosen, it may be necessary to try more than one assessment instrument.

For an initial assessment of acute pain the full multidimensional McGill Pain Questionnaire (MPQ) is useful; however, it requires 15 to 20 minutes to complete and may not be practical or necessary to successfully manage acute pain on an ongoing basis. In general, a visual analogue scale (VAS) and other short instruments that measure only the intensity of pain, such as the verbal descriptive Present Pain Intensity portion of the MPQ, are adequate for ongoing assessment of acute pain following trauma or surgery. These instruments are inexpensive, easy to use, and easily understood by most patients; they place little response burden on fatigued patients, require only a few minutes to explain and administer, and can be repeated as needed. However, when using scales that measure only pain intensity, it is important to remember that data on the location of the pain, its quality, temporal aspects, and factors that increase or relieve the pain also need to be elicited.

For patients with chronic nonmalignant pain both the VAS and the full multidimensional MPQ are appropriate, as are measures of functional ability and activity. The MPQ is also appropriate for assessing chronic malignant pain if the patient's physical condition permits, while VASs or short verbal descriptors that measure intensity and distress may be most useful for patients who are physically debilitated or fatigued. In such patients, observing functional ability and activity would also be helpful.

Clearly, pain is a multidimensional private experience and those of us on the outside can appreciate it most accurately through the subjective verbal report of the patient. However, there are some patients who are unable to complete instruments that quantify various components of pain because they require an understanding of degree or level. Further, patients may be unable to verbally communicate their suffering because of language barriers, low educational level, or cognitive impairments. In particular, as the elderly population increases, we will find more cognitively impaired adults experiencing the acute pain associated with surgery or the chronic pain of cancer. We were acutely reminded of this problem recently when reviewing the chart of a severely cognitively impaired patient (senile dementia of the Alzheimer's type) who received no pain medication following a below-the-knee amputation. Research in assessing pain perception in this special population is sorely needed; clinical reports of case studies would enrich our understanding.

In pain management the clinician must make many decisions between assessment and intervention. Perhaps most important is deciding what outcome is desired. The studies of Krokosky and Reardon and of Wilkie and colleagues document that many patients continue to experience significant pain during hospitalization. In Wilkie and colleagues' study, most of the patients reported pain that was constant; yet all were on a prn analgesic schedule, most were in pain, and many had not received an analgesic within 4 hours of each of the four measurement periods. Krokosky and Reardon found that over half the patients reported moderate to severe pain. Nurses and doctors underestimated the amount of severe pain present, which was described by patients as "horrible and excruciating," words that connote powerful suffering. One-fourth of Krokosky and Reardon's patients reported minimal or no relief of pain. These findings support Donovan's statement that caregivers do not have total relief of pain as a goal for patients in pain. They also lend support to the notion that patients may have woeful misconceptions about the amount of relief that is a reasonable expectation and that caregivers and patients often have different views of the pain experience.

Pharmacological therapy is a mainstay in the treatment of pain; findings in the studies presented in this volume indicate that we do not use this therapy well, though nurses have significant influence over the doses ordered and control over dosing intervals. Clinically we can turn this situation around. Relief of pain is possible; the window between pain relief and ability to function is not as narrow as we imagine— should drowsiness occur, analgesic doses can be reduced. A few hours of drowsiness "endured" until the most therapeutic analgesic dose is titrated seems less harmful than days of unrelieved pain. Patients and their families have a right to information about desired pain relief and professional action to see that such an outcome is attained.

The studies on adult pain reported in this volume primarily examined the effectiveness of nonpharmacological interventions for pain management. The one study that examined pharmacological intervention compared the effectiveness of two methods of narcotic administration, patient-controlled analgesia (PCA) and nurse-administered analgesia. Using a sample of burn patients during a tubbing procedure, Moyer found that there was no difference in pain perception between the two methods of analgesic administration, but other studies of postoperative patients (Jones, 1987) and terminal cancer patients (Baumann, Batenhorst, Graves, Forster, & Bennett, 1986) report contrary results. In Moyer's study the nurse was with the patient during the tubbing procedure and administered the narcotic as the procedure began. This immediate delivery of the needed medication in the same dose that could be obtained using PCA may explain why no difference between treatment groups was discovered. It also raises the question of whether PCA has been found more effective in decreasing pain in other studies because it gives patients "control," or because the patient is able to receive the analgesic immediately, without having to wait for the nurse.

Wilkie et al. reported that patients use self-selected behaviors to help control their pain and that nurse observation and validation with the patient will reveal more of these behaviors than will simply asking the patient. In the clinical setting we can observe patient behaviors and have the patient confirm when they are being used to control pain, and whether they are helpful. If they are, nurses can give "permission" to use them, reinforce their use when needed, and make the environment conducive to their use. We can also determine if some of the behaviors being used have harmful secondary effects (e.g., pressure sores) and suggest other interventions the patient might use to control the pain.

Several chapters in this section reported a variety of adjunctive therapies, usually in a multimodal approach to managing acute or chronic pain. When one thinks of the model presented by Donovan, which suggests at least four points in the body where interventions can be used to modulate or reduce pain, the advantage of a multimodal approach is obvious. Five studies examined the effectiveness of reducing pain perception using cognitive-behavioral interventions, including relaxation (studied by Laframboise and by Dulski and Newman), imagery (examined by Moran), biofeedback (studied by Duchene), and music (explored by Angus and Faux). Nelson and Planchock studied another type of adjunctive pain relief therapy, transcutaneous electrical nerve stimulation (TENS). In each of these studies pain decreased for the experimental group—though not always for each person in that group, and not always to the same degree: for some the decrease was small, while for others it was large. In some of the studies other variables were positively affected; fewer narcotics were used by the experimental group or the length of hospital stay was shorter. None of the interventions had any adverse effects on patient well-being.

From a clinical perspective it is clear that the adjunctive therapeutic interventions presented in the studies in this volume can improve patient outcomes through pain relief. Yet there are many unanswered questions. Which of these therapies should be used for which patients? How do we decide who should and who shouldn't try a particular therapy? What abilities, situations, or environments are conducive to successful implementation of a particular therapy? How long should we try a particular therapy before we say, "this one is effective for this patient," or "this one doesn't work for this patient" so we need to try something else? We do have some knowledge to help us with some of these questions. We know, for example, that current TENS models are most effective for relief of cutaneous pain and that relaxation and imagery require some degree of cognitive integrity; they will not work with the confused. But not knowing the answers to *all* of these questions may lull us into waiting for more research so that we will have the "perfect" answer. In response to this kind of thinking Donovan says:

> Patients can't wait. They hurt. And I suggest an alternative, called successive approximation. Assess the patient; find out if he's in pain; find out what he's used before, what he thinks will work, what he's willing to try, and try it. Then evaluate. Evaluate relief. I did four studies on pain before I remembered to evaluate relief. I used lessened pain— that's not relief. See if it worked, revise your intervention, try again. Evaluate that intervention. And keep going. Clinicians must move ahead in applying what we already know, while those of us who are doing research keep learning more. Otherwise, patients have to wait until we have the perfect answer. And if what we already know about pain is true at all, it's that we will never have the perfect answer to such a complex phenomenon (Donovan, 1988).

After reading the chapters in this section we should be sensitized to the fact that many under our care continue to suffer, with little relief of their pain. As individual practitioners we can examine our goals for pain relief, let the patient and family know that relief is possible and how it can be attained, use a variety of approaches or interventions to relieve pain, and evaluate the effectiveness of our approach. We can also affect the way pain is managed in the units or agencies in which we work. Krokosky and Reardon's paper illustrates one organizational approach taken to increase awareness of problems and to improve pain management.

With the support of your unit coordinator or head nurse, surveys or chart reviews could be used on your unit to determine the state of pain management. Staff meetings can be used to share your findings and other literature. Inservice education can be used to introduce assessment instruments and to teach how they are used. Adjunctive therapies such as relaxation, imagery, TENS, or music can be reviewed to determine if they seem appropriate for your patient population. Researchers can be contacted to answer special questions such as the cost of any equipment involved, staff time required, or ways one might go about learning a particular technique. If certain interventions seem costly to implement, target their use for patients in greatest need.

Tackle one therapy at a time. Relaxation therapy may seem foreign or magic at first, but once it is learned and used, it may become a trusted ally. Evaluate the effectiveness of the intervention in providing patient relief or perhaps in reducing length of stay, increasing functional ability, or activity. Along the way, if you meet some resistance in implementing these innovations, remember even Einstein once remarked that "great spirits have always encountered violent opposition from mediocre minds." Some of the strategies suggested by Cronenwett may help you overcome the opposition to new approaches. Pain control is one area where nurses can make a difference, and that difference means less suffering and better patient outcomes.

References on Pain in Adults

Ahles, T. A., Blanchard, E. B., & Ruckdeschel, J. C. (1983). The multidimensional nature of cancer related pain. *Pain, 17,* 277–288.

Ali, J., Yaffe, C. S., & Serrette, C. (1981). The effect of transcutaneous electric nerve stimulation on postoperative pain and pulmonary function. *Surgery, 89*(4), 507–512.

Averill, J. R. (1973). Personal control over aversive stimuli and its relationship to stress. *Psychological Bulletin, 80*(4), 286–303.

Bailey, L. (1985). Music's soothing charms. *American Journal of Nursing, 85,* 1280.

Barbour, L. A., McGuire, D. B., & Kirchhoff, K. T. (1986). Nonanalgesic methods of pain control used by cancer outpatients. *Oncology Nursing Forum, 13,* 56–60.

Basbaum, A. I., & Fields, H. L. (1984). Endogenous pain control systems: Brainstem spinal pathways and endorphin circuitry. *Annual Review of Neuroscience, 7,* 309–338.

Basmajian, J. (Ed.). (1983). *Biofeedback: Principles and practice for clinicians.* Baltimore: Williams & Wilkins.

Baumann, T. J., Batenhorst, R. L., Graves, D. A., Foster, T. S., & Bennett, R. L. (1986). Patient-controlled analgesia in the terminally ill cancer patient. *Drug Intelligence and Clinical Pharmacy, 20,* 279–301.

Benson, H. (1975). *The relaxation response.* New York: Avon.

Blitz, B., & Dinnerstein, A. J. (1971). Role of attentional focus in pain perception: Manipulation of response to noxious stimulation by instructions. *Journal of Abnormal Psychology, 77,* 42–45.

Bonica, J. (1980). *Sympathetic nerve blocks for pain diagnosis and therapy.* Philadelphia: Breon Laboratories Publications, 1.

Bonica, J. (1980). Pain research and therapy: Past and current status and future needs. In L. K. Ng & J. Bonica (Eds.), *Pain, discomfort and humanitarian care* (pp. 1–46). New York: Elsevier.

Bonica, J. (1986, May). *Magnitude of the problem and the epidemiology of pain.* Consensus Conference on the Integrated Approach to Management of Pain. National Institutes of Health, Bethesda, MD.

Bowers, K. S. (1968). Pain, anxiety, and perceived control. *Journal of Consulting and Clinical Psychology, 32,* 596–602.

Bresler, D. E. (1979). *Free yourself from pain.* New York: Simon and Schuster.

Bressler, L. R., Hange, P. A., & McGuire, D. B. (1986). Characterization of the pain experience in a sample of cancer outpatients. *Oncology Nursing Forum, 13*(6), 51–55.

Brown, J. H., Kazis, L. E., Spitz, P., Gertman, P., Fries, J., & Meenan, K. (1984). The dimensions of health outcomes: A cross-validated examination of health status measurement. *American Journal of Public Health, 74*(2), 159–161.

Brucker, M. (1984). Nonpharmaceutical methods for relieving pain and discomfort during pregnancy. *MCN, 9,* 390–394.

179

Bussey, J. G., & Jackson, A. (1981). TENS for postsurgical analgesia. *Contemporary Surgery, 18*(3), 35–41.

Chapman, C., & Cox, J. (1977). Determinants of anxiety in elective surgery patients. In C. Spielberger & I. Sarason (Eds.), *Stress and anxiety: Vol. 4* (pp. 269–290). New York: John Wiley & Sons.

Chapman, C. R., Casey, K. L., Dubner, R., Foley, K. M., Gracely, R. H., & Reading, A. E. (1985). Pain measurement: An overview. *Pain, 22*, 1–31.

Clark, C. C. (1983). Women and arthritis: Holistic/wellness perspectives. *Topics in Clinical Nursing, 4*(4), 45–55.

Cook, J. (1986). Music as an intervention in the oncology setting. *Cancer Nursing, 9*, 23–28.

Copp, L. A. (1974). The spectrum of suffering. *American Journal of Nursing, 74*, 491–495.

Donovan, M. I. (1988, March). *Adult pain research discussion.* Comments made at a national conference on Key Aspects of Comfort: Management of Pain, Fatigue, and Nausea, Chapel Hill, NC.

Donovan, M. I., & Dillon, P. (1987). Incidence and characteristics of pain in a sample of hospitalized cancer patients. *Cancer Nursing, 10*(2), 85–92.

Donovan, M. I., Dillon, P., & McGuire, D. (1987). Incidence and characteristics of pain in a sample of medical-surgical inpatients. *Pain, 30*, 69–78.

Donovan, M. I., Slack, J., & Wright, S. (1988). *Factors predictive of large patient–nurse and patient–physician disagreements regarding the patient's pain.* Manuscript submitted for publication.

Endler, N., Edwards, J., & Vitelli, R. (1985). *Situation-Response General Trait Anxiety Inventory (S-R GTA) and Present Affect Reactions Questionnaire (PARQ IV): A manual for state and trait anxiety measures.* (Research Report #152). Toronto: York University, Department of Psychology Reports.

Fagerhaugh, S. Y. (1974). Pain expression and control on a burn care unit. *Nursing Outlook, 22*, 645–650.

Fagerhaugh, S. Y., & Strauss, A. (1977). *Politics of pain management: Staff–patient interaction.* Menlo Park, CA: Addison-Wesley.

Feldman, H. R. (1984). Psychological differentiation and the phenomenon of pain. *Advances in Nursing Science, 6*(2), 50–57.

Fezler, W. D. (1980). *Just imagine: A guide to materialization using imagery.* Hollywood, CA: Laurinda Books Publishing Company.

Fields, H. L., (1981). An endorphin-mediated system: Experimental and clinical observations. In J. B. Martin & K. L. Bick (Eds.), *Neurosecretion and brain peptides: Implications for brain function and neurological disease* (pp. 199–209). New York: Raven Press.

Fields, H. L., & Levine, J. D. (1984). Pain—mechanisms and management. *Western Journal of Medicine, 141*, 347–357.

Fisher, S., & Greenberg, R. (1972). Selective effects upon women of exciting and calm music. *Perceptual and Motor Skills, 34*, 987–990.

Flaherty, G., & Fitzpatrick, J. (1978). Relaxation technique to increase comfort level of postoperative patients: A preliminary study. *Nursing Research, 27*, 352–355.

Fowler-Kerry, S., & Lander, J. (1987). Management of injection pain in children. *Pain, 30*, 169–175.

Gal, R., & Lazarus, R. S. (1975). The role of activity in anticipating and confronting stressful situations. *Journal of Human Stress, 1*, 4–20.

Geer, J. H., Davison, G. C., & Gatchel, R. I. (1970). Reduction of stress in humans through nonveridical perceived control of aversive stimulation. *Journal of Personality and Social Psychology, 16,* 731.

Glass, D. C., Singer, J. E., Skipton, L., & Krantz, D. (1973). Perceived control of aversive stimulation and the reduction of stress responses. *Journal of Personality, 41,* 581–595.

Goldstein, A., & Hilgard, E. R. (1978). Lack of influence of the morphine antagonist nalorone on hypnotic analgesia. *Proceedings of the National Academy of Sciences, 72,* 2041–2043.

Graffam, S., & Johnson, A. (1987). A comparison of two relaxation strategies for the relief of pain and its distress. *Journal of Pain and Symptom Management, 2,* 229–231.

Gregg, R. (1983). Biofeedback and biophysical monitoring during pregnancy and labor. In J. Basmajian (Ed.), *Biofeedback: Principles and practice for clinicians* (2nd ed.), (pp. 238–242). Baltimore: Williams & Wilkins.

Guyton, A. C. (1986). *Textbook of medical physiology* (7th ed.). Philadelphia: W.B. Saunders & Company.

Halvorson, M., & Page, G. G. (1988, March). *The assessment and control of pain in preverbal infants.* Paper presented at a national conference on Key Aspects of Comfort: Management of Pain, Fatigue, and Nausea, Chapel Hill, NC.

Hay, H., O'Brien, C., & Jeans, M. E. (1986). The measurement of pain intensity in children and adults—A methodological approach. In S. Stinson, J. Kerr, J. Giovannetti, H. Field, & J. McPhail (Eds.), *New frontiers in nursing research: Proceedings of the International Nursing Research Conference* (p. 169). Edmonton, Alberta: University of Alberta.

Herth, K. (1978). The therapeutic use of music. *Supervisor Nurse, 9,* 22–23.

Hymes, A. C., Raab, D. E., Yonehiro, E. G., Nelson, G. D., & Printy, A. L. (1973). Electrical surface stimulation for control of acute postoperative pain and prevention of ileus. *Surgical Forum, 24* (12), 447–449.

Hymes, A. C., Raab, D. E., Yonehiro, E. G., Nelson, G. D., & Printy, A. L. (1974). Acute pain control by electrostimulation: A preliminary report. In J. J. Bonica (Ed.), *Advances in neurology: Vol 4* (pp. 761–767). New York: Raven Press.

It's over Debbie. (1988, January 8). Letter to the editor. *Journal of the American Medical Association, 259,* 272.

Jacob, S., & Beyerman, K. (1986). Soothing the ragged edge of pain: bring on the music . . . bring back the dream lady. *American Journal of Nursing, 86,* 1034.

Jacox, A. K. (Ed.) (1977). *Pain: A source book for nurses and other health professionals.* Boston: Little, Brown & Company.

Johnson, J., & Rice, V. (1974). Sensory and distress components of pain: Implications for the study of clinical pain. *Nursing Research, 23,* 203–209.

Jones, L. (1987). Patient-controlled oral analgesia. *Orthopaedic Nursing, 6*(1), 38–41.

Kavanaugh, C. K. (1984). Should children participate in burn care? *American Journal of Nursing, 84,* 601.

Kilwein, J. H. (1983). Valium and values. *American Pharmacy, NS23(12),* 5–7.

Kim, S. (1980). Pain: Theory, research and nursing practice. *Advances in Nursing Science, 2,* 44–59.

Kroger, W. S., & Fezler, W. D. (1976). *Hypnosis and behavior modification: Imagery conditioning.* Philadelphia: J. B. Lippincott.

Levin, R., Malloy, G., & Hyman, R. (1987). Nursing management of postoperative pain: Use of relaxation techniques with female cholecystectomy patients. *Journal of Avanced Nursing, 12,* 463–472.

Livingston, J. (1979). Music for the childbearing family. *JOGN Nursing, 8,* 363–367.

Locsin, R. (1981). The effect of music on the pain of selected postoperative patients. *Journal of Advanced Nursing, 6,* 19–25.

Loesser, J. D. (1986). *Pain and its management: An overview.* Consensus Development Conference on the Integrated Approach to Management of Pain, National Institutes of Health, Bethesda, MD.

Long, L., & Johnson, J. (1978). Using music to aid relaxation and relieve pain. *Dental Survey, 54,* 35–38.

MacDonald, M., & Kuiper, N. (1983). Cognitive-behavioral preparations for surgery: Some theoretical and methodological concerns. *Clinical Psychology Review, 3,* 27–39.

Mandler, G., & Watson, D. L. (1966). Anxiety and the interruption of behavior. In C. D. Spielberger (Ed.), *Anxiety and behavior.* New York: Academic Press.

Marks, R. M., & Sachar, E. J. (1973). Undertreatment of medical inpatients with narcotic analgesics. *Annals of Internal Medicine, 78,* 173–181.

Martinez-Urrutia, A. (1975). Anxiety and pain in surgical patients. *Journal of Consulting and Clinical Psychology, 43,* 437–442.

McCaffery, M. (1972). *Nursing management of the patient with pain.* Philadelphia: J.B. Lippincott.

McCaffery, M. (1979). *Nursing management of the patient with pain* (2nd ed.). Philadelphia: J.B. Lippincott.

McGuire, D. B. (1987). The multidimensional phenomenon of cancer pain. In D. B. McGuire & C. H. Yarbro (Eds.), *Cancer pain management* (pp. 1–20). Orlando, Florida: Grune & Stratton.

McGuire, L. (1981). A short, simple tool for assessing your patient's pain. *Nursing 81, 11*(3), 48–49.

Meinhart, N. T., & McCaffery, M. (1983). *Pain: A nursing approach to assessment and analysis.* Norwalk: Appleton-Century-Crofts.

Melzack, R. (1973). *The puzzle of pain.* New York: Basic Books.

Melzack, R. (1975). The McGill Pain Questionnaire: Major properties and scoring methods. *Pain, 1,* 277–299.

Melzack, R. (1983). The McGill Pain Questionnaire. In R. Melzack (Ed.), *Pain measurement and assessment* (pp. 41–75). New York: Raven Press.

Melzack, R., & Wall, P. D. (1965). Pain mechanisms: A new theory. *Science, 150,* 971–979.

National Institutes of Health. (1986). *Consensus development conference statement. The integrated approach to the management of pain.* USHHS, 6(3) (document no. 491–292; 41148).

Nigl, A. (1984). *Biofeedback and behavioral strategies in pain treatment.* New York: Medical and Scientific Books.

Olness, K., Wain, H. J., & Ng, L. (1980). A pilot study of blood endorphin levels in children using self hypnosis to control pain. *Developmental and Behavioral Pediatrics, 1*(4), 187–188.

Orem, D. E. (1971). *Nursing: Concepts of practice.* New York: McGraw-Hill.

Oriol, N., & Warfield, C. (1984). Pain relief during labor. *Hospital Practice, 19*(9), 151–166.

Peck, C. (1986). Psychological factors in acute pain management. In M. J. Cousins & G. D. Phillips (Eds.), *Acute pain management*. New York: Churchill Livingstone.

Pelletier, K. (1977). *Mind as healer: mind as slayer*. New York: Delta.

Peretti, P. (1975). Changes in galvanic skin response as affected by musical selection, sex, and academic discipline. *The Journal of Psychology, 89*, 183–187.

Pert, C., & Snyder, S. (1973). Opiate receptor: Demonstration in nervous tissue. *Science, 179*, 1001–1004.

Porter, J., & Jick, H. (1980). Addiction rate in patients treated with narcotics. *New England Journal of Medicine, 302*, 123.

Rankin, M. A., & Snider, B. (1984). Nurses' perception of cancer patients' pain. *Cancer Nursing, 7*, 149–155.

Rosenberg, M., Curtis, L., & Bourke, D. L. (1978). Transcutaneous electrical nerve stimulation for the relief of postoperative pain. *Pain, 5* (2), 129–133.

Rosenstiel, A. K., & Keefe, F. J. (1983). The use of coping strategies in chronic low back pain patients: Relationship to patient characteristics and current adjustment. *Pain, 17*, 33–44.

Sandidge, C. H., Marvin, J. A., & Heinbach, D. M. (1987, April & May). *Patient controlled analgesia (PCA) in treating pain in burn patients*. Paper presented at the meeting of the American Burn Association, Washington, D.C.

Sandroff, R. (1983). When you must inflict pain on a patient. *RN, 46*(1), 35–39, 112.

Schomburg, F. L., & Carter-Baker, S. A. (1983). Transcutaneous electrical nerve stimulation of postlaparotomy pain. *Physical Therapy, 63* (2), 188–193.

Schuster, G. D., & Infante, M. C. (1980). Pain relief after low back surgery: The efficacy of transcutaneous electical nerve stimulation. *Pain, 8* (3), 299–302.

Scott, D. S., & Barber, T. X. (1977a). Cognitive control of pain: Effects of multiple cognitive strategies. *Psychology Record, 2*, 373–383.

Scott, D. S., & Barber, T. X. (1977b). Cognitive control of pain: Four serendipitous results. *Perceptual and Motor Skills, 44*, 569–570.

Scott, L., Clum, G., & Peoples, J. (1983). Preoperative predictors of postoperative pain. *Pain, 15*, 283–293.

Shatin, L. (1970). Alteration of mood via music: A study of the vectoring effect. *The Journal of Psychology, 75*, 81–86.

Shearn, M. A., & Fireman, B. H. (1985). Stress management and mutual support groups in rheumatoid arthritis. *The American Journal of Medicine, 78*, 771–775.

Simonton, D. C., & Simonton, S. S. (1974). Belief systems and management of the emotional aspects of malignancy. *Journal of Transpersonal Psychology, 7*, 29–47.

Smith, M. (1986). Human-environment process: A test of Rogers' principle of integrality. *Advances in Nursing Science, 9*(1), 21–28.

Snyder, M. (1985). *Independent nursing interventions*. New York: John Wiley & Sons.

Spielberger, C. (1972). Conceptual and methodological issues in anxiety research. In C. Spielberger (Ed.), *Anxiety: Current trends in theory and research: Vol. 2* (pp. 481–493). New York: Academic Press.

Spielberger, C., Gorsuch, R., Lushene, R., Vagg, P., & Jacobs, G. (1983). *Manual for the State-Trait Anxiety Inventory*. Palo Alto, CA: Consulting Psychologists Press.

St. James-Roberts, I., Hutchinson, C., Haran, F., & Chamberlain, G. (1983). Biofeedback as an aid to childbirth. *British Journal of Obstetrics and Gynaecology, 90,* 56–60.

Staub, E., Tursky, B., & Schwartz, G. E. (1971). Self-control and predictability: Their effects on reactions to aversive stimulation. *Journal of Personality and Social Psychology, 18,* 157–162.

Sternbach, R. A. (1968). *Pain: A psychophysiological analysis.* New York: Academic Press, Inc.

Stewart, M. L. (1977). Measurement of clinical pain. In A. K. Jacox (Ed.), *Pain: A source book for nurses and other health care professionals.* Boston: Little, Brown, & Co.

Stoudenmire, J. (1975). A comparison of muscle relaxation training and music in the reduction of state and trait anxiety. *Journal of Clinical Psychology, 31,* 490–492.

Strauss, A., Fagerhaugh, S., & Glaser, B. (1974). Pain: An organizational-work-interactional perspective. *Nursing Outlook, 22,* 560–566.

Taylor, A. G., West, B. A., Simon, B., Skelton, J., & Rowlingson, J. C. (1983). How effective is TENS for acute pain? *American Journal of Nursing, 83,* 1171–1174.

Taylor, S. E. (1982). Hospital patient behavior: Reactance, helplessness, or control? In H. S. Friedman & M. R. DiMatteo (Eds.), *Interpersonal issues in health care.* New York: Academic Press.

Turk, D., & Meichenbaum, G. (1983). *Pain and behavioral medicine: A cognitive-behavioral perspective.* New York: Guilford Press.

Tyler, E. T., Caldwell, C., & Ghia, J. N. (1982). Transcutaneous electrical nerve stimulation: An alternative approach to the management of postoperative pain. *Anesthesia and Analgesia, 61* (5), 449–456.

Wagner, M. (1977). Pain and nursing care associated with burns. In A. K. Jacox (Ed.), *Pain: A source book for nurses and other health care professionals.* Boston: Little, Brown, & Co.

Wells, N. (1982). The effect of relaxation on postoperative muscle tension and pain. *Nursing Research, 31,* 236–373.

Whidden, A., & Fidler, M. R. (1977). Pathophysiology of pain. In A. K. Jacox (Ed.), *Pain: A source book for nurses and other health professionals* (pp. 27–56). Boston: Little, Brown, & Company.

Wilson, J. (1981). Behavioral preparation for surgery: Benefit or harm? *Journal of Behavioral Medicine, 4,* 99–102.

Wolman, R. L., Lasecki, M. H., Alexander, L. A., & Luterman, A. (1987, April and May). *Clinical trial of patient controlled analgesia in burn patients.* Paper presented at the meeting of the American Burn Association, Washington, D. C.

Worthington, E. L., Jr. (1978). The effects of imagery content, choice of imagery content, and self verbalization on the self-control of pain. *Cognitive Therapy and Research, 2*(3), 225–240.

Worthington, E. L., Jr., & Shumate, M. (1981). Imagery and verbal counseling methods in stress inoculation training for pain control. *Journal of Counseling Psychology, 28*(1), 1–6.

Yaksh, T. L., & Hammond, D. L. (1982). Peripheral and central substrates involved in the rostrad transmission of nociceptive information. *Pain, 13,* 1–85.

Part III

FATIGUE

[24]

Fatigue:
Current Bases for Practice

Barbara F. Piper

HISTORICAL OVERVIEW

In the 1920s Muscio suggested that the term fatigue be abandoned altogether since what was called fatigue was not a single entity, but a variety of unrelated phenomena (Bartley, 1965). Others challenged this view, believing that the difficulty in defining fatigue lay in a failure to appreciate its complexity (Bartley, 1965, 1976; Cameron, 1973). The first scale to measure tiredness was developed during the 1920s (Poffenberger, 1928) and the seminal text on fatigue was published by Bartley and Chute in 1947.

During the 1950s, several milestones occurred: Merton's paper led to the physiological theory that fatigue is caused by central and peripheral nervous system mechanisms (1954); Pearson and Byars (1956; Pearson, 1957) developed a tiredness scale for airmen that later was used in several nursing studies (Davis, 1984; Freel & Hart, 1977; Hart, 1978; Haylock & Hart, 1979; Reiger, 1987); Dorpat and Holmes linked the occurrence of fatigue with pain for the first time (1955); and anecdotal intervention reports began appearing in the literature (Kurland, Hamolsky, & Freedberg, 1955; Snow, Machlan, Warnell, & Utt, 1959). During the 1960s, the first international fatigue conference was held (Hashimoto, Kogi, & Grandjean, 1971). Speakers included Dr. Grandjean, a noted psychologist and fatigue theorist (1968, 1970), and members of the Japanese Industrial Research Committee on Fatigue. Yoshitake conducted several studies using the Fatigue Symptom Checklist developed by the Committee (1969, 1971, 1978), and this checklist was also used in several nursing studies (Davis, 1984; Freel & Hart, 1977; Hart, 1978; Haylock & Hart, 1979).

Nurses began to investigate fatigue in 1972 when Hart compared fatigue patterns in multiple sclerosis (MS) patients and healthy controls. She found that MS patients experienced more severe fatigue throughout the day than did the healthy controls, and the severity of fatigue was related to the patient's mobility status (1978). Hart later collaborated with Freel to identify indicators of fatigue in MS patients (1977), and with Haylock (1979) to identify fatigue indicators in radiation therapy patients. In 1977, Putt published the first study examining the relationship between an environmental stimulus, noise, and fatigue. During the 1970s, several classic works were published in other disciplines (Kinsman & Weiser, 1976; Meyerwitz, Sparks, & Sparks, 1979; Rose & King, 1978).

The number of nursing studies of fatigue has increased dramatically in the 1980s (Davis, 1984; Pardue, 1984; Potempa, Lopez, Reid, & Lawson, 1986; Reiger, 1987). Several factors have contributed to this surge in nursing research. Key publications summarizing the fatigue literature have made it easier for nurses new to this body of knowledge to master its complexities quickly (Atkinson, 1985; Ciba Foundation, 1981; Kellum, 1985; Norris, 1982; Piper, 1986; Piper, Lindsey, & Dodd, 1987a; Potempa et al., 1986; Valdini, 1985; Varricchio, 1985). Also, fatigue has recently been accepted for clinical testing as a nursing diagnosis by the North American Nursing Diagnosis Association (see Table. 24.1).

Further, consumers have brought a new syndrome to the attention of health care professionals—the "chronic fatigue syndrome." There is even a national "Chronic Fatigue Syndrome Society" in Portland, Oregon. Clearly, fatigue now is recognized as a bona fide area of research by consumers, nurses, and other disciplines.

CLASSIFICATIONS/TYPES OF FATIGUE

Many classification systems for fatigue are found in the literature. For example, there are the *central* and *peripheral* models put forth by physiologists (Gibson & Edwards, 1985). *Central* fatigue may be caused by lack of motivation, impaired transmission down the spinal cord, impaired recruitment of motor neurons (Gibson & Edwards, 1985), and by ". . . an exhaustion or malfunctioning of brain cells in the hypothalamic region" (Poteliakhoff, 1981, p. 94). *Peripheral* fatigue may be due to impaired functioning of the peripheral nerves, neuromuscular junction transmission, or fiber activation (Gibson & Edwards, 1985). Little

TABLE 24.1   NANDA Nursing Diagnosis for Fatigue

DEFINITION

An overwhelming sustained sense of exhaustion and decreased capacity for physical and mental work.

DEFINING CHARACTERISTICS

Major: verbalization of an unremitting and overwhelming lack of energy; inability to maintain usual routines.

Minor: perceived need for additional energy to accomplish routine tasks; increase in physical complaints; emotionally labile or irritable; impaired ability to concentrate; decreased performance; lethargic or listless; disinterest in surroundings/introspection; decreased libido; accident prone.

RELATED FACTORS

Decreased/increased metabolic energy production; overwhelming psychological or emotional demands; increased energy requirements to perform activities of daily living; excessive social and/or role demands; states of discomfort; altered body chemistry (e.g., medications, drug withdrawal, chemotherapy).

---

is known about how these normal physiological mechanisms may be affected by abnormal processes such as disease states. Both central and peripheral mechanisms may be involved in chronic fatigue. Another system categorizes fatigue as either *normal, pathologic, situational*, or *psychological* in its origins (Kellum, 1985).

The classification system that is most useful to nursing practice characterizes fatigue as *acute* or *chronic* depending on duration (Bartley & Chute, 1947; Piper, 1986; Piper, 1988). The literature suggests that differences exist between these two states (Bartley & Chute, 1947; Cameron, 1973; McFarland, 1971; Muncie, 1941; Piper, in press; Poteliakhoff, 1981; Potempa et al., 1986; Riddle, 1982; Rockwell & Burr, 1977). These differences are summarized in Table 24.2.

MECHANISMS OF FATIGUE

Fatigue Framework

Various theories have been proposed to explain how fatigue occurs (Cameron, 1973; Ciba Foundation Symposium '82, 1981; Grandjean, 1968, 1970; Morris, 1982). The actual mechanisms that produce fatigue, even at the muscle level, are unknown (Piper et al., 1987a). Using the framework depicted in Figure 24.1, mechanisms that most probably cause fatigue in clinical populations are discussed below. With this framework, the nurse can assess possible causes of fatigue in specific

TABLE 24.2 Acute and Chronic Fatigue: Distinguishing Characteristics[a]

Characteristic	Acute Fatigue	Chronic Fatigue
Purpose/Function	Protective	Unknown, may no longer be protective May be nonfunctional
Population at Risk	Primarily healthy	Primarily clinical populations
Etiology	Usually identifiable Usually involves a single mechanism or cause Often experienced in relation to some form of activity or exertion	May not be identifiable Usually multiple & additive causes Often is experienced with no relation to activity or exertion
Perception	Normal, usual Expected/anticipated with respect to specific activities or forms Primarily localized to a specific body part or system Pleasant or unpleasant	Abnormal, unusual Excessive or disproportionate to past experience Generalized, whole body-mind sensation Unpleasant
Time Dimension Onset	Rapid	Insidious, gradual Cumulative Threshold model
Duration	Short; days or weeks	Long; persists over time More than 1 month
Relief Dimension	Usually alleviated by a good night's sleep, adequate rest, proper diet, exercise program, or stress management techniques Resolves quickly	Not completely dispelled by these methods A combination of approaches may be needed Does not resolve quickly
Impact on Activities of Daily Living & Quality of Life	Minor, minimal	Major

[a]Reprinted with permission from Piper (1988).

FIGURE 24.1 Fatigue framework.

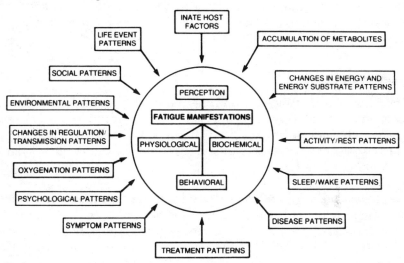

Figure reprinted from the article by Piper, Lindsey, and Dodd in the November/December 1987 (Vol. 14, No. 6) issue of the *Oncology Nursing Forum* with permission from the Oncology Nursing Press, 10/88.

patient situations and select appropriate nursing interventions to test. When fatigue becomes a chronic sensation, management may become more complex and a combination of strategies may be needed.

Manifestations of Fatigue

In the center of the framework are the subjective (perceptual) and objective (physiological, biochemical, and behavioral) indicators of fatigue that have been reported (Atkinson, 1985; Freel & Hart, 1977; Gibson & Edwards, 1985; Hart, 1978; Haylock & Hart, 1979; Kinsman & Weiser, 1976; Kogi, Saito, & Mitsuhashi, 1970; Komoike & Horiguchi, 1971; Piper & Dodd, 1987; Putt, 1977; Reiger, 1987; Rhodes, Watson, & Hanson, 1988; Rhoten, 1982; Saito, Kogi, & Kashiwagi, 1970; Valdini, 1985; Yoshitake, 1969, 1971, 1978). Sign and symptom patterns may vary according to the primary cause of the fatigue, such as stimulation or overwork of a specific muscle group, type of occupational activity, or emotional depression (Piper, 1986; Saito et al., 1970). When fatigue becomes chronic, a combination of mechanisms may be involved. Since it is not known how the subjective and objective indicators may correlate with one another, further research is needed to clarify these relationships. Currently the best way to assess fatigue in clinical populations is to determine the person's own perception of the fatigue experience (Piper et al., 1987a).

Changes in Usual Patterns

Since changes in biological and psychosocial patterns can influence signs and symptoms of fatigue, it is important for the nurse to assess whether changes in pre-existing patterns have occurred as a result of illness or treatment. These patterns surround the center of the framework in Figure 24.1.

• *Accumulation of metabolites.* Accumulations of various metabolites have been associated with fatigue. Whether these products cause fatigue or merely parallel its occurrence remains unknown. In clinical populations, the accumulation of lactate (Morris, 1982), hydrogen ions (Karlsson, Sjodin, Jacobs, & Kaiser, 1981) and cell destruction end products (Haylock & Hart, 1979) are likely mechanisms. Increasing fluid intake in patients with cell destruction end products may promote more rapid dilution of excretion of these products and prevent fatigue.

• *Changes in energy and energy substrate patterns.* Changes in energy production and substrates can influence human performance and fatigue. These changes may result from abnormalities in energy expenditure, cancer cachexia (Lindsey, 1986), anorexia (Atkinson, 1985), infection (Valdini, 1985; Straus et al., 1985), fever (Edwards et al., 1972) and imbalances in thyroid hormones (Axelrod et al., 1983).

• *Activity/rest patterns.* Activity and rest patterns can play significant roles in the prevention, cause, and alleviation of fatigue. Negative changes in activity patterns are common and may lead to a vicious cycle of decreased mobility, increased physical dependence and increased patient and caregiver fatigue. How systematic changes in activity/rest patterns may positively affect fatigue also needs investigation.

• *Sleep/wake patterns.* The relationship between sleep disorders and fatigue needs to be examined.

• *Disease patterns.* Fatigue precedes, accompanies, or follows many diseases; it may be a universal precursor and sequela of a disease process. Fatigue patterns need to be documented and compared across studies to generate practice theory.

• *Treatment patterns.* Various medical treatments are associated with fatigue such as chemotherapy (Brown, Carrieri, Jansen-Bjerklie, & Dodd, 1986; McCorkle & Young, 1978; Meyerwitz et al., 1979; Meyerwitz, Watkins, & Sparks, 1983; Nerenz, Leventhal, & Love, 1982;

Rhodes et al., 1988); radiation therapy (Haylock & Hart, 1979; King, Nail, Kreamer, Strohl, & Johnson, 1985; Kobashi-Schoot, Hanewald, Van Dam, & Bruning, 1985); biological response modifiers (Davis, 1984); beta blockers (Potempa et al., 1986); surgery (Rose & King, 1978); and diagnostic testing. The nurse can play an important role in preventing and alleviating fatigue in patients receiving such treatments by reducing anxiety through patient teaching and counseling and by providing adequate rest periods (Piper et al., 1987a).

• *Symptom patterns.* Assessment and control of symptoms that may precede, accompany, or follow fatigue may reduce or prevent its occurrence (Brown et al., 1986; Dorpat & Holmes, 1955; Norris, 1982).

• *Oxygenation patterns.* Any factor that alters or interferes with the ability to maintain adequate oxygen levels, such as anemia or respiratory muscle fatigue, can influence whole body fatigue (Piper et al., 1987a).

• *Changes in regulation/transmission patterns.* Fluid and electrolyte imbalances or changes in neurohormone levels can affect neurotransmission and muscle force resulting in fatigue (Akerstedt, Gillberg, & Witterberg, 1982; Arendt, Borbely, Franey, & Wright, 1984).

• *Psychological patterns.* Several psychological patterns, such as usual response to stressors (coping strategies), depression, anxiety, degree of motivation, beliefs and attitudes may influence fatigue (Wittenborn & Buhler, 1979).

• *Other related patterns.* Other factors that may contribute to fatigue include *environmental* patterns, such as noise (Putt, 1977), temperature, and allergens; *social* patterns, such as perceived social support, cultural beliefs, and economic factors; *life event* patterns, such as the common transitional events associated with growth and development; and innate host factors, such as age, sex, genetic makeup (e.g., type of muscle fibers and their predisposition to fatigue) (Karlsson et al., 1981), and unique biorhythms.

MEASUREMENT OF FATIGUE

The sensation of fatigue has four dimensions: subjective, physiologic, biochemical, and behavioral (Piper et al., 1987a; Piper, Lindsey & Dodd, 1987b). The subjective dimension is key to understanding how fatigue may differ in healthy and ill populations.

Subjective Dimension

In the past, the subjective dimension of fatigue was measured as the unidimensional feeling of tiredness (Heuting & Sarphati, 1966; McCorkle & Young, 1978; McNair, Lorr, & Droppleman, 1971; Pearson, 1957; Pearson & Byars, 1956; Rhoten, 1982). Only recently has fatigue, like pain, been conceptualized and measured as a multidimensional construct using the statistical procedures of factor and key cluster analyses (Kinsman & Weiser, 1976; Piper, Lindsey, & Dodd, 1984; Yoshitake, 1978). Various subdimensions have been identified. In healthy subjects symptoms seem to cluster around factors such as general fatigue (which includes tiredness), mental fatigue, and localized fatigue.

Unfortunately, many of the instruments that measure subjective fatigue are limited by their dimensions or by their reliability and validity estimates. This is an important area for tool development (Reiger, 1987; Varricchio, 1985). At this time, the Symptom Distress Scale (McCorkle & Young, 1978), the Rhoten Fatigue Scale (Rhoten, 1982), and the Pearson Byars Fatigue Feeling Checklist (Pearson & Byars, 1956; Pearson, 1957; Reiger, 1987) may be the best instruments to measure feelings of tiredness.

Objective Dimensions

A variety of *physiological indicators* and methods have been used to measure fatigue. These include melatonin (Akerstedt et al., 1982; Arendt et al., 1984), the electromyogram (Malmquist, Ekholm, Lindstrom, Petersen, & Ortengen 1981), heart rate, and oxygen consumption (Burton, 1980). Others that might be studied include rates and degrees of anemia, changes in the levels of blood glucose, thyroid hormones, and serum electrolytes, and temperature changes. Several *biochemical indicators* and methods have been studied. These include hydrogen ions or pH changes (Karlsson et al., 1981), muscle biopsies, magnetic resonance spectroscopy (Miller et al., 1987), and lactate and pyruvate (Rennie, Johnson, Park, & Sularman, 1973). The existence of a fatigue receptor has even been postulated (Steve Lehman, personal communication, August, 1986). Nurses have begun to identify *behavioral indicators* of fatigue (Freel & Hart, 1977; Putt, 1977; Rhoten, 1982) through behavioral checklists (Rhoten, 1982) and task performance indicators (Freel & Hart, 1977; Heuting & Sarphati, 1966; Putt, 1977; MacVicar & Winningham, 1986). While Rhoten's observational checklist has not been tested in other studies, its categories, which include general appearance, communication, activity, and attitude, can be used to guide patient validated nursing assessments. This is a fertile area for nursing research.

ASSESSMENT AND MANAGEMENT OF FATIGUE

Assessment

The nurse's assessment needs to include all *subjective and objective data* that may influence fatigue for an individual. *Subjective data* should include an assessment of fatigue's location (muscular/physical, mental or emotional, or a combination of these), pattern, intensity, onset, and duration; aggravating and alleviating factors; and associated symptoms such as pain (Engel & Morgan, 1973), as well as changes in usual patterns. Family members may be more sensitive than the patient to changes in the patient's usual pattern of fatigue. Additional information should be collected about the meaning of the fatigue and the degree of distress (Rhodes et al., 1988). Maintaining a daily fatigue diary for one week often can reveal previously unrecognized patterns of fatigue and relief measures (Piper, 1986).

Objective data should include a physical examination and a review of laboratory data and medical and drug histories to reveal coexisting factors contributing to the fatigue (Kellum, 1985). Environmental factors should be assessed (Putt, 1977); frequently the use of assistive devices or furniture rearrangement can prevent fatigue by reducing unnecessary expenditure of energy. Behaviorally, the nurse needs to assess for any changes in the patient's physical appearance, performance status, and ways of moving, talking, or interacting that may indicate fatigue (Rhoten, 1982).

Management of Fatigue

Management of fatigue involves a wide range of nursing activities that span the treatment continuum, from preventing chronic fatigue (Kellum, 1985; Piper, 1986) and screening high risk individuals, to tailoring therapies to fit specific etiologies and initiating referrals. Unfortunately, there is little in the research literature on interventions at this time. Anecdotal and case studies abound, however, particularly about drug treatments (Cheraskin, Ringsdorf, & Medford, 1976; Clark, 1978; Cohen, 1973; Ellis & Nasser, 1973; German & Stampfer, 1979; Hargreaves, 1977; Hicks, 1964; Kaye, 1980; Kruse, 1961; Kurland et al., 1955; Snow et al., 1959; Tracy, 1960; Young, 1959).

A few well-designed studies suggest that certain interventions may be helpful under certain conditions. For example, Amantadine, an antiviral agent, may be helpful in treating fatigue in MS patients. Like all drugs, it is not without side effects (Murray, 1985). Several studies

TABLE 24.3 Perceived Causes of Fatigue in Cancer Patients

PSYCHOLOGICAL PATTERNS
  Stress
  Worry
  Depression
  Anxiety
  Emotional strain
TREATMENT PATTERNS
  Radiation
  Surgery
  Chemotherapy
  Medical
ACTIVITY/REST PATTERNS
  Work
  Everyday activities
  Hospital/RT travel
SLEEP/WAKE PATTERNS
  Insomnia
DISEASE PATTERNS
  Cancer
  Other
OTHER PATTERNS
  Symptoms
  Environment
  Nutrition
  Innate host factors

suggest that exercise may be beneficial. In one study, a 10-minute brisk walk was associated with longer lasting and higher perceived energy levels than those following ingestion of a candy bar (Thayer, 1987). Pardue (1984) found that a five-week, three-times-per-week pulmonary rehabilitation program decreased fatigue and improved exercise tolerance in chronic obstructive pulmonary patients. MacVicar & Winningham (1986) found that a structured 10-week exercise program reduced fatigue, stabilized weight, and reduced nausea in Stage II breast cancer patients being treated with chemotherapy.

Until additional well-designed studies test interventions in specific populations, patients may be our best teachers. Table 24.3 summarizes the preliminary data on cancer patient responses (Piper et al., 1984) to an open-ended question: "What do you believe most directly contributes to or causes your fatigue?" The responses are listed in descending order of frequency. The average repondent identified more than one reason for fatigue.

Changes in psychological patterns were most common, with "stress"

TABLE 24.4 Patient-Initiated Fatigue Interventions

ACTIVITY/REST PATTERNS*
Rest*
Nap*
Alter activities*
Sit/lie down
Read
Walk/exercise*
PSYCHOLOGICAL PATTERNS
Distraction
Relaxation
SLEEP/WAKE PATTERNS*
Sleep
OTHER PATTERNS
Nutritional*
Environmental
Social
Symptoms

*Piper & Dodd, 1987.

being the most frequently identified cause. This underscores the importance of using therapeutic listening, counseling, and patient education to reduce anxiety and increase a patient's sense of control. Controlling or preventing symptoms related to medical therapies also is very important. Skin reactions and other symptoms such as pain, shortness of breath, and headaches were frequent causes of fatigue in these patients.

Table 24.4 summarizes patient responses, again in descending order of frequency, to an open-ended question about what they did to relieve fatigue (Piper & Dodd, 1987; Piper et al., 1984). Distraction techniques included going to work, taking car rides, and listening to tapes or soft music. Rhodes and associates (1988) found that prescheduling essential activities and avoiding nonessential ones were helpful to cancer patients. Decreasing unnecessary energy expenditure by increasing dependence on others was also helpful. Clearly, there is value in determining what patients perceive will work for them.

SUMMARY AND RECOMMENDATIONS

Table 24.5 lists recommendations for future practice and research. Under assessment and measurement of fatigue, the concepts tiredness, weakness, fatigue, and exertion need to be differentiated since nursing

TABLE 24.5   Recommendations for Future Research and Practice

---

ASSESSMENT/MEASUREMENT
  Concept clarification
  Circadian rhythmicity
  Subjective/objective
  Reliability/validity
DOCUMENTATION OF PATTERNS
  Basic research
  Acute vs. chronic
  Healthy vs. ill populations
  Cultural patterns
  Incidence data
  Risk factors
  Longitudinal studies
INTERVENTION STUDIES
  Activity/rest patterns
  Psychological patterns
  Symptom patterns
  Environmental patterns
  Others

---

management of these states may vary (Piper et al., 1987b; Rhodes et al., 1988). Correlations between subjective and objective indicators of fatigue need to be explored. Instruments need to be valid and reliable, and basic research is needed to identify normal fatigue mechanisms and learn how these mechanisms may be affected by disease or treatment states. Incidence and prevalence data on fatigue are needed to target nursing interventions for those patients at high risk for chronic fatigue. Lastly, intervention studies are needed, particularly in the areas in which nursing can make a difference in patient outcomes.

[25]

The Development
of an Instrument to Measure
the Subjective Dimension
of Fatigue

Barbara F. Piper, Ada M. Lindsey,
Marylin J. Dodd, Sandra Ferketich,
Steven M. Paul, and Steve Weller

This chapter describes a new instrument that measures multiple dimensions of subjective fatigue, the Piper Fatigue Self-Report Scale; reports the initial psychometric properties of the scale; and describes baseline patterns of fatigue experienced by radiation therapy patients who participated in a pilot study using the new scale.

PIPER FATIGUE SELF-REPORT SCALE (PFS)

The design and selection of PFS items and dimensions were guided by the clinical experience of the authors and by the literature on the conceptualization and measurement of symptoms in general (Engel & Morgan, 1973; McCorkle & Young, 1978) and the symptoms of fatigue and pain in particular (Akerstedt, Gillberg, & Witterberg, 1982; Arendt,

The authors would like to acknowledge the nurses who served as expert reviewers, the radiation therapy staff who facilitated patient access, and Sigma Theta Tau, Alpha Eta Chapter, for a research award that partially defrayed the expenses associated with this pilot study.

Borbely, Franey, & Wright, 1984; Atkinson, 1985; Davis, 1984; Freel & Hart, 1977; Gibson & Edwards, 1985; Grandjean & Kogi, 1971; Hart, 1978; Haylock & Hart, 1979; Heuting & Sarphati, 1966; Kinsman & Weiser, 1976; Kogi, Saito, & Mitsuhashi, 1970; Komoike & Horiguchi, 1971; McCorkle & Young, 1978; McGuire, 1984; Melzack, 1983; Pardue, 1984; Pearson, 1957; Pearson & Byars, 1956; Poffenberger, 1928; Putt, 1977; Rhoten, 1982; Rose & King, 1978; Saito, Kogi, & Kashiwagi, 1970; Yoshitake, 1969, 1971, 1978). Fatigue was defined as a subjective feeling of tiredness that is influenced by circadian rhythm; it can vary in unpleasantness, duration, and intensity. When acute, fatigue serves a protective function; when it is excessive or chronic, its function is unknown (Piper, 1986).

The PFS is in two forms, a baseline form (PFS-B) and a current form (PFS-C). The PFS-B is designed to measure usual patterns of fatigue and any changes experienced during the six months prior to a medical diagnosis or the start of medical treatment. The PFS-C determines fatigue patterns "now" or "for that day." Fatigue symptoms are measured using a 100-millimeter horizontal visual analogue scale (VAS) anchored at each end by the verbal descriptors "none" and "a great deal." Subjects are asked to place an "x" at the point on the scale that best indicates the degree to which they are experiencing the symptom. Thus, scores for each symptom can range from "0" to "100." The PFS is designed to be self-administered; questions may be read aloud but the person must be able to mark the scale himself. Items are grouped together according to the fatigue dimension that they represent. The seven subscales on the PFS-B and a representative item from each are shown in Table 25.1.

The *Temporal Subscale* measures time patterns or the timing of fatigue (e.g., when and how long it occurs). This dimension is essential since differences in the perception of fatigue may occur as a function of the frequency, duration, and pattern of fatigue (e.g., intermittent or continuous). Ten items represent this dimension on the PFS-B and six on the PFS-C. The *Intensity/Severity Subscale* reflects the severity of the fatigue, the degree of distress and interference with activities of daily living. There are 12 items on this subscale. The *Affective Subscale* reflects the emotional meaning of the fatigue. Meaning is important since actions taken to relieve fatigue may differ vastly depending on whether the fatigue is perceived as normal or usual or as abnormal or unusual. Five items measure this dimension. The *Sensory Subscale* measures the physical, emotional, and mental sensations attributable to fatigue. There are 18 items on this subscale. The *Evaluative Subscale* assesses what the person believes is causing the fatigue. Beliefs about cause can influence the emotional meanings ascribed to the experience and thus

TABLE 25.1   Piper Fatigue Self-Report Scale–Baseline Form (PFS-B) Subscales with a Representative Subscale Item

---

TEMPORAL DIMENSION
  How long do you usually experience fatigue?
  Days_____Weeks
INTENSITY/SEVERITY DIMENSION
  Overall, how would you describe the intensity/severity of the fatigue you usually experience?
  Mild_____Severe
AFFECTIVE DIMENSION
  To what degree would you describe the fatigue you usually experience as being:
  Normal_____Abnormal
SENSORY DIMENSION
  When I am fatigued, I usually feel:
  Refreshed_____Exhausted
EVALUATIVE DIMENSION
  To what degree do you believe too much stress usually contributes to or causes your fatigue?
  Not all all_____A great deal
ASSOCIATED SYMPTOMS DIMENSION
  When I am fatigued, I usually am in pain.
  No pain_____Severe pain
RELIEF DIMENSION
  To what degree does sleep usually relieve your fatigue?
  No relief_____Complete Relief

---

also can influence the selection and perceived effectiveness of fatigue interventions. Thirteen items measure this dimension (one is open-ended). The *Associated Symptom Subscale* measures physical signs and symptoms that may occur concurrently with fatigue and may influence or intensify the fatigue experience (Feuerstein, Carter, & Papciak, 1987). There are 11 items on this subscale. The last subscale is the *Relief Subscale* measuring perceived effectiveness of actions taken to relieve fatigue. Seven items make up this subscale including one open-ended item.

METHOD

Subjects

The study was conducted in a radiation therapy (RT) department in a 450-bed northern California community hospital between December

1985 and September 1987. To participate, patients had to be newly diagnosed with breast or lung cancer, have disease confined to the chest region and/or immediately adjacent nodes, and be starting their first week of outpatient RT to the chest region. Patients were ineligible if they were receiving concurrent chemotherapy, steroids, or antidepressants.

Instruments

In addition to the PFS, all patients completed a Demographic Profile, the Profile of Mood States (POMS) and the Fatigue Symptom Checklist (FSCL). The *Demographic Profile* measured usual demographic data, caffeine intake, and changes in weight, appetite, sleep, rest, exercise, and nap patterns. The *POMS*, a standardized 65-item, five point adjective rating scale that has acceptable reliability and validity (McNair, Lorr, & Droppleman, 1971), measures six mood or affective states: tension-anxiety, depression-dejection, anger-hostility, vigor-activity, confusion-bewilderment, and fatigue-inertia. A total mood disturbance score can be calculated, with the vigor-activity scale negatively weighted. The *FSCL* is a 30-item instrument that measures three symptom dimensions: general feelings of incongruity, mental symptoms, and specific feelings of incongruity. Acceptable reliability and validity estimates are available for this instrument (Hart, 1978; Pardue, 1984; Kogi et al., 1970; Komoike & Horiguchi, 1971; Saito et al., 1970; Yoshitake, 1969, 1971, 1978). Patients were asked to indicate the degree to which each symptom was experienced "at that moment" using a five point scale (1 = absence of, 2 = a little, 3 = moderate amount, 4 = quite a bit, 5 = a great deal). The number of symptoms and their intensities were calculated for each subscale and for the instrument as a whole. Additional information was gathered from the medical record.

Procedures

Patients were identified from weekly simulation schedules and by chart review. All patients were asked to fill out the instruments at a "convenient" time of day (week one) and to fill out the instruments at the same approximate time for the duration of the study (weeks two and three of RT). Patients completed the Demographic Profile, the FSCL, the POMS and the PFS-B during the first week of RT; they completed the FSCL, the POMS, and the PFS-C during the second and third weeks of RT. Only data from the first week are reported here.

RESULTS

Data were collected on 50 patients (35 breast and 15 lung cancer patients). Forty-seven additional patients refused to participate in the study. The most commonly volunteered reason was "not wanting to think about my disease any more than I already have to." Twelve of the 50 patients, or 24%, experienced difficulties in responding to the visual analogue scales used in the PFS-B. Their difficulties included marking the lines only at the extreme end points; writing in word responses; and placing both an "x" and a check mark. These same subjects commonly had unanswered questions. Eight patients who left more than nine per cent of the questions unanswered and also evidenced difficulties with the VAS were dropped from the study. Thus, the analysis is based on a final sample of 42 patients. The eight subjects who were dropped did not differ significantly from the final sample in age, education, or income levels (Mann-Whitney U).

The majority of the sample were Caucasian (88%) females (90%) with Stage I breast cancer (60%), 60 years old (range = 41–77 yrs.) and with a Karnofsky Performance Status of 80 or above (normal activity with effort; some signs or symptoms of disease [Schag, Heinrich, & Ganz, 1984]). RT was designed to be curative and commonly involved three treatment sites (breast or chest wall plus adjacent nodes). Most subjects had completed high school and part of college; 38% were retired; and 31% were working outside the home, with the majority of these subjects working between 20 and 40 hours per week. Over half (62%) had experienced an unintentional weight change during the previous six months; 38% had gained weight and 24% had lost weight, for a mean change of 11 pounds. Despite this change in weight, the majority of patients reported no changes in appetite, sleep, or nap patterns during this time period.

Reliability and Validity of the PFS-B

A measure of internal consistency, Cronbach's alpha, was chosen to assess reliability. The reliability coefficients for the PFS-B subscales ranged from an alpha of .69 for the associated symptoms dimension to .95 for the sensory dimension. The reliability estimate for the total fatigue score (calculated on the basis of four subscales: temporal, severity, affective and sensory) was .85.

To determine validity of the PFS-B, all PFS-B items were reviewed by 11 fatigue experts. Items were considered to be relevant and essential to the measurement of subjective fatigue if 78% of the experts agreed that this was the case (Waltz & Bausell, 1981). The experts were asked to indicate whether each item needed revision and to classify each item by the dimension it best represented. Items that measured the temporal, severity, affective, and sensory dimensions equalled or surpassed the preset 78% criterion level; items on the associated symptoms, evaluative, and relief dimensions did not, and were not considered by the experts to be essential to the measurement of subjective fatigue. Therefore, the total fatigue score was calculated solely on the basis of the scores from the four subscales representing the temporal, severity, affective, and sensory dimensions of subjective fatigue. The other three subscales, evaluative, associated symptoms, and relief, were considered to constitute a useful "planning index" for nursing care, but were not included in the calculation of the total fatigue score. The PFS-B subscales were correlated with the POMS and FSCL subscales to determine convergent validity; discriminant validity was determined by negative correlations between the PFS-B subscales and the POMS vigor-activity subscale. The statistically significant positive and negative correlations found between these instrument subscales are given in Table 25.2.

A significant negative correlation was found between the POMS vigor-activity scale and the PFS-B scale for the sensory dimension. Two of the PFS-B scales, affective and total fatigue score, positively correlated with five POMS subscales including the fatigue-inertia subscale. The PFS-B intensity/severity and relief dimensions did not show significant correlations with the POMS fatigue-inertia subscale. In contrast two PFS-B scales and the PFS-B total fatigue score were correlated significantly with the POMS total mood disturbance score, and the affective dimension correlated significantly with the FSCL general and specific symptoms and their intensities, and with total number of symptoms and mean intensities. Thus, moderate evidence for discriminant and convergent validity of the PFS-B was found. Using the average linkage between groups method of cluster analysis (Aldenderfer & Blashfield, 1984; Mishel, 1983), ten clusters were formed, providing evidence for the multidimensionality of the PFS-B. Three clusters confirmed the presence of the relief, evaluative, and sensory dimensions. The remaining seven clusters contained the items from the four remaining dimensions: temporal, affective, severity, and associated symptoms.

Baseline Fatigue Patterns

During the first week of RT (mean = 4.1 days), the average number of FSCL symptoms reported by patients was 6.36; only 4 patients re-

TABLE 25.2 Significant Convergent and Discriminant Validity Coefficients Between PFS-B, POMS, and FSCL Subscales

Piper Fatigue Self-Report Scale	Profile of Mood States: Subscales (n = 40)							Fatigue Symptom Checklist: Subscales & Intensities (n = 42)							
	Depression/ Dejection	Tension/ Anxiety	Anger/ Hostility	Vigor/ Activity	Fatigue/ Intertia	Confusion/ Bewilderment	Total Mood Disturbance	General Symptoms	Mental Symptoms	Specific Symptoms	Total No. of Symptoms	General Mean Intensity	Mental Mean Intensity	Specific Mean Intensity	Total Mean Intensity
Temporal															
Intensity/ Severity															
Affective	.42*	.36*	.37*		.37*	.37*	.43*	.54***		.42*	.46**	.55***		.38*	.47**
Sensory				−.57***		.33*	.41*								
Evaluative				.33*				−.31*	−.34*		−.34*		−.36*		
Associated Symptoms															
Relief															
Total Fatigue Score	.46**	.44*	.44**		.42*	.33*	.50**								

*p < .05; **p < .01; ***p < .001

ported no symptoms of fatigue. Most patients reported specific fatigue symptoms ($n = 30$, mean $= 1.64$), followed by general symptoms ($n = 28$, mean $= 2.29$), and mental symptoms ($n = 26$, mean $= 2.43$). The mean average intensities of these symptoms fell in the "little to moderate" range. The most frequent general symptoms were "tired legs," "tired over my whole body," and "wanting to lie down." Feeling "anxious," "nervous," or "impatient" were the most frequent mental symptoms; "feeling thirsty," "having back pain," and "stiff shoulders" were the most frequent specific symptoms. Stage of disease did not affect the number, type, or intensity of fatigue symptoms significantly (one-way ANOVA), but the intensity of specific symptoms was influenced by sex and diagnosis variables. Intensities were more likely to be higher in males than in females [$t(40) = 2.38$, $p < .05$] and higher in lung cancer patients than in breast cancer patients [$t(40) = 2.20$, $p < .05$]. The mean fatigue score on the POMS was 7.10, which is lower than the norms reported for male and female psychiatric patients and healthy college students (McNair et al., 1971). No statistically significant relationships were found between fatigue scores and stage of disease (one-way ANOVA), sex, or diagnosis (student's t).

The majority of patients had experienced an increase in fatigue as scored by the PFS-B during the six months prior to diagnosis (VAS mean $= 61.19$, maximum possible score $= 100$). Most experienced fatigue infrequently (VAS mean $= 39.77$), and the fatigue was more likely to be intermittent (VAS mean $= 20.19$) and perceived as acute (VAS mean $= 40.68$) rather than continuous or chronic. The usual patterns of fatigue were considered by most patients to be mild (VAS mean $= 19.27$); they were not associated with other physical symptoms such as pain and did not interfere with activities of daily living (VAS mean $= 25.01$). Affective VAS means were all less than 45. Fatigue was not imbued with any negative emotional meaning for patients who were beginning their first week of radiation therapy. The usual fatigue sensations included "tired," "unenergetic," "sluggish," "listless," "unmotivated," "drowsy," "weak," and "sleepy" (VAS means all above 70). Most patients believed that illness or disease was the cause of their fatigue (VAS mean $= 51.79$). Too much stress (VAS mean $= 49.92$), exercising too little (VAS mean $= 44.81$) and inadequate rest and sleep (VAS mean $= 43$ for both) were also major causes of fatigue. For these patients, sleep (VAS mean $= 78.22$) and lying down for short periods of time (napping; VAS mean $= 64.81$) were effective in relieving fatigue. The majority of patients were not fatigued at the time they completed the PFS-B (VAS mean $= 26.80$).

Average PFS-B Subscale Scores

Subscale item scores were averaged for each patient and subscale means calculated for the entire sample (see Table 25.3). The sensory dimension had the highest mean, and severity the lowest. Interestingly, the relief subscale mean indicated that these subjects reported at least moderate relief from their fatigue. Mean scores were not significantly affected by stage of disease (one-way ANOVA), sex, or diagnosis (student's t), although breast cancer patients were more likely to use effective fatigue relief measures than were lung cancer patients [t (40) = 2.19; $p < .05$].

DISCUSSION

While the PFS-B shows excellent reliability and moderate construct validity for a new instrument, the results cannot be generalized to other clinical or RT populations. Further studies are needed to reduce the number of PFS-B items, provide evidence for reliability and validity in other samples, and simplify the instrument's scoring.

The PFS was designed as a research instrument to measure subjective fatigue patterns in a variety of populations. It was not designed to be an instrument that would be used clinically to assess fatigue, although its seven dimensions can be used as a general guide for fatigue assessments and interventions. A shorter, more easily analyzed scale is needed for the practice setting. Knowledge about patients' baseline fatigue patterns however can help nurses to identify high risk patients

TABLE 25.3   PFS-B Mean Subscale Scores

Subscale	Mean Scores[a]	Number of Items
Temporal	37.23	7
Severity	18.22	12
Affective	36.62	5
Sensory	63.52	18
Fatigue Total[b]	44.94	42
Evaluative	36.04	12
Assoc. Sx.	12.06	11
Relief	55.17	6

[a] Possible range for all subscale means = 0–100.
[b] The "Fatigue Total" scale is the average of the items on the temporal, severity, affective, and sensory subscales.

and to tailor nursing assessments and interventions. This study confirmed that lung cancer patients tend to begin radiation therapy at higher fatigue levels than breast cancer patients (Haylock & Hart, 1979). Some investigators suggest that higher fatigue levels in these patients may be a function of the diagnostic workup and surgical treatments that precede radiation therapy (King et al., 1985). Clearly the lack of perceived relief effectiveness also may be a contributing factor. Periodic reassessment is needed particularly for patients who are likely to experience cumulative fatigue due to medical therapies such as radiation therapy or disease states such as cancer.

[26]

Fatigue in Patients with Catastrophic Illness

Felissa L. Cohen and Sally B. Hardin

On October 15, 1983, the third largest outbreak of botulism ever reported in the United States struck in Peoria, Illinois. This outbreak was distinguished from others by the rapid diagnosis of the first cases, the low case-fatality rate, an unusual vehicle for the poisoning, early implementation of systematic longitudinal research (five days after the

This research was supported in part by the Division of Nursing, Bureau of Health Professions, Health Resources and Services Administration, U.S. Public Health Service, under grant # R01 NU 01220.

first case was diagnosed), and the professional background of the research team—nurses. Botulism is a life-threatening, catastrophic illness caused by the action of neurotoxin produced by *Clostridium botulinum*. *C. botulinum* spores are widely distributed in the environment
and can be found in the soil, in fish, and on the surface of fruits and
vegetables. The spores form toxin only under certain conditions, and it
is this lethal toxin that leads to clinical signs and symptoms.

Conditions that favor the production of toxin from *C. botulinum*
spores include an anaerobic environment; a low degree of acidity (pH
over 4.6); the presence of a solution with a low solute concentration; a
warm temperature (spores are very heat resistant and can survive up
to two hours in boiling water); and adequate nutrients (CDC, 1984;
MacDonald, Spengler, Hatheway, Hargrett, & Cohen, 1985). *C. botulinum* produces a total of eight toxin types, A through G. In humans,
toxins A, B, and E have been associated with disease; only infrequent
outbreaks have been attributed to F and G. Type A toxin,found most
commonly west of the Mississippi River, was the type responsible for
the Peoria outbreak. Type A toxin causes more severe disease than all
the others.

There are four major types of botulism—foodborne, wound, infant,
and unclassified (CDC, 1984). In foodborne botulism, the toxin is
formed in contaminated food and this preformed toxin is then ingested
and absorbed. Wound botulism occurs when spores gain entry into a
wound, form toxins, and are absorbed. Infant botulism, first described
in 1976, occurs when the organism is ingested, colonizes the G.I. tract,
and produces toxin in the infant's intestine. The unclassified category
of botulism was developed by the Centers for Disease Control in 1978
to include those cases in which affected persons were over one year of
age and it was not possible to implicate a specific vehicle of infection
(CDC, 1979). While most adults regularly ingest *C. botulinum* spores
without harm, recently cases of botulism have been described in which
toxin is produced *in vivo*, often secondary to intestinal surgery, gastro-
achlorhydria, or antibiotic therapy. Spores have also been found in
adults dying suddenly from no apparent cause.

In foodborne botulism, the food containing the preformed toxin is
ingested and the toxin is transported across the intestinal epithelium to
the lymphatics and serum. The toxin binds to receptors on the external
surface of the neuronal membrane where it is translocated through it.
The toxin then binds irreversibly to the neuronal membrane receptors
where it selectively inhibits the release of the neurotransmitter acetylcholine from peripheral nerves. This blockade causes impairment in
cranial nerves, in autonomic nerves, and at neuromuscular junctions
(Arnon & Chin, 1981; Cherrington, 1974; Sellin, 1981; Simpson, 1979).

Formerly, foodborne botulism most commonly resulted from improperly canned vegetables that were contaminated with spores and inadequately prepared, allowing toxin to be produced. However, in the three largest outbreaks, all occurring in the past decade, the contaminated food was served in commercial establishments (CDC, 1979, 1984).

In the Peoria outbreak, sauteed onions served on patty melt sandwiches were the vehicle for *C. botulinum* type A toxin (MacDonald et al., 1985). The CDC was able to discover this source because one of the victims had not yet thrown out a "doggie bag" containing the remnants of a patty melt sandwich. As the CDC reconstructed the event, the onions had been sliced and cooked for about 10 minutes and then covered by a thick layer of melted margarine. A pan of warm, "smothering" onions was then set on a grill for use all during the day on patty melt sandwiches. The CDC hypothesized that the raw onions were contaminated with spores from the soil (especially because the onions had been transported from the west coast where large amounts of spores are found in the soil) and these spores germinated and formed toxin in the warm anaerobic environment caused by keeping the pan on the grill, with the smothering effect of the margarine (CDC, 1984).

Signs and symptoms from foodborne botulism usually begin 12–48 hours after the ingestion of contaminated food, although ranges from 2 hours to 8 days have been reported. In the Peoria victims, the range of time for symptom occurrence was 12.5 to 114.5 hours with an overall mean of 34.2 hours (Cohen et al., 1981, 1984). Major signs and symptoms (resulting from blocked acetylcholine release) include symmetrical impairment of cranial nerves, followed by muscle weakness involving upper and lower extremities in a descending pattern. In severe cases, the neuromuscular blockade eventually affects neurotransmitter release from the phrenic nerve to the diaphragmatic musculature, leading to respiratory failure. Mental clarity is usually not affected (Sanders, Seifert, & Kobernick, 1983; Schmidt-Nowara, Samet, & Rosario, 1983). In this particular outbreak, the Centers for Disease Control defined a case as an illness in a person who had eaten at the Skewer Inn Restaurant on October 14 through October 16, 1983, and reported diplopia and any two of the following signs or symptoms: dry mouth, blurred vision, dysphagia, or dysphonia, or any one of these symptoms in combination with cranial nerve dysfunction, extremity weakness, or respiratory failure.

That foodborne botulism is a catastrophic illness is substantiated by the Peoria statistics: length of hospital stay ranged from 4 to 190 days with a mean of 50 days; ICU stay ranged from 0 to 175 days with a mean of 30 days. For those requiring intensive care, the mean stay was

35 days. Twelve patients received mechanical ventilation for periods from 14 to 172 days (mean = 68). One patient died. One suffered a psychotic depression. The time period between admission and return to work ranged from 6 to 690 days with a mean of 298 days.

In previous case reports of patients recovering from botulism (Terranova, Breman, Locey, & Speck, 1978; Sanders et al., 1983), patients have complained of residual fatigue over varying amounts of time, but this has not been assessed with objective instruments nor has it been examined over a long period. Nevertheless, the literature reports that fatigue is a major clinical feature in botulism; it is probably due, at least in part, to the impaired release and transmission of acetylcholine at the myoneural junction.

Questions concerning the nature and duration of fatigue in botulism patients arose during the Peoria outbreak. Therefore, this research explored the length of time after botulism that fatigue feelings persisted among the Peoria victims, and the times of day at which these patients experienced greatest fatigue.

METHOD

Eight males and 20 females were involved in the Peoria outbreak. Ages ranged from 20 to 73 years (mean = 42.5). Two of the 27 living patients chose not to participate in the study on the advice of their attorneys. Therefore, most of the data came from a sample of 25 patients; 24 of these completed the three-year study.

There are few scientific instruments that measure subjective feelings of fatigue. Most of these measures have been developed for industry and measure the quality of work performance, productive output, or accident rates. In this study, fatigue was measured in two ways—by self-report and by use of the Pearson Byars Fatigue Feeling Checklist (PBFFC) (Pearson & Byars, 1956) (see Table 26.1). This tool measures fatigue feelings at different times of day—upon awakening, one hour after awakening, midday, afternoon, early evening/after work, and just before retiring. Respondents select the phrase that most closely reflects how they feel at the designated time of day. These phrases are written in lay terms and range on a continuum from 1(extremely peppy) to 10 (ready to drop). The numbers are summed to provide a Total Fatigue Score, ranging from 10 to 60, that is a measure of tiredness for an entire day.

The botulism patients completed the PBFFC at eight data collection periods: before hospitalization (recalled retrospective data), during hospitalization, and during home visits made by a team of clinical

TABLE 26.1 Pearson Byars Fatigue Feeling Checklist

Which phrase below best describes your feelings at the indicated times of day? Please place a check (√) in the box that best describes how you feel at the times indicated. Answer according to *how you felt yesterday*.

		Time of Day				
Feeling	Upon Awakening	One Hour After Awakening	Midday	Afternoon	After Work or Early Evening	Just Before Retiring
Extremely Peppy	——	——	——	——	——	——
Very Lively	——	——	——	——	——	——
Very Refreshed	——	——	——	——	——	——
Quite Refreshed	——	——	——	——	——	——
Somewhat Refreshed	——	——	——	——	——	——
Slightly Pooped	——	——	——	——	——	——
Fairly Well Pooped	——	——	——	——	——	——
Petered Out	——	——	——	——	——	——
Extremely Tired	——	——	——	——	——	——
Ready to Drop	——	——	——	——	——	——

nurse specialists at regular intervals from onset to 36 months post onset. A total fatigue score was obtained for each botulism patient, and a mean total fatigue score for all patients at each of the eight data collection periods was then calculated.

A second method used to measure fatigue was the Symptom Checklist, which patients completed at each data collection period. The Symptom Checklist is a list of symptoms presented with a dichotomous (yes–no) response format. Patients circled "yes" for each fatigue symptom they experienced.

RESULTS

Figure 26.1 shows a line graph of the mean total fatigue scores for all patients at each data collection period. The before-botulism data (collected retrospectively) were compared with a matched control group. There was no significant difference in the pre-botulism total fatigue scores of the control group and the botulism group, although the control group had slightly higher scores. (That is, the botulism group retrospectively recalled being less fatigued and more energetic).

As Figure 26.1 illustrates, the total fatigue score before botulism was 21.5 and, in the hospital, it more than doubled to 48.9, indicating a serious level of fatigue. Three years after the outbreak, the total fatigue

FIGURE 26.1 Line graph of patients' mean total fatigue scores at eight observations over a three-year period. (Mean total fatigue scores can range from a low of 10 to a high of 60.)

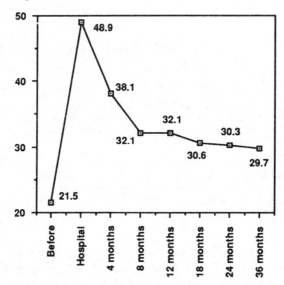

score was still higher than before botulism, at 29.7. Repeated measures ANOVA showed that the total fatigue score was significantly higher during hospitalization and at each of the other data collection periods, up to three years after the onset of botulism [$F(7,140) = 31.96$; $p < .0001$; Dunnett's tests between pre- and all postbotulism scores were significant, $p < .01$]. Thus, excessive feelings of fatigue persisted in these patients.

The mean total fatigue scores for all of the botulism patients at different times of day were also calculated. Six times of day were ranked from least tired (1) to most tired (6). When the botulism patients' fatigue rankings were compared to those of a control group and to the normal population in Hart's (1978) study of fatigue in multiple sclerosis patients, the rank order of daily fatigue for controls, Hart's normals, and subjects before botulism was the same (see Table 26.2). The normal fatigue pattern is that persons are most alert one hour after waking and become steadily more fatigued throughout the day.

Once the botulism patients were hospitalized, the normal fatigue trajectory was disrupted entirely. During hospitalization, botulism patients were highly fatigued throughout the day. The traditional time at which nursing staff "put the unit to sleep" was the third most alert time of the day for botulism patients. The normal pattern of daily fa-

TABLE 26.2 Rank Order of Fatigue Scores at Six Times of Day by Control, Normal, and Sample Subjects[a]

			Sample Subjects			
Time of Day	Control	Hart's Normals[b]	Before	Hospital	4 Months	24 Months
Awakening	4	4	4	5	3	4
One Hour Later	1	1	1	4	1	1
Midday	2	2	2	1	2	2
Afternoon	3	3	3	2	4	3
Early Evening	5	5	5	6	5	5
Before Retiring	6	6	6	3	6	6

[a]1 = least tired; 6 = most tired
[b]Hart (1978)

tigue was not restored for botulism patients until two years after the onset of illness. Figure 26.2 illustrates this daily fatigue trend before botulism, during hospitalization, and at home visits at 4, 12, and 24 months. Before botulism, a partial "U" curve of daily fatigue was seen; this disappeared at hospitalization, began to reform at 4 months, and *gradually* built until it was again present at 18 months.

Total fatigue scores were also examined in relation to clinical severity and mechanical ventilation status. The total fatigue scores for mild, moderate, or severe clinical status during hospitalization and at 4, 8, and 36 months were examined. Although the mild group was consistently less fatigued, the difference in total fatigue scores was never statistically significant.

Twelve of the patients were on mechanical ventilation for an average of 68 days (range, 14–172 days). There was no significant difference in fatigue between botulism patients who received mechanical ventilation and those who did not. This was a surprising finding because respiratory muscle fatigue might be expected to contribute to a higher total fatigue score. On the other hand, perhaps botulism toxin causes a degree of fatigue in all patients that is not significantly exacerbated by mechanical ventilation. Nonventilated patients may also have been fatigued from the efforts involved in difficult breathing and ambulatory movement that mechanically ventilated patients did not experience.

At three years postonset, 50% of the participating patients still noted on the symptom checklist that they were experiencing fatigue. The mean duration of fatigue as reported by these botulism patients was

FIGURE 26.2 Daily fatigue trend before illness, at hospitalization, and at three post-illness observations. (Mean total fatigue scores can range from a low of 1 to a high of 10.)

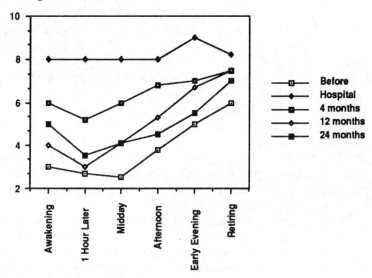

25.16 months and this was the top-ranked symptom at the three-year observation period.

DISCUSSION

Nurses need to continue systematic research on fatigue and on the long-term impact of catastrophic illness in order to plan more effective early and ongoing interventions. These findings illustrate, in a specific way, the intensity, duration, pattern, and trajectory of fatigue in the Illinois patients who suffered from the catastrophic illness of botulism. Because fatigue has been reported as a primary long-term symptom for botulism victims and this fatigue can be attributed, at least in part, to disturbance in the neurotransmitter acetylcholine, there are questions about the applicability of the findings to patients who suffer from other catastrophic illnesses. Qualitative findings, derived from audio- and videotaped structured interviews with the botulism patients and families, indicate that aspects of the botulism victims' fatigue may have been unique (Hardin & Cohen, in press). For example, patients described their fatigue as swift and severe. "I would be home in the kitchen and I couldn't unscrew a soda cap," said one. Another patient reported, "It was awful. I was pulling into the garage and couldn't get my foot to the brake—I hit the wall!"

Nonetheless, some aspects of these patients' fatigue are likely to be applicable to patients suffering from other catastrophic illnesses. One patient described her exhaustion after not being allowed to sleep in the ICU: "After 10 weeks, I wrote in my diary, 'Slept for four hours for the first time.'" Indeed, all of the 24 patients who were in the ICU (with a mean stay of 35 days) described the experience as physically and psychologically exhausting.

The psychological aspects of fatigue also need to be considered. Qualitative data not reported here (Hardin & Cohen, in press) show that the Peoria patients experienced severe depression and anger up to two years after their illness; probably not coincidentally, this was also the period of high fatigue. One wife glibly summarized her husband's psychological and physical fatigue level at two years postillness: "He was a regular couch potato!"

These botulism patients were most alert from midday to just before retiring. An educated guess about the antecedents of this alertness hinges on clues given by the patients in interviews: "I was terrified I would die in my sleep." "We all knew we had to be alert and watch our ventilators all the time." "Sleeping was the most difficult." These quotes offer evidence that the patients' lack of fatigue at the traditional hospital bedtimes was related to their heightened anxiety. Nighttime, the loud stillness interrupted by rhythmic respirator sounds and the hushed voices of nurses, may have been related to patients' hypervigilance.

Nursing staff could begin now to use the Pearson Byars Fatigue Feeling Checklist to assess both ICU and regular unit patients' fatigue levels. The tool is a brief, simple, reliable method to measure precisely the level, time of occurrence, and duration of fatigue. Various types of patients, units, illnesses, and phases of illness could be measured in this way and then compared. The goal of precisely measuring fatigue is, of course, to determine its pattern and peaks so that it can be prevented. For while nurses from Nightingale on intuitively sense that Shakespeare was correct in describing sleep and rest as "nature's gentle nurse," they also realize how difficult it is to ensure that patients do, in fact, rest and thus cure themselves.

[27]

Fatigue in End-Stage Renal Disease Patients

Rani Hajela Srivastava

Chronic fatigue is a common problem in patients with renal failure, and fatigue in End Stage Renal Disease (ESRD) patients is well documented. Fatigue has been identified among the top three stressors experienced by hemodialysis as well as CAPD (continuous ambulatory peritoneal dialysis) patients (Baldree, Murphy, & Powers, 1982; Eichel, 1986). The symptom is also prevalent among patients who have received a successful kidney transplant (Parfrey, Vavasour, Henry, Bullock, & Gault, in press). The toxic effects of uremia combined with low hemoglobin levels readily explain why renal patients might feel fatigued. However, fatigue is more than just a physiological phenomenon and all the fatigue seen in this population is not due to renal disease per se (Srivastava, 1986). Fatigue can arise as a result of various physiologic and psychologic processes. Fatigue that is worse in the morning and tends to improve during the day is commonly found in persons who are emotionally upset. Fatigue that increases with the progression of the day is probably due to organic causes or may simply be the effect of exertion (Cardenas & Kutner, 1982). The latter type of fatigue is often relieved by sleep and rest.

Dialysis is the only treatment available to ESRD patients. Although their well-being improves tremendously once the treatment is initiated, complaints of fatigue generally continue. It is imperative for health professionals to realize that symptoms such as fatigue can have major adverse effects on quality of life.

The nonspecific nature of fatigue makes it difficult to study, and investigations of fatigue in renal patients are scarce. Cardenas & Kutner

217

(1982) found that 58.3% of their sample of dialysis patients experienced moderate or severe fatigue; in Parfrey et al.'s (in press) study the prevalence of moderate or severe fatigue was 47.4%. Both studies, however, documented only the magnitude of the problem; they did not explore the specific characteristics of fatigue. It is essential to document both the overall feeling of fatigue and its specific symptoms in order to plan interventions that will improve patients' quality of life.

Hart (1978) studied fatigue in multiple sclerosis patients and Haylock and Hart (1979) studied it in patients receiving localized radiation. Both studies were exploratory and were designed to identify specific symptoms of the fatigue experience in these populutions. The purpose of this study was to identify characteristics of the fatigue experienced by ESRD patients (specifically, fatigue level and symptoms). The study was part of a larger group of studies of nonspecific symptoms in End-Stage Renal Disease patients conducted by Dr. P. Parfrey and his colleagues in the division of Nephrology at the Health Sciences Centre, St. John's, Newfoundland.

METHOD

Subjects

Subjects were obtained from one of the two teaching hospitals in St. John's, Newfoundland, which offer dialysis facilities. Twenty-seven hemodialysis patients (22 in-center and 5 in minimal care) were interviewed over a three-week period by the investigator. All patients who had been on hemodialysis for at least two months and were mentally competent to participate in an interview were approached for consent. Patients who were experiencing severe physical instability were not approached. All interviews were conducted in the dialysis units while the patients were being dialyzed.

The environment for the interviews was less than ideal. In addition to the usual noise of a dialysis unit, there was little privacy from other patients and the interview was subject to interruptions from staff for routine checks and medications. While the patients did not seem to mind these conditions, their responses may have been influenced by the environment. The interviews usually took 20 to 30 minutes. Patients were generally glad to have someone to talk to and were quite receptive to questions about their tiredness.

Instruments

A semistructured interview schedule was used to collect data. Areas of measurement included (a) patients' activity level, (b) subjective quality of life, (c) level of fatigue, (d) symptoms of fatigue, and (e) mood status. Additional data on physiological indices (such as hemoglobin), treatment, and demographics were obtained from the chart.

Activity was measured using the Karnofsky Performance Index (cited in Parfrey et al., in press). This scale is simple and has been widely used with both cancer and renal patients. The scale provides an activity score ranging from 1 (normal activity) to 5 (moribund).

Subjective quality of life was measured using a visual analogue scale. Patients were asked to grade their quality of life on a scale of 0 to 100, 0 being completely dependent upon others, seriously troubled mentally, unaware of surroundings and in a hopeless position, and 100 being mentally and physically independent, communicating well with others, able to do most of the things they enjoyed, pulling their own weight, and with a hopeful, realistic attitude (Spitzer et al., 1981). This tool was devised for use with cancer patients and was selected here because of its simplicity and established validity and reliability. Some patients had difficulty understanding the concept of quality of life and were reluctant to mark the visual analogue scale. However, they were able to translate quality into a percentage where 0 was feeling cheated or as bad as things could get and 100 was feeling great or 100%.

Level of fatigue was measured in three ways: by a graded linear scale, a clinical aggregate score, and the Pearson Byars Fatigue Feeling Checklist. The linear scale is a line ranging from 0 to 100, with 0 corresponding to total exhaustion, 25 = very tired, 50 = mediocre, 75 = good, and 100 = great or no fatigue. Patients were shown the scale and asked to mark the place on the line that best described how tired they had been feeling for the past month. This scale has previously been used to measure fatigue of dialysis patients (Cardenas & Kutner, 1982) but it requires further testing for validity and reliability.

The clinical aggregate score is a measure of several dimensions of a symptom. The original tool was developed by Spitzer et al. (1981) and adapted for use with ESRD patients by Parfrey et al. (in press). Patients were asked to rate the severity of their tiredness with regard to its being a problem, and to identify the frequency of occurrence, duration, effects on daily living, activity, and thought, and impact of symptom relief on quality of life (see Table 27.1).

Level of fatigue was also measured using the Pearson Byars Fatigue Feeling Checklist, a list of 10 easily understood adjective phrases that define the feeling of fatigue. The 10 phrases are listed in order of in-

TABLE 27.1 Calculation of Aggregate Fatigue Scores

A. Patient's perception of fatigue being a problem	0.	Not at all
	1.	A little
	2.	Somewhat
	3.	Very bad
	4.	Extremely bad
B. Frequency	+ 1	Occurs every day
C. Duration	+ 1	Lasts > 6 hours
D. Sleep	+ 1	Not relieved by sleep
E. Daily living/thought	+ 1	Interferes with normal activities or ability to think clearly
F. Activity	+ 1	Has some effect on being able to go out and do the things you want to do
G. Subjective quality of life	+ 1	Relief will improve quality of life ≥ 10%
	TOTAL _____	
	(Range = 0 - 10)	

creasing fatigue: extremely peppy, very lively, very refreshed, quite refreshed, somewhat refreshed, slightly pooped, fairly well pooped, petered out, extremely tired, and ready to drop (cited in Hart, 1978). The checklist has been used to measure fatigue in patients with multiple sclerosis and patients receiving localized radiation (Hart, 1978; Haylock & Hart, 1979). The reliability and validity of this tool are reported elsewhere (Hart, 1978). In the present study subjects were asked to identify the phrase that best described their feeling of fatigue at four different times during the day: upon awakening, one hour after awakening, at midday, and just before retiring. An overall fatigue score was obtained by summing the four ratings.

Symptoms of fatigue that are expressions of specific complaints have been identified and compiled into a 30-item Fatigue Symptom Checklist by the Japanese Association of Industrial Health. Yoshitake (1971) placed these symptoms in three categories: (a) general feelings of incongruity in the body, (b) decline of motivation or mental symptoms, and (c) specific feelings of incongruity in the body. The development, validity, and reliability of the tool are discussed elsewhere (Haylock & Hart, 1979; Yoshitake, 1971). In this study patients were asked to check all symptoms experienced when they felt tired.

Mood status was measured using the Beck Depression Inventory

(BDI). The BDI is a 22-item, self-report questionnaire that requires the respondent to indicate the relative presence of emotional, behavioral, and physical symptoms associated with depression (Beck, Ward, Mendelson, Mock, & Erbauch, 1961). Each item contains four response alternatives of different intensity. The BDI has been widely used and has established validity and reliability.

RESULTS

The sample consisted of 17 men and 10 women ranging in age from 25–81 years (mean = 59.3). The duration of hemodialysis ranged from 3 to 201 months, with a mean of slightly over 4 years (50 months). Four subjects had previously been on CAPD and six had previously had a transplant. Most patients were being dialyzed three times a week for four hours each treatment.

The scores on the Karnofsky Performance Index (KPI) ranged from 1 (no complaints) to 4 (requiring at least some assistance for care of bodily needs). The majority of the patients (78%) had scores of either 1 or 2, suggesting that they were able to carry out normal physical activity at least part of the time. However, during the course of the interviews it became apparent that for some patients there had been a considerable reduction in activity since beginning dialysis. Responses like "I can't do anything anymore" and "doing anything at all makes me tired" were not uncommon. Thus it is debatable as to what is "normal activity." This finding emphasizes the need to consider the patient's perspective. It would be better to measure activity more objectively and to compare the present level to the patient's previous desired activity level.

The range of scores for subjective quality of life (SQL) was 0 to 95 (mean = 61) out of a possible 100. Significant relationships were noted between the SQL score and level of fatigue as measured by the analogue scale, aggregate score, and Pearson-Byars overall score ($r = .80$, $p < .01$; $r = -.71$, $p < .01$; and $r = -.39$, $p < .05$, respectively). The greater the level of fatigue, the lower the perceived quality of life. Most people who reported a SQL of lower than 90% also felt that their quality of life would improve significantly if their tiredness were somehow relieved.

All three measurements of fatigue revealed similar results. The correlations between the measures were .87 or higher (significant at the $p < .01$ level). Although there was considerable variation between subjects, the average fatigue level was approximately 49 out of 100 on the linear scale. Only the Pearson Byars Checklist was used to delineate fatigue at various times in the day. In general, the fatigue level was lowest approximately an hour after awakening and highest just before going to bed.

In addition to measuring fatigue levels, the investigator asked subjects if they could identify things that made them feel more tired or less tired. Fifteen of the 27 patients said yes to both questions. Things that made people feel more tired tended to involve overexertion or physical activity, such as doing something outdoors or working. Things that made patients feel less tired included rest periods, particularly in the afternoon, and spacing out activities. However, one subject stated that lying down often made him feel more tired and he was able to get relief by doing something he enjoyed such as going for a drive. These findings could be shared with other patients so that they too might try these techniques of alleviating fatigue.

An overall fatigue symptom score was calculated for each patient by adding the number of symptoms experienced. Similarly, subscores were calculated for each category of symptoms (i.e., general incongruities, mental symptoms, and specific incongruities). Symptoms reflecting general incongruities were experienced most frequently, followed by mental symptoms and symptoms reflecting specific incongruities. Table 27.2 shows the 12 most commonly experienced symptoms. It is interesting that 7 of the 12 symptoms reflect general incongruity.

Nine of these top 12 symptoms were also experienced by cancer patients receiving localized radiation (Haylock & Hart, 1979), although

TABLE 27.2   Rank Ordering of Top 12 Fatigue Symptoms Experienced by ESRD Patients

Fatigue Symptoms	Frequency	Rank	Category[a]
Want to lie down	27	1	GI
Become rigid or clumsy	21	2	GI
Feel tired in legs	20	3	GI
Feel tired in body	20	3	GI
Lack patience	20	3	MS
Become weary while talking	18	6	MS
Unable to concentrate	17	7	MS
Become drowsy	16	8	GI
Give a yawn	16	8	GI
Feel unsteady while standing	15	10	GI
Lack self-confidence	15	10	MS
Feel stiff in shoulders	15	10	SI

[a]GI = general incongruity; MS = mental symptom; SI = specific incongruity.

the rankings differed. Symptoms such as becoming weary while talking, inability to concentrate, and lack of self-confidence were infrequent among cancer patients but frequent among ESRD patients, suggesting that the fatigue associated with ESRD differs from that experienced by patients receiving radiation. "Being tired" appears not to be the same for everyone.

Study subjects were also asked if there were symptoms other than those on the checklist that they experienced when they felt tired. Six additional symptoms were identified: pain in heel, tired in back, pressure in ears, tense neck, cramps/pain under ribs, and pain in legs. Each of these symptoms was mentioned only once.

A statistically significant relationship was found between level of fatigue and the overall symptom score ($r = .7$, $p < .01$). The more numerous the symptoms, the greater the feeling of fatigue. According to Yoshitake (1971), this is because symptoms are the most dominant expression of the feeling of fatigue.

This study did not ask whether certain symptoms contribute more than others to the overall feeling of fatigue. Haylock and Hart (1979), in their study of patients receiving radiation therapy, identified six symptoms that were significantly related to the level of fatigue. These symptoms were feeling tired in body, feeling tired in legs, yawning, wanting to lie down, feeling heavy in the head, and feeling ill. Clearly, this is an area that requires further study.

For the most part the study subjects were not suffering from clinical depression. No relationships were noted between depression scores and scores on either the subjective quality of life or the overall fatigue level.

The lack of depression and the fact that most subjects felt an increase in fatigue as the day progressed suggest that the fatigue experienced by this group of patients was physiological rather than psychological. This idea is further supported by the frequency of symptoms categorized as physical symptoms—for example, tired in body, want to lie down, tired in legs, and yawning (Yoshitake, 1971).

DISCUSSION

While the fatigue experienced by hemodialysis patients seems to be largely physiological, the components of the fatigue remain unknown. Further study of physiological indices, medications, and other illness may provide some answers, but in the meantime interventions must focus on symptom management and relief. With the identification of specific symptoms, fatigue does not have to remain an ambiguous, nonspecific phenomenon for ESRD patients. Central to the management of fatigue is the recognition by patients and staff that fatigue can be alleviated, at least to some extent. Patients can be encouraged to plan their day in ways that allow for adequate rest as well as activities they enjoy.

Although emotional fatigue was not prevalent in this study sample, depression can go hand in hand with chronic illnesses such as ESRD, and it has been seen in renal patients by other researchers (Cardenas & Kutner, 1982). Therefore, as practitioners we must continue to assess for the psychological as well as physiological components of fatigue.

Level of fatigue has been shown to be strongly correlated with patients' quality of life. Since improving the quality of life is a major goal in the management of chronic illness, fatigue in ESRD patients can no longer be ignored.

[28]

Fatigue in Women Receiving Chemotherapy for Ovarian Cancer

Susan Christensen Jamar

Fatigue is a frequent complaint among persons receiving chemotherapy: oncology clinicians who were informally surveyed reported the occurrence of fatigue in 75–95% of patients receiving chemotherapy (Christensen, 1987). Further, fatigue can be a frustrating and distressing side effect, affecting many aspects of the individual's life and leading some persons to question whether therapy is worth completing (Nerenz, 1979). Fatigue associated with cancer and cancer treatment may persist over time, interfering with quality of life. Feelings of tiredness are intensified, and in addition to physical symptoms, the person may demonstrate increased irritability, decreased motivation, and a tendency toward depression (Grandjean, 1970).

Fatigue has been reported as a major side effect in persons receiving radiation therapy (Haylock & Hart, 1979; King, Nail, Kreamer, Strohl, & Johnson, 1985; Kobashi-Schoot, Hanewald, Van Dam, & Bruning, 1985), but there is little literature on the fatigue experienced by individuals receiving chemotherapy. Additionally, it is not well understood what changes in activity level and lifestyle of either population may occur with fatigue.

Most of the literature on fatigue has focused on acute fatigue in healthy subjects, as related to motivation, work productivity, and skill performance (Cameron, 1973; Pearson & Byars, 1956; Yoshitake, 1971). Acute fatigue, usually of brief duration, may be related to specific events such as strenuous exercise or loss of sleep, and can be relieved by nourishment or sleep (Burkhardt, 1956; Hart & Freel, 1982; Potempa, Lopez, Reid, & Lawson, 1986). Acute fatigue, unlike chronic fatigue, is an expected part of the stress and strain of normal life (Chen, 1986).

Many factors may contribute to chronic fatigue in persons receiving chemotherapy. The side effects caused by antineoplastic agents (e.g., anemia secondary to bone marrow suppression or gastrointestinal toxicities that compromise nutritional status, protein and calorie malnutrition, and accumulation of cellular waste products) contribute to fatigue (Brager & Yasko, 1984; Britton, 1983; Haylock & Hart, 1979; Kokal, 1986; Leite & Hoogstrateen, 1977; Nunnally, Donoghue, & Yasko, 1982). Also, characteristics of the individual such as age, sex, and treatment response, and variables associated with the disease such as disease stage, specific treatment regimen, and length of therapy may affect fatigue.

Psychological responses to the illness and/or therapy, including mood changes, stress, and sleep pattern changes, and physical responses such as chronic pain, cachexia, and malnutrition can contribute to overall weakness and result in fatigue (Beszterczey & Lipowski, 1977; Eidelman, 1980; Foley, 1978; Haylock & Hart, 1979; Kisner & Dewys, 1981; Lamb, 1982; MacBryde & Blacklow, 1980).

The common occurrence of fatigue in persons receiving chemotherapy and the lack of research on this problem point to the need for descriptive studies to examine the fatigue experience. The purposes of this exploratory study, therefore, were to obtain descriptions of the phenomenon of fatigue in individuals receiving chemotherapy, to determine if there is an identifiable fatigue pattern related to the chemotherapy cycle, and to determine the effect of fatigue on activity level and lifestyle of the individual.

METHOD

Data for the study were collected using self-report measures and a semistructured interview conducted in an ambulatory oncology clinic of a large Midwestern teaching hospital. The sample included 16 women who were receiving chemotherapy for treatment of ovarian cancer. Symptom distress, mood state, sleep pattern changes, and activity level were examined as potential indicators of fatigue. Accounts of fatigue experiences were also obtained as the basis for an initial description of the fatigue experience.

The instruments used to collect data included the Pearson Byars Fatigue Feeling Checklist (PBFFC) (Pearson & Byars, 1956), the Symptom Distress Scale (SDS) (McCorkle & Young, 1978), the Profile of Mood States–short form (POM-S) (Shacham, 1983), and a semistructured interview. Demographic data and information on the specific chemotherapy regimen were collected from the subject's chart.

Pearson and Byars (1956) developed the Fatigue Feeling Checklist to measure subjective fatigue in aviation pilots. This adjective checklist defines the fatigue continuum in 10 short phrases ranging from "extremely peppy" to "ready to drop." In this study, subjects indicated whether they felt better than, the same as, or worse than the specific feeling described. This scale was chosen over other fatigue scales because of its previous use in illness states (Cohen et al., 1987; Davis, 1987; Haylock & Hart, 1979).

The Symptom Distress Scale (McCorkle & Young, 1978) was developed to facilitate the measurement of degree of discomfort, as perceived by the patient, associated with identified symptoms. The 10 symptoms that make up the tool were major concerns noted by persons actively undergoing treatment for cancer. The tool has been used extensively with oncology patients.

The Profile of Mood States (short form) is a 37-item scale that measures six distinct transient mood states: anxiety, anger, confusion, fatigue, depression, and vigor. It was adapted by Shacham (1983) from the original 65-item Profile of Mood States (McNair, Lorr, & Droppleman, 1971), to be used with patients under stress or pain.

The interview, developed by the investigator, consisted of nine open-ended questions that asked about the subject's personal experience with fatigue, the pattern of fatigue, sleep pattern changes, activity level, and strategies used to relieve fatigue.

RESULTS

The sample consisted of 16 Caucasian females. Subjects' ages ranged from 36 to 66 years. Ten of the women (63%) lived with a spouse or in a nuclear family setting, while 2 (13%) were single parents. Four (25%) lived alone. Almost half of the subjects (44%) stated they had assistance with home responsibilities. Disease stage ranged from I to IV. Subjects were at various points in their chemotherapy regimens at the time of the interview.

Subjects' responses produced rich descriptive data on the fatigue experience in a clinical population. Twelve of the 16 women (75%) reported a pattern of fatigue related to the chemotherapy cycle. Fatigue was worse the first week following chemotherapy, but lessened during the subsequent three weeks of the cycle, only to return again the first week of the next cycle. Three types of fatigue descriptions were identified from the interviews: physical descriptors, emotional descriptors, and descriptors related to changes in energy level. Physical descriptors included physical and somatic symptoms, physical incongruities, and changes in physical functions. Physical descriptors used by subjects to describe the fatigue experience included "weak in the body," "sick to my stomach," "weary talking," and "sleepy." Emotional descriptors incuded items related to emotional and psychological state, such as "frustrating," "decreased self-esteem," "lonely," and "bored." Descriptors related to changes in energy level included items related to alteration in activity, changes in motivation, and impairment of activity level—for example, "decreased energy," "exhausted," and "lethargic." Physical descriptors and descriptors related to changes in energy level were used most often by subjects to describe fatigue.

Eleven women (69%) reported a change in their sleep pattern. Six of these reported changes in the quality of their sleep, primarily needing naps during the day and more sleep at night. Twelve of the 16 women (75%) described activities that they had to give up or change because of fatigue. The primary and most frequent loss named by the subjects was social activities. None of the women reported giving up personal self-care activities or family activities, and in most cases restrictions on activities were limited to the first week following chemotherapy. Subjects tried a variety of activities to relieve their fatigue including diversional activities, exercise, and naps. Some of the women mentioned the importance of maintaining a positive outlook on the problem.

Fifty-six percent of the women ($n = 9$) had below normal hemoglobin (Hgb) and hematocrit (Hct) levels. There was a negative correlation between fatigue and the Hct level ($r = -.9650$, $p = .001$).

Subjective fatigue as measured by the Pearson Byars Fatigue Feeling Checklist was significantly correlated with total symptom distress as measured by the Symptom Distress Scale ($r = .6249$, $p = .01$) and with the subscales of nausea ($r = .5811$, $p = .01$) and fatigue ($r = .8656$, $p = .01$). Fatigue was also positively correlated with the Profile of Mood States (short form) total score ($r = .6405$, $p = .01$) and with three of the subscales: Depression-Dejection ($r = .9408$, $p = .001$), Anger-Hostility ($r = .4541$, $p = .05$), and Fatigue-Inertia ($r = .4844$, $p = .05$); it was negatively correlated with the Vigor-Activity subscale ($r = -.8260$, $p = .001$). Levels of fatigue were significantly related to living arrangements and assistance with home responsibilities; single parents and women without assistance at home generally had higher levels of fatigue ($p = .01$).

DISCUSSION

Although the sample was small, these findings indicate that fatigue is a pervasive experience in women receiving cancer chemotherapy. The pattern of fatigue experienced by these women, with worse fatigue at the beginning of the chemotherapy cycle and less fatigue in the later weeks of the cycle, has implications for clinicians. Informing clients about this potential pattern and assisting them to adjust activities to the pattern may help them in making appropriate plans for daily activities. Although these women reported being more tired since the initiation of their therapy, their activity level and lifestyle were not significantly affected. However, many women said they had to give up social activities, particularly during the first week of a chemotherapy cycle.

The complexity of fatigue and the numerous factors that may influence fatigue make it imperative for the nurse to perform ongoing physical, psychological, and psychosocial assessments of the client. The subjective nature of fatigue requires questions on how the individual perceives her/his experience with fatigue, how the person interprets the fatigue, and what effect fatigue has on lifestyle. Nursing interventions can then be developed to meet the needs of the person experiencing fatigue.

[29]

Chronic Fatigue: Directions for Research and Practice

Kathleen Potempa

Chronic fatigue was first described in the literature over a century ago. Since that time, numerous reports of the symptom have been published. Research efforts have been aimed at various aspects of fatigue such as acute muscle fatigue (Jones & Bigland-Ritchie, 1986) and job-related and mental fatigue (Bartley, 1964). Except for those interested in muscle fatigue, however, most researchers have abandoned the construct as too difficult to measure.

But patients have a way of being tenacious despite the literature. They continue to come to us with their complaints of fatigue. Many of the people who complain of chronic fatigue also have chronic illnesses that require prolonged therapy. Fatigue has been associated with various therapies as a side effect. Moreover, a clinical syndrome currently receiving attention, the Epstein Barr syndrome, is characterized primarily by fatigue. Because of the difficulties in describing and measuring fatigue, it is impossible to estimate its true prevalence. It has occurred often enough, however, to receive sustained, albeit controversial, attention in the literature.

Nurses are often the only patient care providers to give the symptom serious recognition. Perhaps this is because there is so little known about what it is and how to treat it. The symptom is begging for our attention. This is the challenge and the opportunity for the nursing community. Chronic fatigue has recently been accepted as a nursing diagnosis by the North American Nursing Diagnosis Association, giving formal backing for study of the phenomenon. This also establishes the responsibility of nurses to diagnose and treat fatigue adequately.

The four chapters on fatigue in this section show clear progress in delineating the symptom, perhaps because of their clinical focus. It is easier to describe a phenomenon when it is drastically represented—as in people who have cancer or end-stage renal disease or who are recovering from catastrophic illness, such as botulism.

Three main issues must be addressed in carrying the work forward if our understanding of fatigue is to advance in a clinically relevant manner. First, it is imperative that we develop valid and reliable ways to measure the presence and intensity of fatigue. This will allow applications that are useful to patients and also foster further understanding of the construct fatigue. It is essential that practicing nurses be part of this descriptive process, for it is clinicians who have access to the rich patient data that keep measurement clinically appropriate. Second, we must describe the patient characteristics that are correlated with fatigue. In determining these, we can assess the impact of the phenomenon on people's lives. Finally, we need to learn what interventions are effective in reducing or eliminating fatigue. Treatments need to be developed that are specific to different patient populations and situational contexts.

As we grow in our understanding, we will be able to predict who is vulnerable to fatigue, in what situations, and to what degree. In addition, we will be able to make preventive as well as curative prescriptions for chronic fatigue.

THE MEASUREMENT OF FATIGUE

The current research on fatigue emphasizes measurement. From a clinical perspective, the ability to describe and quantify symptoms is a prerequisite for diagnosis and treatment. In this case, diagnosis means not only understanding the characteristics of fatigue that make it a syndrome, but also recognizing what factors differentiate it from related syndromes.

Fatigue was first described as a "generalized neurasthenia" or weakness of the body. However, many of the early cases, if described today, would be characterized as depression. A major clinical question is whether fatigue is a distinct syndrome or whether its characteristics can be subsumed under other disease states such as depression. Because fatigue is often associated with chronic illness, as is depression, this differentiation is critical to the care and treatment of chronically ill patients.

The answer to this question lies with our patients and the way we choose to measure their experience of fatigue. To be clinically valid, measures must analyze patients' descriptions, yet most of the fatigue instruments currently available were developed for nonclinical populations. Further, the emphasis on the single dimension of tiredness seen in these measures limits our understanding of fatigue in clinical populations.

The work of Piper et al., presented in this volume, is the most sophisticated attempt to date to capture the fatigue experience of patients. Her focus on cancer patients is particularly germane because of the incidence of fatigue symptoms in cancer patients undergoing radiation treatment.

Others have field tested existing instruments, most notably the Pearson Byars Fatigue Feeling Checklist, with clinical populations. The data from these studies are impressive. For example, Cohen and Hardin provide estimates of the incidence and course of fatigue in people with botulism, Srivastava in patients with end-stage renal disease, and Jamar in patients receiving chemotherapy. This information gives us a perspective that can be immediately applied to care of these patients. We know that fatigue is a bona fide symptom of serious proportions in these patients and that interventions need to be designed to control or alleviate the symptom.

Although continued testing is required using larger samples and different patient populations, the data presented in this volume thus represent a major step forward in our ability to measure fatigue in clinical populations. To further determine their clinical validity, the instruments need to be widely tested in subjects highly likely to experience fatigue. Concurrent testing with instruments to measure related phenomena such as depression is needed to help us understand the divergence or convergence of these symptoms.

In the meantime, clinicians can use available measures to interpret patient complaints. Visual analogue scales of fatigue, depression inventories, and measures of anxiety, for example, can be used when patients complain of chronic fatigue. Carefully kept records on many patients can be a rich source of information for case reports. The case reports of practicing clinicians will be invaluable not only to other clinicians but to methodologists attempting to discern the nature of fatigue.

SYMPTOMS RELATED TO FATIGUE

An understanding of the significance of fatigue in the daily life of patients requires identification of the range of symptoms associated with fatigue. There may be similarities as well as differences in the symptoms in different patient populations. These symptoms may reflect subjective or objective characteristics of patients. Objective characteristics include sleep and exercise performance as well as job or role performance. Several recent studies have explored the correlates of fatigue in various populations.

For example, Srivastava reports a negative correlation between fatigue and subjective quality of life in patients with end-stage renal disease. Although this relationship is intuitively expected, its statistical strength suggests the importance of fatigue in the total life experience of these patients. Nursing measures to reduce fatigue are crucial at this stage of the disease.

Further information needs to be gathered about the relationship of subjective fatigue to objective indicators of performance. This relationship, furthermore, may be related to the intensity of the fatigue experienced. This information is highly clinically relevant. Preventive interventions may need to be developed at certain stages of fatigue to delay or offset its impact on the daily life of the patient. This is particularly important when fatigue is an inevitable part of a disease or treatment. We must learn the range of fatigue and the situations that exacerbate or alleviate it.

INTERVENTIONS FOR FATIGUE

The greatest knowledge gap to date is in our understanding of when and how to intervene when fatigue occurs. Our current ability to manage fatigue can be described as "educated intuition." Because of what we are learning now about the phenomenology of fatigue in the populations sampled, clinical judgment can be more sophisticated. For example, fatigue appears to be multidimensional with some specificity to disease state. This emphasizes the need to clearly assess each patient's fatigue experience. Individualized interventions can be designed to fit their needs. It is important, however, that clinicians report these trial and error experiences so that they can be systematized and intervention studies planned. As mentioned earlier, the case report is an invaluable tool for clinicans to share clinical wisdom.

The data presented within this volume suggest that patient perceptions are key mediators of fatigue. The effects of feedback regarding the severity of disease or the situational context of the patient are fertile areas for research. Although it is tempting to say that patients should be given objective feedback regarding these variables, there are many potential problems with this approach. First, the "objective" view of the clinician is actually often as subjective as the patient's, being a clinical judgment extrapolated from data that may have limited predictive ability. Further, feedback of any kind from a health care provider may or may not alter patient expectations. Individual personality factors are potentially influential in patient suggestibility. For now, it is prudent for nurses to be aware of the influence of expectations on the fatigue experience and use clinical judgment regarding whether to intervene with feedback. Again, anecdotal reports of this approach will be an asset to the literature.

SUMMARY

We are in an exciting era of clinically relevant fatigue research. We have made significant strides in instrument development and clinical testing. This affords us the opportunity to describe fatigue in patient populations that are primary targets for our interventions. We must move forward in the development of theoretically sound intervention studies that will give specific information on patient characteristics, situational contexts, and disease types. We are at the beginning of very fruitful research.

References On Fatigue

Akerstedt, T., Gillberg, M., & Witterberg, L. (1982). The circadian covariation of fatigue and urinary melatonin. *Biological Psychiatry, 17* (5), 547–554.

Aldenderfer, M. S., & Blashfield, R. K. (1984). *Cluster analysis.* Sage Publications: Beverly Hills.

Arendt, D., Borbely, A. A., Franey, C., & Wright, J. (1984). The effects of chronic, small doses of melatonin given in the late afternoon on fatigue in man: A preliminary study. *Neuroscience Letters, 45,* 317–321.

Arnon, S. S., & Chin, J. (1981). Botulism. In P. F. Wehrle and F. L. Top, Sr. (Eds.), *Communicable and infectious diseases* (9th ed.) (pp. 125–137). St. Louis: The C.V. Mosby Co.

Atkinson, H. (1985). *Women and fatigue.* New York: G. P. Putnam.

Axelrod, L., Halter, J. B., Cooper, D. S., Aoki, T. T., Roussell, A. M., & Bagshaw, S. L. (1983). Hormone levels and fuel flow in patients with weight loss and lung cancer. Evidence for excessive metabolic expenditure and for an adaptive response mediated by a reduced level of 3,5,3'-Triiodothyronine. *Metabolism, 32* (9), 924–937.

Baldree, K. S., Murphy, S. P., & Powers, M. J. (1982). Stress identification and coping patterns in patients on hemodialysis. *Nursing Research, 31,* 107–112.

Bartley, S. H. (1964). Some things to realize about fatigue. *Journal of Sports Medicine and Physical Fitness, 4,* 153–157.

Bartley, S. H. (1965). *Fatigue: Mechanism and management.* Springfield, IL: Charles C. Thomas.

Bartley, S. H. (1976). What do we call fatigue? In E. Simonson & P. C. Weiser (Eds.), *Psychological aspects and physiological correlates of work and fatigue* (pp. 409–414). Springfield, IL: Charles C. Thomas.

Beck, A. T., Ward, C. H., Mendelson, M., Mock, J., & Erbauch, J. H. (1961). An inventory for measuring depression. *Archives of General Psychiatry, 4,* 561–571.

Beszterczey, A., & Lipowski, Z. (1977). Insomnia and cancer patients. *Canadian Medical Journal, 77,* 335.

Brager, B. L., & Yasko, J. (1984). *Care of the client receiving chemotherapy.* Reston, VA: Raven Publishing Company.

Britton, D. (1983). Fatigue. In J. Yasko (Ed.), *Guidelines for cancer care: Symptom management* (pp. 33–37). Reston, VA: Raven Publishing Company.

Brown, M. L., Carrieri, V., Janson-Bjerklie, S., & Dodd, M. J. (1986). Lung cancer and dyspnea: The patient's perception. *Oncology Nursing Forum, 13* (5), 19–24.

Burkhardt, E. A. (1956). Fatigue: Diagnosis and treatment. *New York State Journal of Medicine, 56,* 62–67.

Burton, R. R. (1980). Human responses to repeated high G stimulated aerial combat maneuvers. *Aviation, Space, and Environmental Medicine, 51,* 1185–1192.

Cameron, C. (1973). A theory of fatigue. *Ergonomics, 16,* 633–646.

Cardenas, D. D., & Kutner, N. G. (1982). The problem of fatigue in dialysis patients. *Nephron, 30,* 336–340.

Centers for Disease Control (1979). *Botulism in the United States, 1899–1977.* Handbook for Epidemiologists, Clinicians and Laboratory Workers.

Centers for Disease Control (1984). Foodborne botulism—Illinois. *Morbidity and Mortality Weekly Report, 33*(2), 22–23.

Chen, M. K. (1986). The epidemiology of self-perceived fatigue among adults. *Preventive Medicine, 15,* 74–81.

Cheraskin, E., Ringsdorf, W. M., & Medford, F. H. (1976). Daily vitamin C consumption and fatiguability. *Journal of the American Geriatrics Society, XXIV* (3), 136–137.

Cherrington, M. (1974). Botulism. *Archives of Neurology, 30,* 432–437.

Christensen, S. (1987). [Informal survey of oncology nurse clinicians regarding fatigue in patients receiving chemotherapy]. Unpublished raw data.

Ciba Foundation Symposium 82. (1981). *Human muscle fatigue: Physiological mechanisms.* London: Pittman Medical.

Clark, A. N. G. (1978). Morale and motivation. *The Practitioner, 220,* 735–737.

Cohen, F. L., Hardin, S. B., Nehring, W. M., Foreman, M. D., Kim, K, & Tse, A. (1987). *Measurement of fatigue feelings over a 2 year span in patients with catastrophic illness.* Paper presented at the meeting of the 11th annual Midwest Nursing Research Society, St. Louis.

Cohen, F. L., Scovill, N., Doyle, S., Alms-Duboise, J., Hardin, S., Maloney, J., Ruthman, J., Schmitt, M., Wetter, P., & Wyss, K. (1984). *The short-term impact of botulism on patients and their families.* Paper presented at 12th Annual Nursing Research Conference, University of Arizona, Tucson.

Cohen, F. L., Ruthman, J., Maloney, J., Doyle, S., Alms-Buboise, J., Hardin, S., Schmitt, M., Scovill, N., Clark, C., McNabb, J., Weber, C., Wetter, P., & Wyss, K. (1981). *Botulism patients' perceptions of hospitalization problems: Discussion and nursing case study.* Paper presented at research conference, St. Louis University, St. Louis.

Cohen, H. M. (1973). Fatigue caused by vitamin E? (Letter to the editor). *California Medicine, 119* (1), 72.

Davis, C. A. (1984). Interferon-induced fatigue. (Abstract No. 72). *Oncology Nursing Forum, 11* (Suppl.).

Davis, L. (1987). Patient care and education in interferon induced fatigue. *Oncology Nurse Bulletin, 2,* Lederle Laboratories.

Dorpat, T. L., & Holmes, T. H. (1955). Mechanisms of skeletal muscle pain and fatigue. *Archives of Neurology & Psychiatry, 74* (1), 638–640.

Edwards, R. H. T., Harris, R. C., Hultman, E., Kaijser, L., Koh, D., & Nordesjo, L. O. (1972). Effect of temperature on muscle energy metabolism and endurance during successive isometric contractions, sustained to fatigue, of the quadriceps muscle in man. *Journal of Physiology, 220* (2), 335–352.

Eichel, C. J. (1986). Stress and coping in patients on CAPD compared to hemodialysis patients. *ANNA Journal, 13*(1), 9–13.

Eidelman, D. (1980). Fatigue: Towards an analysis and a unified definition. *Medical Hypotheses, 6,* 517–526.

Ellis, F. R., & Nasser, S. (1973). A pilot study of vitamin B12 in the treatment of tiredness. *British Journal of Nutrition, 30* (2), 277–283.

Engel, G. L., & Morgan, W. L. (1973). *Interviewing the patient*. Philadelphia: W. B. Saunders & Co..

Foley, K. M. (1978). Pain syndrome in patients with cancer. In J. J. Bonica & V. Ventafridda (Eds.), *Advances in pain research and theory: Vol. 1* (pp. 59–75). New York: Raven Press.

Freel, M. I., & Hart, L. K. (1977). *Study of fatigue phenomena of multiple sclerosis patients* (Grant No. 5R02-NU-00524-02). Division of Nursing, USDHEW.

Fuerstein, A. l. A., Carter, R. L., & Papciak, A. S. (1987). A prospective analysis of stress and fatigue in recurrent low back pain. *Pain, 31,* 333–344.

German, G. A., & Stampfer, H. G. (1979). Hypothalamic releasing factor for reactive depression. (Letter to the editor). *The Lancet, 2,* (8146), 789.

Gibson, H., & Edwards, R. H. T. (1985). Muscular exercise and fatigue. *Sports Medicine, 2* (2), 120–132.

Grandjean, E. P. (1968). Fatigue: Its physiological and psychological significance. *Ergonomics, 11,* 427–436.

Grandjean, E. P. (1970). Fatigue. *American Industrial Hygiene Association Journal, 31,* 401–411.

Grandjean, E., & Kogi, K. (1971). Introductory remarks. In K. Hashimoto, K. Kogi, & E. Grandjean (Eds.), *Methodology in human fatigue assessment* (pp. xvii–xxx). London: Taylor & Francis, Ltd.

Hardin, S. B., & Cohen, F. L. (in press). Psychosocial effects of a catastrophic botulism outbreak. *Archives of Psychiatric Nursing.*

Hargreaves, M. (1977). The fatigue syndrome. *The Practitioner, 218,* 841–843.

Hart, L. K. (1978). Fatigue in the patient with multiple sclerosis. *Research in Nursing and Health, 1*(4), 147–157.

Hart, L. K., & Freel, M. I. (1982). Fatigue. In C. M. Norris (Ed.), *Concept clarification in nursing* (pp. 241–161). Rockville, MD: Aspen Systems Corporation.

Hashimoto, K., Kogi, K., & Grandjean, E. (Eds.) (1971). *Methodology in human fatigue assessment*. London: Taylor & Francis, Ltd.

Haylock, P. J., & Hart, L. K. (1979). Fatigue in patients receiving localized radiation. *Cancer Nursing, 2,* 461–467.

Heuting, J. E., & Sarphati, H. R. (1966). Measuring fatigue. *Journal of Applied Physiology, 50* (6), 535–538.

Hicks, J. T. (1964). Treatment of fatigue in general practice: A double blind study. *Clinical Medicine, 71* (1), 85–90.

Jones, D. A., & Bigland-Ritchie, B. (1986). Electrical and contractile changes in muscle fatigue. In B. Sattin (Ed.), *Biochemistry of exercise* (pp. 377–392). Champaign, IL: Human Kenetics Publishers.

Karlsson, J., Sjodin, B., Jacobs, I., & Kaiser, P. (1981). Relevance of muscle fiber type to fatigue in short intense and prolonged exercise in man. In *Ciba Foundation Symposium 82. Human muscle fatigue: Physiological mechanisms* (pp. 59–74). London: Pittman Medical.

Kaye, P. L. (1980). Fatigue: Pervasive problem. *New York State Journal of Medicine, 80*(8), 1225–1229.

Kellum, M. D. (1985). Fatigue. In M. M. Jacobs & W. Geels (Eds.), *Signs and symptoms in nursing: Interpretation and management* (pp. 103–118). Philadelphia: J. B. Lippincott Co.

King, K. B., Nail, L. M., Kreamer, K., Strohl, R., & Johnson, J. E. (1985). Patients' descriptions of the experience of receiving radiation therapy. *Oncology Nursing Forum, 12*(4), 55–61.

Kinsman, R. A., & Weiser, P. C. (1976). Subjective symptomatology during work and fatigue. In E. Simonson & P. C. Weiser (Eds.), *Psychological aspects and physiological correlates of work and fatigue* (pp. 336–405). Springfield, IL: Charles C. Thomas.

Kisner, D. L., & Dewys, W. D. (1981). Anorexia and cachexia in malignant disease. In G. R. Newell & N. M. Ellision (Eds.), *Nutrition and cancer: Etiology and treatment.* New York: Raven Press.

Kobashi-Schoot, J. A. M., Hanewald, G., Van Dam, F., & Bruning, P. F. (1985). Assessment of malaise in cancer patients treated with radiotherapy. *Cancer Nursing, 8,* 306–313.

Kogi, K., Saito, Y., & Mitsuhashi, T. (1970). Validity of three components of subjective fatigue feelings. *Journal of the Science of Labor, 46*(5), 251–270.

Kokal, W. A. (1986). Effects of antineoplastic therapy on nutritional status: Surgery, chemotherapy, and radiation therapy. *Clinics in Oncology, 5,* 277–292.

Komoike, Y., & Horiguchi, S. (1971). Fatigue assessment on key punch operators, typists and others. *Ergonomics, 14*(1), 101–109.

Kruse, C. A. (1961). Treatment of fatigue with aspartic acid salts. *Northwest Medicine, 60*(6), 597–603.

Kurland, G. S., Hamolsky, M. W., & Freedberg, A. S. (1955). Studies in nonmyxedematous hypometabolism. *Journal of Clinical Endocrinology and Metabolism, 15,* 1354–1366.

Lamb, M. A. (1982). The sleeping patterns of patients with malignant and nonmalignant diseases. *Cancer Nursing, 5,* 389–396.

Leite, C., & Hoogstrateen, B. (1977). Differential diagnosis of anemia and cancer. *Ca-A Cancer Journal for Clinicians, 27,* 88–89.

Lindsey, A. M. (1986). Cancer cachexia: Effects of the disease and its treatment. *Seminars in Oncology Nursing, 2*(1), 19–29.

MacBryde, C., & Blacklow, R. (1980). *Signs and symptoms* (5th ed.). Philadelphia: J. B. Lippincott Co.

MacDonald, K. L., Spengler, R. F., Hatheway, C. L., Hargrett, N. T., & Cohen, M. L. (1985). Type A botulism from sauteed onions. *Journal of the American Medical Association, 253,* 1275–1278.

MacVicar, M. G., & Winningham, M. L. (1986). Promoting functional capacity of cancer patients. *The Cancer Bulletin, 38*(5), 235–239.

Malmquist, B., Ekholm, I., Lindstrom, L., Petersen, I., & Ortengren, R. (1981). Measurement of localized muscle fatigue in building work. *Ergonomics, 24*(9), 695–709.

McCorkle, R., & Young, K. (1978). Development of a symptom distress scale. *Cancer Nursing, 1,* 373–378.

McFarland, R. A. (1971). Understanding fatigue in modern life. *Ergonomics, 14*(1), 1–10.

McGuire, D. B. (1984). The measurement of clinical pain. *Nursing Research, 33,* 152–156.

McNair, D. M., Lorr, M., & Droppleman, L. F. (1971). *POMS: Manual for Profile of Mood States.* San Diego: Educational and Industrial Testing Service.

Melzack, R. (Ed.). (1983). *Pain measurement and assessment.* New York: Raven Press.

Merton, P. A. (1954). Voluntary strength and fatigue. *Journal of Physiology, 123,* 553–564.

Meyerwitz, B. E., Sparks, F. C., & Sparks, I. K. (1979). Adjuvant chemotherapy for breast cancer. *Cancer, 43,* 1613–1618.

Meyerwitz, B. E., Watkins, I. K., & Sparks, F. C. (1983). Quality of life for breast cancer patients receiving adjuvant chemotherapy. *American Journal of Nursing, 83*(2), 232–235.

Miller, R. G., Giannini, D., Milner-Brown, H. S., Layzer, R. B., Koretsky, A. P., Hooper, D., & Weiner, M. W. (1987). Effects of fatiguing exercise on high-energy phosphates, force, and EMG: Evidence for three phases of recovery. *Muscle & Nerve, 10,* 810–821.

Mishel, M. H. (1983). Adjusting the fit: Development of uncertainty scales for specific clinical populations. *Western Journal of Nursing Research, 5,* 355–370.

Morris, M. L. (1982). Tiredness and fatigue. In C. M. Norris (Ed.), *Concept clarification in nursing* (pp. 263–275). Rockville, MD: Aspen Systems Corporation.

Muncie, W. (1941). Chronic fatigue. *Psychosomatic Medicine, 3*(3), 277–285.

Murray, T. J. (1985). Amantidine therapy for fatigue in multiple sclerosis. *Le Journal Canadien Des Sciences Neurologiques, 12*(3), 251–254.

Nerenz, D. (1979). *Control of emotional distress in cancer chemotherapy.* Unpublished doctoral dissertation, University of Wisconsin, Madison.

Nerenz, D. R., Leventhal, H., & Love, R. R. (1982). Factors contributing to emotional distress during cancer chemotherapy. *Cancer, 50,* 1020–1027.

Norris, C. M. (1982). Synthesis of concepts: Evolving an umbrella concept— Protection. In C. M. Norris (Ed.), *Concept clarification in nursing* (pp. 385–403). Rockville, MD: Aspen Systems Corporation.

Nunnally, C., Donoghue, M., & Yasko, J. M. (1982). Nutritional needs of cancer patients. *Nursing Clinics of North America, 17,* 557–578.

Pardue, N. H. (1984). *Energy expenditure and subjective fatigue of chronic obstructive pulmonary disease patients before and after a pulmonary rehabilitation.* Unpublished doctoral dissertation, Catholic University, Washington, D.C.

Parfrey, P., Vavasour, H., Henry, S., Bullock, M., & Gault, M. (in press). Clinical features and severity of nonspecific symptoms in dialysis patients.

Pearson, R. G. (1957). Scale analysis of a fatigue checklist. *Journal of Applied Psychology, 41*(3), 186–191.

Pearson, R. G., & Byars, G. E. (1956). *The development and validation of a checklist for measuring subjective fatigue.* (Report No. 56–115). School of Aviation Medicine, USAF, Randolph AFB, TX.

Piper, B. F. (1986). Fatigue. In V. K. Carrieri, A. M. Lindsey, & C. W. West (Eds.), *Pathophysiological phenomena in nursing: Human responses to illness* (pp. 219–234). Philadelphia: W. B. Saunders & Co.

Piper, B. F. (1987). [Perceptions of fatigue in cancer patients who are receiving radiation and chemotherapy]. Unpublished raw data.

Piper, B. F. (1988). Fatigue in cancer patients: Current perspectives on measurement and management. Fifth National Conference on Cancer Nursing. *Monograph on nursing management of common problems: State of the art.* New York: American Cancer Society .

Piper, B. F., & Dodd, M. J. (1987). [Fatigue analysis of chemotherapy and radiation therapy self-care behavior logs]. Unpublished raw data, University of California, San Francisco.

Piper, B. F., Lindsey, A. M., & Dodd, M. J. (1984). [Fatigue: The measurement of a multidimensional concept]. Unpublished raw data.

Piper, B. F., Lindsey, A. M., & Dodd, M. J. (1987a). Fatigue mechanisms in cancer patients: Developing nursing theory. *Oncology Nursing Forum, 14*(6), 17–23.

Piper, B. F., & Lindsey, A. M., & Dodd, M. J. (1987b). Measurement issues related to fatigue in cancer patients (Abstract No. 190A). *Oncology Nursing Forum, 14*(Suppl.).

Poffenberger, A. T. (1928). The effects of continuous work upon output and feelings. *Journal of Applied Psychology, 12*(5), 450–467.

Poteliakhoff, A. (1981). Adrenocortical activity and some clinical findings in acute and chronic fatigue. *Journal of Psychosomatic Research, 25*(2), 91–95.

Potempa, K., Lopez, M., Reid, C., & Lawson, L. (1986). Chronic fatigue. *Image: Journal of Nursing Scholarship, 18*(4), 165–169.

Putt, A. M. (1977, March). Effects of noise on fatigue in healthy middle-aged adults. *Communicating Nursing Research, 8*, 24–34.

Reiger, P. T. (1987, November 10). Interferon-induced fatigue: A study of fatigue measurement (Abstract A163). *Sigma Theta Tau International 29th Biennial Convention Book of Proceedings.*

Rennie, M. J., Johnson, R. H., Park, D. M., & Sularman, W. R. (1973). Inappropriate fatigue during exercise associated with high blood lactates. *Clinical Science, 45*(1), 5.

Rhodes, V. A., Watson, P. M., & Hanson, B. M. (1988). Patients' descriptions of the influence of tiredness and weakness on self-care abilities. *Cancer Nursing, 11*(3), 186–194.

Rhoten, D. (1982). Fatigue and the postsurgical patient. In C.M. Norris (Ed.), *Concept clarification in nursing* (pp. 277–300). Rockville, MD: Aspen Systems Corporation.

Riddle, P. K. (1982). Chronic fatigue and women: A description and suggested treatment. *Women & Health, 7*(1), 37–47.

Rockwell, D. A., & Burr, B. D. (1977). The tired patient. *Journal of Family Practice, 5*(5), 853–857.

Rose, E. A., & King, T. C. (1978). Understanding postoperative fatigue. *Surgery, Gynecology, & Obstetrics, 147*, 97–101.

Saito, Y., Kogi, K., & Kashiwagi, S. (1970). Factors underlying subjective feelings of fatigue. *Journal of Science and Labour, 46*(4), 205–224.

Sanders, A. B., Seifert, S., & Kobernick, M. (1983). Botulism: Clinical report. *Journal of Family Practice, 16*, 987–1000.

Schag, C. C., Heinrich, R. L., & Ganz, P. A. (1984). Karnofsky performance status revisited: Reliability, validity, and guidelines. *Journal of Clinical Oncology, 2*(3), 187–193.

Schmidt-Nowara, W. W., Samet, J. M., & Rosario, P. A. (1983). Early and late pulmonary complications of botulism. *Archives of Internal Medicine, 143*, 451–456.

Sellin, L. C. (1981). The action of botulism toxin at the neuromuscular junction. *Medical Biology, 59*, 11–20.

Shacham, S. (1983). A shortened version of the Profile of Mood States. *Journal of Personality Assessment, 47*, 305–306.

Simpson, L. (1979). The action of botulinal toxin. *Reviews of Infectious Diseases, 1*(4), 656–659.

Snow, E. W., Machlan, L. O., Jr., Warnell, C. E., & Utt, T. P. (1959). The tired patient. *Medical Times, 87*, 1500–1504.

Spitzer, W. O., Dobson, A. J., Hall, J., Chesterman, E., Levi, J., Shepherd, R., Battista, R. N., & Catchlove, B. R. (1981). Measuring the quality of life of cancer patients: A concise QL-index for use by physicians. *Journal of Chronic Diseases, 34*, 585–597.

Srivastava, R. H. (1986). Fatigue in the renal patient. *ANNA Journal, 13*(5), 246–249.

Straus, S. E., Tosato, G., Armstrong, G., Lawley, T., Preble, O. T., Henle, W., Davey, R., Pearson, G., Epstein, J., Brus, I., & Blaese, M. (1985). Persisting illness and fatigue in adults with evidence of Epstein-Barr virus infection. *Annals of Internal Medicine, 102*(1), 7–16.

Terranova, W., Breman, J. G., Locey, R. P., & Speck, S. (1978). Botulism type B: Epidemiologic aspects of an extensive outbreak. *American Journal of Epidemiology, 108*(2), 150–156.

Thayer, R. E. (1987). Energy, tiredness, and tension effects of a sugar snack versus moderate exercise. *Journal of Personality and Social Psychology, 52*(1), 119–125.

Tracy, F. E. (1960). The cyclic psychosomatic fatigue syndrome. *Connecticut Medicine, 24*(6), 357–359.

Valdini, A. F. (1985). Fatigue of unknown etiology—A review. *Family Practice, 2*(1), 48–53.

Varricchio, C. G. (1985). Selecting a tool for measuring fatigue. *Oncology Nursing Forum, 12*(4), 122–123; 126–127.

Waltz, C. F., & Bausell, R. B. (1981). *Nursing research: Design, statistics, and computer analysis.* Philadelphia: F. A. Davis.

Wittenborn, J. R., & Buhler, R. (1979). Somatic discomforts among depressed women. *Archives of General Psychiatry, 36*(4), 465–471.

Yoshitake, H. (1969). Rating the feelings of fatigue. *Journal of the Science of Labour, 45*(7), 422–432.

Yoshitake, H. (1971). Relations between the symptoms and the feeling of fatigue. *Ergonomics, 14,* 175–186.

Yoshitake, H. (1978). Three characteristic patterns of subjective fatigue symptoms. *Ergonomics, 21*(3), 231–233.

Young, Z. O. (1959). Deaner: A new stimulant for office practice. *Clinical Medicine, 6*(10), 1801–1809.

Part IV

NAUSEA

[30]

Management of Nausea: Current Bases for Practice

Patricia H. Cotanch

Though it has existed for as long as there have been human beings, the symptom of nausea has never received much attention in health care practice or research. In fact, until recently the sensation of nausea was frequently dismissed as "just a passing thing." Perhaps the rationale for the dismissal was the understanding that nausea is (1) self-limiting (it always passes with time); (2) never life-threatening in itself; (3) probably psychogenic in nature (at least to some degree); and (4) being subjective, very difficult to measure. In addition, in the past the most predictable nausea was pregnancy-related, and that may also explain the lack of attention given to it.

This chapter focuses on the recent surge of clinical research on nausea, with attention to the milestones already achieved and the areas of research and practice that remain to be rigorously investigated. Attention will also be given to modes of adopting the research findings on nausea in the practice of providing comfort. Finally, suggestions for scrutinizing our practices will be given since these are the launch pad for future research on the symptom of nausea.

NAUSEA AS A SYMPTOM

As noted above, nausea, by itself, has never received much attention. Indeed, even vomiting—an observable behavior—has received very little attention in the history of clinical research. Considering that vomiting is a primitive neurologic process that has remained almost unchanged in the evolution of animals, it is surprising that mechanisms that regulate the behavior remain virtually unknown (McCarthy & Bouson, 1983). In the last 15 years, there has been a noticeable increase in research on nausea as a drug side effect because it was so frequently seen in cancer chemotherapy clinical trials sponsored by the National Cancer Institute and the American Cancer Society. As more powerful chemotherapy agents and aggressive combinations were clinically investigated, patients began to experience severe, potentially life-threatening nausea and vomiting. Yet it was still the symptom of "vomiting" that began to receive attention. Nausea was either coupled with the investigation of vomiting and the two were treated as a unit or it remained ignored. Still, efforts continued to improve antiemetic drugs and finally, nausea began to be seen as possibly a separate yet related symptom. Interestingly, there is still little research on the nausea associated with pregnancy, though it is a common symptom.

CURRENT THINKING: NAUSEA— A PSYCHOPHYSIOLOGICAL CONNECTION

The sensation of nausea is believed to have a strong psychogenic component (Andrykowski, 1988). One only has to look at our language to gain insight into the connection between the gut and the affect. In fact, to grossly simplify the work of Beck (1979), human emotion can be classified into four broad categories—mad, sad, glad, and scared. All the broad categories have "gut metaphors" associated with them.

Here are some examples: scared sick, yellow belly, gutless, gut in a vice (to express fright); heaviness in the gut, sick with sadness (to express loss, grief); fire in the gut, spitting mad, hissing mad (to express anger); iron gut, gutsy (to express bravery, courage). It is interesting to note that adults are more likely to express emotions of mad, sad, or scared using "gut" metaphors, while children are more likely to include the emotion of "glad" along with the others. Gut metaphors for glad include these: "my belly was jumping . . quivering, happiness bubbles in my belly, I have butterflies in my stomach."

Considering the connections described by our language, it is not so surprising that the sensation of nausea has often been reduced by interventions that affect our minds, specifically behavioral interventions and psychotropic pharmacological interventions.

ANTIEMETIC THEORY

While our language has given us rich evidence of the connection between affect and the gut, this was not taken seriously by "hard" science investigators until recently. As antiemetic drug trials increased in frequency to keep pace with aggressive combination chemotherapy drug trials, certain findings became clearer. For example, all antiemetics share a common feature of sedation. Therefore, all antiemetics are consciousness altering drugs. To illustrate, Ativan, which is a sedative, is frequently used as an antiemetic in cancer chemotherapy, and at large doses it has the effect of making patients forget any nausea and vomiting they experience—which is useful in avoiding the development of conditioned responses. It is very possible that antiemetic drugs and behavioral interventions are effective because they produce alterations in neurotransmitters in or near the specific areas of the brain responsible for nausea and vomiting, e.g., the chemotherapy trigger zone, the nucleus of the tractus solitarius, and area postrema (Armstrong, Pickel, John, Reis, & Miller, 1981; Bouson & Wang, 1949; Karksu, Toth, Kiraly, & Jancso, 1981; McCarthy & Bouson, 1983; Scott & Huskisson, 1976).

Of special interest to those of us who are proponents of a "hard wiring" mind-body connection, the neurotransmitters mentioned above also affect the physiology of the gastrointestinal system, e.g., vasoactive intestinal peptide (VIP), gastrin, somatostatin, neurotensin, and vasopressin, to name but a few (Bouson & Wang, 1949). While these connections are of interest, it is currently impossible to determine specific causes and effects and resultant emetic or antiemetic activity, let alone determine these for the subjective symptom of nausea; it is still almost impossible to measure the occurrence of nausea.

Since 1980 there have been a number of antiemetic trials, and various combinations of antiemetics have been used to treat chemotherapy-related nausea and vomiting. Currently the common drugs used to treat nausea related to antineoplastic chemotherapy are Metoclopramide, Lorazopam, Thorazine, Phenergan, Dalmane, and Haldol. The goal is to get the person sedated, then bring the nausea down, and then use distraction.

A second major group of interventions are the behavioral interventions such as relaxation and self-hypnosis. Nurses have had a big impact on behavioral interventions to treat chemotherapy-related nausea and vomiting. Time and time again, we have found that a behavioral intervention is almost always better than nothing at all, and very often better than the self-care that patients would initiate on their own.

Some patients for example say, "I ate crackers and crackers helped me get over the nausea." And sometimes self-care, the patient-generated intervention, works, but more often the behavioral intervention works better.

WHERE DO WE GO FROM HERE?

Nausea has many parallels with pain. Both are hard to objectively assess; both are often self-limiting; both are symptoms and therefore warnings. Since more research exists on pain than on nausea, perhaps we can borrow from the pain research that has already been accomplished. This is especially true for assessment. Visual analogue scales (Scott & Huskisson, 1976), psychophysical scaling techniques (Tursky, Jammer, & Friedman, 1982), and symptom distress adaptation scales (Rhodes, Watson, & Johnson, 1984) have already been adapted to assess nausea. One symptom distress scale adapted from Tursky's Pain Perception Profile (Tursky et al., 1982) tries to tease out the different components of nausea, the suffering component and the intensity component. This kind of psychophysical scaling uses different words that describe the intensity (how much nausea you have) and the misery (how bad the nausea makes you feel). Scales are now being developed that measure nausea and vomiting (Lundberg & Frankenhaeuser, 1980; Morrow, Arseneau, & Ashbury, 1982).

Perhaps some research will focus on the mechanisms underlying the sensation of nausea. We do not know what actually happens in the gut when someone does or does not respond to an antiemetic drug. When the patient does not respond, does the chemotherapy trigger zone get bathed with the right antiemetic, but the anxiety overrides that? Sometimes we sedate people, so they sleep through the stimulus of nausea and vomiting, only to send them home when we're sure the chemotherapy is cleared out of their system and there's no real reason for them to have nausea and vomiting—and then they have delayed nausea and vomiting. We can keep people asleep for hours on end and they do fine. Three or four days later they call saying that they are deathly ill with delayed nausea and vomiting. Where is that coming from? It's not coming from the chemotherapy trigger zone. This is a rich area for research.

One difficulty in conducting research on nausea is the lack of adequate animal models. There is no way to measure nausea in lower animals. Some lower animals, for example rats, cannot vomit. Is nausea a phenomenon that rats experience? Dogs experience nausea and dogs can expectorate, but humans are the only animals who can describe nausea.

There is some interesting preliminary work being carried out now on the relationship between the perception of chemotherapy as threat or as challenge and nausea as a symptom of distress. The research is based on the view that there are selective responses of the pituitary-adrenal and the sympathetic-adrenal systems to different psychological conditions (Frankenhaeuser, 1980; Frankenhaeuser, Lundberg, & Forsman, 1980). The pituitary-adrenal activation or catecholamines are associated with negative feelings like dread and distress; and the sympathetic-adrenal activation or cortisol is associated with feelings of alertness and readiness for action. In some ways, these activations fit the potentially negative synergistic effect of the "double-bind" deadlock perceived by some patients receiving chemotherapy. The sympathetic adrenal system is activated when the subject is challenged in attempting to control a threat, while the pituitary-adrenal system is activated with the endure ("bear it") response. One 19-year-old patient profoundly described his chemotherapy as the ally that was killing him while his Hodgkins Disease was a comfortable, friendly enemy. It remains to be seen how important cognitive factors and altered states of consciousness are in suppressing or abating the arousal of the adrenal-cortisol system, thereby altering the level of various gut stimulating neuropeptides and changing the degree of nausea experienced by patients. An aspect of this work is currently being done at Duke Medical Center (Bedell, Sowers, & Cotanch, 1988).

As more projects are launched to better understand the mechanisms of nausea and vomiting, better pharmacological and behavioral therapies are being discovered to help improve patient comfort. Future lines of research in the area of patient comfort, specifically with management of nausea, will probably focus on the following:

1. More accurate tailoring of the drug and/or behavioral intervention to the needs and desires of the patient. The focus will be on issues of control to the patient, and ways to increase self-care behaviors for those patients who desire proactive, participant health care.

2. More accurate assessment techniques such as self-reports and observer rated scales. There is also a need for technological interventions such as a way to hardwire the gut in order to get an accurate readout of changes in gut motility in response to antiemetic and behavioral interventions. We also need more accurate assessment of neuropeptide assays and their relationship to patients' mood states, levels of nausea, functional status and quality of life. We can then derive what may be

the most effective coping strategy for a particular patient. Better yet, we can develop a list of effective coping strategies and pharmacological interventions from which patients can select the one(s) that are most appropriate for their lifestyles.

[31]

Postchemotherapy Nausea and Vomiting

Verna A. Rhodes, Phyllis M. Watson,
Mary H. Johnson, Richard W. Madsen,
and Neils C. Beck

In the United States, 85% of the estimated 985,000 new cases of cancer annually will receive antineoplastic treatment, i.e., surgery, chemotherapy, radiation, and/or a combination of these (Silverberg, 1988). For cancer patients undergoing treatment, nausea and vomiting are symptoms that disrupt activities and worsen the quality of life. They are by far the most distressing and uncomfortable side effects of antineoplastic chemotherapy agents with a high emetic potential (Rhodes, Watson, Johnson, Madsen, & Beck, 1987; Rhodes & Watson, 1987a). These two symptoms cause some people to withdraw from treatment that has the potential for cure.

Supported by US PHS Grant #5 R01 NU01154-02.

Management of these disruptive side effects varies and has a limited scientific basis. Clinical assessment of nausea and vomiting has usually focused on the occurrence of vomiting, i.e., the frequency and number of episodes. Nausea, however, is a subjective phenomenon unobservable by another (Rhodes & Watson, 1987b; Rhodes & Watson, 1987c; Rhodes, Watson, & Hansen, 1988; Watson, Rhodes, & Germino, 1987). Few data collection instruments that measure separately the patient's experience of nausea and vomiting and his symptom distress are reported in the literature. In fact, the Rhodes Index of Nausea and Vomiting (INV) Form 2 is the only tool that measures the individual components of nausea, vomiting, and retching (Grant, 1987; Rhodes & Watson, 1987a; Rhodes, Watson, & Johnson, 1983, 1984, 1985, 1986; Rhodes, Watson, Johnson, Madsen, & Beck, 1987).

Although the notion of a pattern in the occurrence of these symptoms has been alluded to (Kennedy, Packard, Grant, & Padilla, 1981; Morrow, 1984; Scofield, 1980; Zenk, 1980), limited information is available about frequency, duration, and distress; most of what we know is in general terms of incidence and onset. In a recent pilot study ($N = 32$) of two successive cycles of postchemotherapy side effects, the investigators found that patterns of posttherapy nausea differed from patterns of posttherapy vomiting, and there were individual differences in the patterns of posttherapy nausea and posttherapy vomiting (Rhodes, Watson, & Johnson, 1985). These data provide additional evidence for the view that the frequency, duration, and distress of nausea and the amount, frequency, and distress of vomiting differ for different patients.

The study reported here, which was part of a larger study of patterns of nausea and vomiting among cancer patients, was designed to delineate patterns of postchemotherapy symptom occurrence and distress during six consecutive cycles of six initial antineoplastic drug protocols; to analyze the relationship of the duration, frequency, and distress from nausea and vomiting to specific antineoplastic drug protocols; and to determine whether the experience of nausea and vomiting changed with repeated cycles of chemotherapeutic drug administration.

Orem's Self-Care Deficit Theory of Nursing was used to guide the study (Orem, 1985). According to this theory, the self-care act is comprised of three elements: the demand or requisite for action, the measure or method appropriate to meet that action, and the capacity for action (self-care agency). The experience of nausea, vomiting, and retching produces new demands for self-care actions. How patients respond to these new demands depends upon their knowledge of what to do when the symptom occurs, their skill, and their capacity to perform the needed self-care measures.

An important aspect of self-care agency is the patient's ability to regulate the response to the symptoms of nausea, vomiting, and retching that produce new demands and require changes in usual self-care practices. The Parallel Process Model proposed by Leventhal and Johnson (1983) suggests that fear or distress behaviors and coping behaviors are the result of two parallel psychophysiological processes that occur simultaneously in the human response to a stressor or threatening event. This model emphasizes the differences between the occurrence of a symptom (e.g., vomiting) and the emotional response to its occurrence (distress). In addition, it is useful in explaining patients' coping responses and the effectiveness of nursing interventions to influence coping or distress responses.

METHOD

Subjects

This time-series study comprised 309 adult patients scheduled to receive an initial six cycles of antineoplastic chemotherapy. The sample was stratified by antineoplastic drug groups and data were collected at 25 sites in two Midwestern states. Study methods have been described in more detail elsewhere (Rhodes, Watson, Johnson, Madsen, & Beck, 1987; Rhodes & Watson, 1987a). Study criteria required subjects to be starting an initial course of therapy (i.e., first chemotherapy ever) with one of the selected drug combinations; receiving the same drug combinations and dosages for a minimum of six cycles of antineoplastic drug therapy; and without intervening complications (e.g., surgery, pathological fractures).

Subjects who met the criteria for inclusion were invited to "participate in a study to determine how they felt." When gaining consent and providing protocol instructions, the words "nausea and vomiting" were omitted to prevent subjects from focusing on these symptoms. Subjects were followed for six cycles of first-time chemotherapy. Figure 31.1 outlines the procedure followed for each cycle.

Data Collection Tools

Five reliable and valid data collection tools were used: The State-Trait Anxiety Inventory (STAI), the Behavior Manifestations of Anxiety Checklist (BMAC), the Adapted Symptom Distress Scale (ASDS) Form 1, the Subject Description Record (SDR), and the Rhodes Index of Nausea and Vomiting (INV) Form 2.

FIGURE 31.1 Nausea, vomiting, and anxiety in cancer patients: Procedure flow sheet.

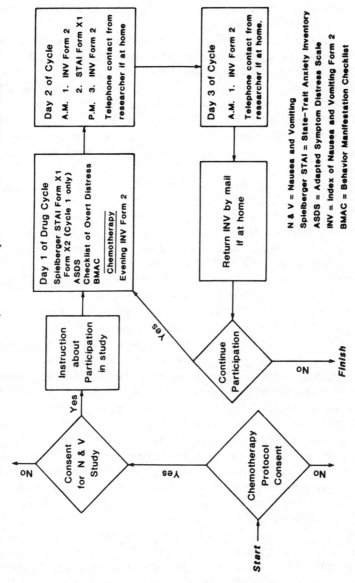

The STAI, developed by Spielberger, is a 20-item, 4-point Likert-type self-report scale for two distinct anxiety concepts, state anxiety (a transitory anxiety) and trait anxiety (a more stable constant anxiety proneness). The STAI has proven useful in clinical situations (Spielberger, Gorsuch, & Lushene, 1970).

The BMAC consists of 10 items that describe the overt behavioral manifestations of anxiety. Each item is scored depending on whether the behavior is or is not observed. Operational definitions for each behavior are provided. The BMAC has been adapted by Beck, Rhodes, and Watson (Rhodes & Watson, 1987a) for this population from a tool developed and used by Fuller, Endress, & Johnson (1978) in a study of anxiety manifested during an aversive health examination. The authors established interrater reliability of .82 to 1.0 for each item (Rhodes & Watson, 1987a).

The ASDS Form is a 16-item, 5-point Likert-type paper and pencil instrument that measures the degree of discomfort reported by patients in relation to their symptoms. The instrument yields a total score for symptom distress, a total score for nausea, a total score for vomiting, and subscale scores for each symptom. The ASDS was adapted by Rhodes and Watson (Haylock, 1987; Rhodes & Watson, 1987a; Rhodes, Watson, & Johnson, 1984) from the Symptom Distress Scale (SDS) originally developed by McCorkle and Young (1978).

The Rhodes INV Form 2 is an 8-item, 5-point Likert-type pencil and paper tool that measures the patient's perception of the duration of nausea, frequency of nausea, distress from nausea, frequency of vomiting, amount of vomiting, distress from vomiting, frequency of retching or dry heaves, and distress from dry heaves (Rhodes, Watson, & Johnson, 1983, 1984, 1985, 1986). The INV total score provides a total symptom experience score for the patient. Symptom experience is defined as the configuration of the frequency, amount, duration, and degree of distress caused by each symptom. Subscale scores can be derived from the INV for nausea experience, vomiting experience, and the experience of dry heaves, as well as total symptom distress, defined as the perceived worry or upset caused by the experience of each symptom. Subscale scores can also be derived for nausea occurrence, vomiting occurrence, the occurrence of dry heaves, and the total occurrence of the three symptoms. Symptom occurrence is the configuration of frequency, amount, and duration of the symptom. Factor analysis supports the three experience subscales as unique and distinct. Psychometric properties have been reported in detail elsewhere (Rhodes & Watson, 1987a; Rhodes, Watson, Johnson, Madsen, & Beck, 1987).

The SDR was designed by Watson and Rhodes to collect the following data from the hospital record: demographics, including age, sex, and geographic location; drugs ordered, including dosage, route, time, and date; drugs administered, including date, time, route, and dosage; and complications experienced during therapy (Rhodes & Watson, 1987a; Rhodes, Watson, Johnson, Madsen, & Beck, 1987).

RESULTS AND DISCUSSION

Patterns of Posttherapy Symptom Experience, Occurrence, and Distress

Contrary to frequent language usage, patients not only can distinguish between the individual symptoms of nausea, vomiting, and retching but can also differentiate the components of each, i.e., frequency, amount, and duration (occurrence) and distress. In fact, in this study, four unique patterns of symptom experience, symptom occurrence, and symptom distress were identified. Detailed information on these is found elsewhere (Rhodes & Watson, 1987a; Rhodes, Watson, Johnson, Madsen, & Beck, 1987).

Nausea Experience Four patterns of posttherapy nausea experience were noted (see Figure 31.2). The predominant pattern was minimal nausea; 71% of the sample had little or no nausea during the 48 hours postchemotherapy. This group apparently responded well to antiemetic drugs. However, 29% of the sample fell into three distinct drug resistant patterns: peak nausea experience ($n = 34$); latent nausea experience ($n = 39$), and intense nausea experience ($n = 18$). Those who reported a high level of discomfort at about 24 hours and lower levels before and after that were considered to experience a peak nausea pattern. Those who experienced latent or delayed nausea reported a low level of discomfort for the first 12–36 hours followed by increasing discomfort. Those who experienced intense or sustained nausea reported a prolonged high degree of discomfort. Individuals who experienced either intense or latent nausea continued to have high levels of nausea at 48 hours posttherapy.

Nausea Distress Four patterns of nausea distress, as distinct from nausea experience, are delineated in Figure 31.3. Although 82% of the sample had low levels of distress from nausea, the remaining 19% fell into three distinct patterns: delayed nausea distress; sustained nausea distress; and declining nausea distress, or a decrease in discomfort

FIGURE 31.2 Nausea experience patterns.

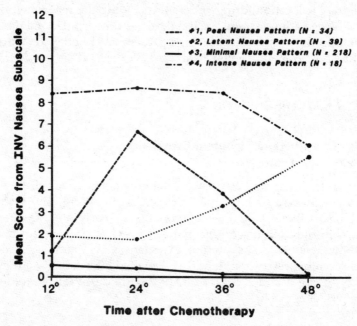

Reprinted from *Oncology Nursing Forum*, 14(4), 1987, with permission from Oncology Nursing Press, March 1988.

from an initial high level. Subjects with all these patterns still experienced some distress at 48 hours posttherapy; scores of the sustained
group remained high.

Vomiting Experience Of the four patterns of posttherapy vomiting experience, the predominant pattern was minimal vomiting, experienced
by 83% of the sample ($n = 257$) (see Figure 31.4). This group had little
or no vomiting in the 48 hours posttherapy. In spite of aggressive antiemetic therapy, however, 17% of the sample experienced severe vomiting postchemotherapy. Still, it is important to note that a larger percentage of the sample experienced nausea than vomiting.

Vomiting Distress Although four patterns of vomiting distress were
seen (see Figure 31.5), the predominant pattern was minimal distress;
82% of the sample ($n = 254$) had little or no vomiting distress in the 48
hours posttreatment. Five percent of the sample ($n = 16$) experienced
the latent distress pattern, i.e., a low amount of vomiting distress for
the first 36 hours, increasing abruptly at 48 hours. Patients in the re-

FIGURE 31.3   Nausea distress patterns.

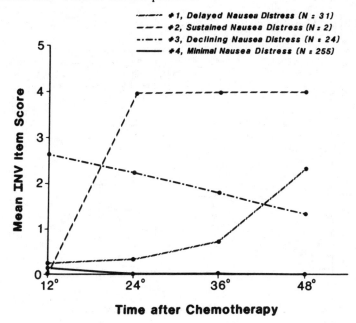

FIGURE 31.4   Vomiting experience patterns.

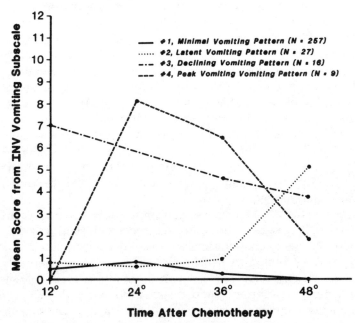

Reprinted from *Oncology Nursing Forum*, 14(4), 1987, with permission from Oncology Nursing Press, March 1988.

FIGURE 31.5 Vomiting distress patterns.

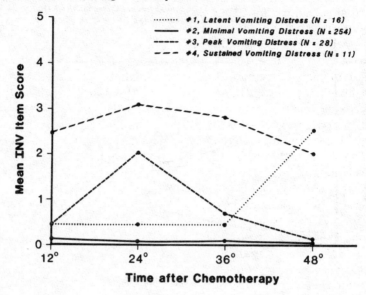

maining two patterns, peak and sustained vomiting distress, had the highest distress at 24 hours with lesser amounts at 36 and 48 hours.

Symptom experience was related to specific antineoplastic drug combinations. The emetic protocols were those containing cyclophosphamide (Cytoxan), doxorubin (Adriamycin), and platinum. Different patterns of symptom experience, symptom occurrence, and symptom distress were identifiable. These patterns were similar to the patterns of postchemotherapy occurrence of symptoms and postchemotherapy distress that have been reported previously (Rhodes & Watson, 1987a; Rhodes, Watson, Johnson, Madsen, & Beck, 1987). In addition, antiemetic drug-resistant patterns of symptom experience were identified. Nausea was disruptive to more people than vomiting. Some individuals indicated that nausea never went away.

As expected, there was a strong, statistically significant relationship ($r = .94$, $p < .001$) between symptom occurrence (stressor) and the distress response. Generally, subjects who experienced minimal nausea, vomiting, and retching also had limited distress. Of special interest, however, were those patients for whom there was not a logical match between symptom occurrence and distress. For example, 27 persons who experienced minimal distress experienced a pattern of peak occurrence of symptoms. In addition, 3 individuals with sustained symptoms experienced minimal distress, whereas 2 patients who experienced minimal symptoms experienced peak distress.

One question is "Why didn't the 27 patients who experienced peak symptoms have a greater amount of distress in response to the symptom experience?" Perhaps the fear/distress response was blocked by an intervention such as accurate sensory information, which reduced fear and facilitated the use of coping behaviors. The 2 individuals who experienced the reverse—minimal symptoms with peak distress—may have expected to experience symptoms (inaccurate sensory preparation) and consequently experienced distress in spite of the absence of symptoms. The authors recommend that patients on antineoplastic drug and antiemetic regimens similar to those which caused few symptoms in this study be told to expect little or no nausea and vomiting posttherapy. In other words, the predominant symptom experience should provide the basis for the development of sensory information protocols. It is important to differentiate informed consent procedures from the procedures designed to prepare patients for chemotherapy. Incorrect messages may be conveyed to patients in attempts to "inform" them of every possible side effect.

Although total symptom experience did not increase with each successive cycle, symptom experience at 12 hours posttherapy did increase with each successive cycle. Strategically timed nursing interventions should be planned to prevent or alleviate this discomfort (Rhodes, Watson, Johnson, Madsen, & Beck, 1987). Consideration must be given to the time sense in planning interventions. In addition, chemotherapy administration oncology nurses should make every effort to provide proactive interventions to alleviate symptom distress prior to, during, and following the first cycle of chemotherapy, since the cycle 1 symptom experience for both nausea and vomiting is predictive of cycles 2 through 6.

Neither pretherapy state nor trait anxiety was predictive of posttherapy nausea, vomiting or retching. This validates findings in two previous studies (Rhodes, Watson, & Johnson, 1985, 1986). However, posttherapy state anxiety was positively correlated with posttherapy nausea and vomiting. This anxiety can serve as a stimulus to use self-care behaviors in an attempt to alleviate nausea and vomiting. Nurses can increase their repertoire of interventions merely by listening or gently inquiring what people do to help themselves feel better. Self-care logs or journals may be useful to gather data.

An important finding is that the pretherapy Adapted Symptom Distress Scale (ASDS) score was predictive of posttherapy nausea and vomiting (Rhodes, 1987a; Haylock, 1987). This self-report tool can be completed by the patient and quickly scored by the nurse in the outpatient facility before chemotherapy. The ASDS score can then help the nurse plan proactive interventions to relieve individual symptom distress.

Antiemetic drugs have been administered in hundreds of patterns and in numerous drug combinations (Rhodes & Watson, 1987a; Rhodes, Watson, & Simms, 1985, 1988). The effectiveness of antiemetics in reducing nausea is not known (Rhodes, Watson, & Simms, 1985, 1988). Until studies of specific antiemetics, using reliable and valid measurement tools, are available, nurses can encourage regular dosage rather than prn, start medications the day prior, and continue for 48 hours or longer as needed.

As members of a caring profession, nurses are concerned with how patients feel. However, our nursing practice has frequently focused on the presence or absence of patients' signs and symptoms, rather than on patients' response to the occurrence of symptoms. Symptoms, strictly speaking, are not observable; i.e., although vomiting occurrence (a sign) can be noted, the distress caused by the occurrence can be noted only by the patient. A major function of nursing practice is to assist patients in coping with symptom distress. To do so, the amount of mental or physical anguish or upset (distress) the patient perceives or feels must be assessed. Assessment tools that measure symptom occurrence and symptom distress separately should be used to inform us of the patient's response to the occurrence. Future experimental research should be conducted on nursing interventions to enhance coping behaviors to reduce distress and promote self-care.

[32]

Nausea and Vomiting in Pregnancy

Colleen K. DiIorio and Donna J. van Lier

Although nausea and vomiting are common complaints of women during the first trimester of pregnancy, few investigators have explored these phenomena. Our knowledge of the characteristics of nausea and vomiting has come primarily from anecdotal reports of pregnant women. The historical lack of interest in nausea and vomiting during pregnancy may be traced to the fact that health care professionals and patients alike have viewed these symptoms as mild and so short lived as not to be of any great importance for study. This attitude, however, has now been eroded by a changing society and the changing health care expectations of women. Today, more pregnant women work outside the home in demanding positions and those who opt to stay at home shoulder jobs previously assumed by members of the extended family. Both lifestyles leave little time for illness.

Retrospective studies including those by Brandes (1967), Fairweather (1968), Jarnfelt-Samsioe, Samsioe, and Velinder (1983), and Klebanoff, Koslowe, Kaslow, and Rhoads (1985) confirm that 50–80% of all pregnant women suffer from nausea or vomiting during pregnancy. Studies conducted by Tierson, Olsen, and Hook (1986) and Jarnfelt-Samsioe et al. (1983) provide additional information on the frequency and duration of the symptoms and the relationship of the nausea and vomiting to pregnancy outcomes. Only a few studies have explored the use of relief measures and their effectiveness in controlling the symptoms, but the findings of these studies, including those by Voda and Randall (1982), Abney (1985), Wilson (1984), and DiIorio (1985), have provided preliminary information on relief.

259

The present study, building on these preliminary studies, examined the experience of nausea and vomiting in a small group of pregnant women using a longitudinal design so as to increase the accuracy of accounts of symptoms and attempts to control them. Specifically, the study looked at patterns of nausea and vomiting (NVP) experienced by women during the first trimester of pregnancy, factors associated with the onset of nausea and vomiting, accompanying symptoms, the frequency with which nausea and vomiting were reported to interfere with concentration or activity, interventions women used to control NVP, and their effectiveness.

METHOD

The sample consisted of pregnant women who were experiencing nausea and/or vomiting during the first trimester of pregnancy. They were recruited from a nurse-midwife/obstetrician practice in a large metropolitan area and from volunteers obtained through snowball sampling (i.e., referrals from earlier subjects). Only individuals meeting the following criteria were asked to participate: minimum of a 12th grade education; married or in a stable relationship; desired pregnancy; between the sixth and twelfth week of pregnancy; accurate date of the last menstrual period or an early ultrasound to determine the length of gestation; English as the first language; and willingness to participate.

Subjects were asked to keep a daily record of their nausea and vomiting for 7 consecutive days, 24 hours a day. For each hour that a participant experienced nausea or vomiting, she was requested to rate the severity of the nausea; identify any precipitating factors and any interventions tried; and rate the helpfulness of the interventions. Space was also available to record daily food intake as well as other symptoms experienced during the day. At the end of each day and the 7-day period, subjects were asked to respond to several short answer questions on their experience with nausea and vomiting.

RESULTS

The 19 subjects who composed the sample ranged in age from 23 to 38 years with a mean age of 31 years. The mean number of years of schooling of subjects was 16.1 years and of their husbands, 16.5 years. Eighteen of the participants worked outside the home and most of these (79%) held full-time jobs. The majority of subjects were nonsmokers; those who did smoke indicated that they had reduced the number of cigarettes smoked after becoming pregnant, now averaging between 2 and 15 per day. Most subjects said they never consumed alcohol or had stopped drinking since becoming pregnant. Those who continued to drink did so only on occasion.

The majority of the women (58%) were pregnant for the second or third time. Most could identify the week when symptoms of nausea and vomiting first became apparent, the majority indicating that this was between the fourth and the sixth week. This is consistent with other studies (Biggs, 1975; Fairweather, 1968), as is the finding that 37% of the subjects experienced nausea and vomiting before confirmation of the pregnancy by a positive pregnancy test (DiIorio, 1985). For several women, nausea and vomiting were a cue to consider the possibility of pregnancy.

The mean number of days the participants reported nausea was 6.25, with a range of 2 to 7 days. The actual hours in which nausea was experienced during the sampled week ranged from between 14 and 122, with an average of 51 hours per week.

Subjects were asked to rate their nausea on a 3-point scale: mild, moderate and severe. Mild nausea was defined as an awareness of nausea without interference with activity or concentration; moderate nausea was nausea that interfered somewhat with the ability to perform tasks and/or concentrate; and severe nausea was defined as inability to perform tasks or to concentrate.

Women rated most of the nausea they experienced as mild (an average of 28 hours per week). However, they experienced moderate nausea an average of 18 hours per week and severe nausea an average of 5 hours per week. When moderate and severe nausea, both of which interfere with concentration and the ability to perform tasks, were combined, it was found that subjects complained of debilitating nausea an average of 23 hours per week. Subjects complained of symptoms as little as 8.3% of the week to as much as 73% of the total hours in the week. When these percentages were recomputed based on a 16-hour standard waking day, the percentages increased to between 12 and 108%. (The one subject who complained of nausea 108% of the time suffered from nausea more than 16 hours per day.) The average percentage of time in which symptoms were experienced, using a 16-hour basis, was 46%. This means that the average woman in this sample experienced nausea approximately half of her waking day. Only a few subjects complained of vomiting, however, and then only on a few occasions.

The nausea of pregnancy is often referred to as "morning sickness" since it has been reported that most women suffer from these symptoms in the morning (Brandes, 1967; DiIorio, 1985). Jarnfelt-Samsioe et

TABLE 32.1 Factors Contributing to Nausea, Rank-ordered by Reported
Frequency

Factor	Frequency	Percent
Fatigue	87	46.0
Eating	34	18.0
Hunger	19	10.1
Odors	13	6.9
Waking	6	3.2
Driving	5	2.6
Stress	5	2.6
Indigestion	5	2.6
Headache	4	2.1
Thoughts of food	3	1.6
Vitamins	3	1.6
Feeling too warm	3	1.6
Exercise	2	1.1

al. (1983), however, found that women complained of several different
patterns of nausea and the findings of the present study support this.

Nausea patterns showed marked variance and unpredictability from
day to day. For some women, there was a morning peak period of nausea, and for others a peak period in the evening. In other cases nausea
was present throughout the day, with a peak period occurring in either
late morning, afternoon, or early evening. Finally, some women had
no specific peak period.

The major factor contributing to nausea was fatigue, which precipi-
tated 46% of all reported instances of nausea (see Table 32.1). Other
major factors were eating, hunger, and odors; the latter two are commonly thought to be major factors contributing to nausea and vomiting
in pregnant women. Other factors that were cited by one or two subjects included driving to work, stress, thoughts of food, and vitamins.

Eating produced the most severe nausea with an average rating of
2.32 on a 3-point scale. Fatigue and odors produced less severe nausea
(1.63 and 1.61) and hunger produced only moderate nausea (1.42).

It was surprising to find that fatigue played such a major role in the
onset of nausea since fatigue had not been identified as a precipitating
factor in any of the previous studies. However, Voda and Randall
(1982) did note that women who were asked about their experience
with nausea during the first trimester reported that fatigue seemed to
contribute to the onset of symptoms. One reason fatigue was not iden-

tified in other studies may have been that the resulting nausea is not as severe as the nausea following eating and therefore women often forget the connection between nausea and fatigue.

Subjects in this study complained of fatigue on an average of 4 out of the 7 days sampled. Only one subject said that she did not experience fatigue during the week. Over the week, subjects experienced an average of 17 hours of fatigue, which was considerably less than the hours of nausea experienced. However, since the focus of the study was on nausea and vomiting, it is possible that subjects did not record all symptoms of fatigue.

In some subjects the relationship between fatigue and nausea was quite striking; in others it was less, but it does appear that in certain women the two symptoms may have a significant relationship, and interventions to reduce fatigue might also be helpful in alleviating nausea.

Lying down was the relief measure these women used most frequently, reported by 18 of the 19 subjects (see Table 32.2). Interestingly, although lying down or resting to relieve nausea is noted in the literature, it is not emphasized as an important intervention. Crackers, toast, and small frequent meals are the three most commonly cited relief measures (Myles, 1985; Neely, 1980). Crackers and toast were used as interventions by 14 subjects, and 7 subjects noted that they tried to eat small frequent meals. Fewer individuals tried carbonated beverages, milk, teas, or medicines. Measures recommended in the literature but not used by this group of subjects include Vitamin B, low fat intake, high carbohydrate intake, increased protein intake, hypnosis, and acupressure.

Subjects were asked to rate the helpfulness of each measure they tried on a 5-point rating scale, where 1 = worse, 2 = no change, 3 =

TABLE 32.2 Frequency of Use of Recommended Measures to Control Nausea in Pregnancy

Recommended Measures	Number of Women Using Measure	Percentage of Sample
Lying/sitting down	18	94.7
Crackers/toast	14	73.7
Small, frequent meals	7	36.8
Carbonated beverages	7	36.8
Milk	2	10.5
Herbal tea	1	5.3
Medicine	1	5.3

mild relief, 4 = moderate relief, and 5 = complete relief. Relief measures were classified into five categories: eating, lying down, sitting, activity, and medicine; and thus it was possible to determine which type of measure proved most helpful (see Table 32.3). Eating made the symptoms worse 14.4% of the time and subjects experienced no change in nausea 23.7% of the time; however, most of the time (combining mild, moderate, and complete relief) the nausea improved (61.7%), and eating completely relieved the symptom 12.7% of the time. In contrast, lying down did not appear to be as effective in controlling nausea. Although the nausea worsened only 1.3% of the time, lying down had no significant impact on the intensity of the nausea over 60% of the time. Although used less frequently as a relief measure, sitting down proved to be more helpful than either eating or lying down; over 80% of the time the nausea improved with this measure.

Resting (the combination of lying down and sitting) was less effective than eating something (62% reported relief of their nausea with eating while 47% reported improvement with resting). Given that fa-

TABLE 32.3 Reported Degree of Helpfulness of Relief Measures to Control Nausea[a]

	Degree of Helpfulness				
Relief Measures	Worse	No Change	Mild Relief	Moderate Relief	Complete Relief
EATING					
%	14.4	23.7	27.9	21.1	12.7
n	34	56	66	50	30
LYING DOWN					
%	1.3	62.5	14.9	10.2	10.9
n	2	92	22	15	16
SITTING DOWN					
%		13.1	42.1	31.5	13.2
n		5	16	12	5
ACTIVITY					
%		33.3	46.6	13.3	6.6
n		5	7	2	1
MEDICINE					
%			100		
n			1		

[a]Table entries are percentage and frequency of times relief measure resulted in each degree of helpfulness

tigue was a major factor contributing to nausea, it is unclear why eating was more effective than resting in bringing relief. This finding may be due, however, to the nature of the sample—women who worked could not lie down for extended periods of time. Lying down seemed to help most on weekends or in the evening when subjects had the opportunity to lie down and nap without interruption.

Most of the primiparas indicated that the experience of nausea was worse than they had anticipated. The multigravidas were divided on this question. As expected, some had experienced more severe nausea with previous pregnancies and therefore were somewhat relieved that the present experience was not as bad. Others, however, found that the present experience was worse than previous pregnancies and acknowledged the distressing nature of the situation.

The major factors that interfered with the ability to use relief measures were work—not being able to lie down; insomnia—not getting enough sleep, which produced a vicious cycle; travel—particularly to work; child care responsibilities, which interfered with resting; shopping and cooking, which forced some women to confront food that they could not tolerate; and decreased appetite, which interfered with eating frequent meals.

Lifestyle changes necessitated by the symptoms included changing eating habits, reducing physical and outside activities, sleeping more, avoiding food or shopping, changing work schedules, and being less productive.

DISCUSSION

These findings point to the need to provide symptomatic women with permission to rest. Among today's active women, a need for rest is often interpreted as being lazy, unproductive, and uncooperative. The pregnant woman may be her harshest critic. Nurses can provide pregnant women with a new interpretation of rest: rest as a form of therapy that may actually relieve nausea and allow for continued performance in work or home life.

Women may need assistance from health care professionals, husbands, and bosses in restructuring their daily activities to ensure proper rest. Only one of these women said her husband was doing more of the housework since her pregnancy began. Most women indicated they were giving up social or other activities to cope with symptoms of nausea and to obtain needed rest.

Some women reported that keeping a diary was useful in determining which interventions were most helpful. Other women had difficulty completing the diary because of strong aversions to the thought of food. Nonetheless, the diaries were helpful in discerning the factors associated with nausea and patterns of nausea.

Recognition of the varying types of nausea may prove helpful in counseling pregnant women—for example, now we know that interventions based on a morning sickness model would not be helpful for women who experience other patterns of nausea.

The interventions these women used relieved the nausea most of the time. However, this finding must be interpreted with caution because the subjects did not or could not use relief measures every time they experienced nausea. Many women waited hours before trying an intervention or tried several that were ineffective before finding one that provided relief. Women at work had difficulty using relief measures such as lying down or eating small frequent meals throughout the day. The subjects also noted that nothing worked for 38% of the time sampled.

In conclusion, the results of this study clearly demonstrate the distressing nature of nausea and its multidimensional impact on the lifestyles of active modern women. We are continuing the study of this phenomenon and hope further studies will reveal more effective means of coping with the symptoms.

[33]

The Effectiveness
of Self-Care Actions
in Reducing "Morning Sickness"

Melinda L. Jenkins and Barbara J. Shelton

Morning sickness remedies are common in lay and professional literature (David & Doyle, 1976). However, only limited research has been
done to assess the effectiveness of nonpharmacological methods to
reduce the discomfort of morning sickness (DiIorio, 1985; Minturn &
Weiher, 1984; Voda & Randall, 1982). The study reported here was a
retrospective survey of pregnant women to describe which self-care actions (Orem, 1980; Woolery, 1983) they used and which they perceived
as effective in reducing morning sickness.

METHOD

Questionnaires were completed by 55 consenting pregnant women enrolled in four different central Missouri prenatal classes. Data collected
included (a) the incidence and timing of symptoms of morning sickness, (b) the degree of distress experienced, (c) sources of information
about remedies, (d) nonpharmacological self-care actions used to reduce symptoms, and (e) perceived effectiveness of the self-care actions
used. Background information on the sample included socioeconomic
status and relevant lifestyle characteristics.

The subjective experience of morning sickness was measured by a
portion of the Adapted Symptom Distress Scale, Form 1, by Rhodes,
Watson, and Johnson (1984), adapted from McCorkle (1981). Reliability

and validity for the instrument were reported in 1984. Symptoms measured were (a) frequency and severity of nausea and vomiting, (b) appetite or desire for food, (c) worry, and (d) fear. Symptoms were scored on a Likert-type scale from 1 (least distress) to 5 (most distress). The total distress score for each subject was calculated by summing an individual's response to each of the seven symptoms. The range of possible scores was 7 to 35.

RESULTS

A majority of the subjects (64%) were pregnant for the first time; most (76%) were younger than age 30. Over half had 13-16 years of education. The total sample contained two subsamples: subjects who did not experience morning sickness in the current pregnancy ($n = 18$), and subjects who did ($n = 37$). Of subjects without morning sickness, 5 had experienced distress in a previous pregnancy. Of the women with morning sickness, 2 had had previous pregnancies without morning sickness. The subsample without morning sickness tended to be multigravidae and older. Similar percentages were reported in both subsamples for planned pregnancy, marital status, and education. Smoking, partner smoking, and intake of alcohol or caffeine drinks were not related to morning sickness.

Of those subjects experiencing morning sickness, over 60% noted the onset of distress between 3 and 6 weeks past the last menstrual period; 46% experienced morning sickness for 6 weeks or less, 35% for 7 to 10 weeks and 19% for more than 11 weeks. Morning sickness did not always occur early in the morning; about a third had symptoms at various times throughout the day. The duration of symptoms varied greatly, from less than 5 minutes to 9 hours or more (see Table 33.1).

The subjective experience of morning sickness was measured by the Adapted Symptom Distress Scale. The symptoms reported most often were "nausea or sickness at my stomach most or all of the time" and "I had to force myself to eat." For most subjects, nausea was of medium severity, though 7 said: "I was as nauseated as I could possibly be." The degree of distress caused by specific symptoms is shown in Table 33.2. Over a third of the women with morning sickness did not vomit. Fear and worry were the least common symptoms. Subjects' total distress scores ranged from 9 to 30, with a mean of 17.22. Seven women with total scores greater than 20 were identified as a subset having a high degree of distress.

Self-care actions attempted by subjects fell into the three broad categories of manipulating diet, adjusting behavior, and seeking emotional

TABLE 33.1 Timing of Symptoms of Morning Sickness

Time Factor	Number of Subjects ($N = 37$)	Percent
Onset		
< 3 weeks past LMP	2	5.4
3-4 weeks past LMP	11	29.7
5-6	12	32.4
7-8	7	18.9
9-10	3	8.1
11-12	2	5.4
Hours duration		
< 5 min.	4	10.8
5-15 min.	9	24.3
16-30 min.	3	8.1
31-45 min.	2	5.4
46-60 min.	2	5.4
1-2 hrs.	3	8.1
3-4 hrs.	1	2.7
5-6 hrs.	2	5.4
7-8 hrs.	2	5.4
> 9 hrs.	3	8.1
Varied	6	16.2
Weeks duration		
< 1	3	8.1
1-2	3	8.1
3-4	3	8.1
5-6	8	21.6
7-8	8	21.6
9-10	5	13.5
> 11	7	18.9
Time of day		
As soon as I wake up	2	5.4
After rising, before breakfast	7	18.9
Between breakfast & lunch	2	5.4
Between lunch & midafternoon	0	0.0
Between midafternoon & supper	2	5.4
After supper, before bedtime	2	5.4
After going to bed	0	0.0
All day long	9	24.3
Varied	13	35.1

TABLE 33.2 Degree of Symptom Distress Caused by Morning Sickness

Symptom	Low (score 1)	Medium (score 2 or 3)	High (score 4 or 5)
	Degree of Distress[a]		
Nausea Frequency	0	23	14
Nausea Severity	0	30	7
Vomiting Frequency	13	19	5
Vomiting Severity	14	18	5
Appetite	2	20	15
Worry	12	21	4
Fear	20	15	2

[a]Entries in the table are the number of subjects reporting that the specified symptom caused low, medium, or high distress.

support. The six most effective self-care actions were (a) getting more rest, (b) eating several small meals rather than three big ones, (c) avoiding bad smells, (d) avoiding greasy or fried food, (e) avoiding cooking, and (f) receiving extra attention from the partner. The rank order of the 29 actions included in the questionnaire and the five actions added by subjects is shown in Table 33.3.

All five remedies ranked most effective by the most distressed women were among the six ranked most effective overall. This fact reinforces the identification of the top self-care actions as most effective. "Eating several small meals" was the action subjects said they would recommend most often to a friend.

Trial and error, noted by over 50% of the 37 subjects with morning sickness, was the most common source of information about morning sickness. The woman's mother and an experienced friend were each noted as information sources by 13.5% of the women. About 10% received information from a doctor, 8% from a nurse practitioner, 5.5% from a nurse, and about 3% from a midwife.

DISCUSSION

This study provides a basis for educating women in the use of self-care actions to reduce morning sickness. Over 70% of the women surveyed were able to manage morning sickness by adjustments in resting, eating, cooking, and increased emotional support. Interestingly, the particular actions identified in this study are not usually mentioned in the literature.

TABLE 33.3   Effective Self-Care Actions to Reduce Morning Sickness

Rank	Self-Care Action	Number of Subjects Reporting "used, helped" ($n = 37$)
1.	Getting more rest	27
2.	Eating several small meals rather than three big ones	24
3.	Avoiding bad smells	21
4.	Avoiding greasy or fried foods	21
5.	Avoiding cooking	19
6.	Receiving extra attention from my partner	19
7.	Avoiding spicy foods	18
8.	Eating whenever I felt nauseous	16
9.	Keeping myself busy	16
10.	Sharing experiences with another mother	13
11.	Eating bland foods, such as baked potato or hot cereal	13
12.	Eating dry toast or crackers before getting out of bed in the morning	11
13.	Cutting down on drinks with caffeine (cola, tea, coffee)	9
14.	Getting more exercise	9
15.	Cetting down on alcoholic drinks	8
16.	Eating a midnight snack	8
17.	Taking some prescription medicine	7
18.	Having someone tell me that morning sickness is normal and will go away soon	7
19.	Eating hard candy	6
20.	Avoiding certain other foods	6
21.	Drinking some herbal tea	5
22.	Taking vitamins at bedtime	5
23.	Cutting down on smoking	5
24.	Avoiding riding in the car	4
25.	Taking extra B vitamins	3
26.	Eating more acid foods, such as grapefruit or pickles	3
27.	Avoiding vitamins with iron	2
28.	Avoiding liquids with meals	1
29.	Taking some over-the-counter medicine	0
Added by subjects in short answer:		
*	Trying to ignore	1
*	Drinking Pepsi	1
*	Keeping my tummy full	1
*	Papaya chewables	1
*	Eating certain foods	2

Nurses in contact with pregnant women have the opportunity to promote self-care by discussing simple lifestyle adjustments that may help to reduce the discomfort of morning sickness. Women who cope well with the early problem of morning sickness may more readily adapt to the further physical, emotional, and social changes of pregnancy.

Further investigation is needed in this area. A large cross-sectional survey of pregnant women to identify self-care actions would improve the list of effective remedies. The safety and effectiveness of specific methods need evaluation through clinical research.

In the meantime, nurses should give pregnant women the list of effective self-care actions identified in this study as soon as pregnancy is confirmed and encourage them to try other lifestyle changes to decrease their discomfort. Further, nurses should keep records to determine which actions work best with clients, or ask groups of women to try a specific action and let them know how it works.

[34]

Relieving Nausea:
A Discussion

Laura E. Pole

The studies on nausea presented in this volume make it clear that nausea and vomiting continue to be significant problems in the oncology and obstetric patient populations. It is possible to identify patterns of nausea and vomiting in these populations; further, patients are able to identify, choose, and evaluate interventions to relieve nausea and vomiting.

Rhodes and colleagues' study indicates that certain chemotherapy protocols are associated with the occurrence of nausea and vomiting as well as with antiemetic resistance patterns. By identifying those chemotherapy protocols, clinical nurses can identify patients who are at risk for developing chemotherapy-related nausea and vomiting. This at-risk profile can then be used in classifying the acuity of chemotherapy patients and the amount of nursing time needed to care for them. The at-risk classification can also serve to determine whether patients should be treated in an ambulatory chemotherapy clinic or as inpatients.

Some patients in Rhodes and colleagues' study experienced peak nausea, vomiting and distress after 12 hours following treatment. Most chemotherapy patients have been discharged home by 12 hours. It is important, then, that clinicians provide patients with measures to manage these symptoms at home. Additionally, a symptom assessment log or the Rhodes Index of Nausea and Vomiting-II filled out at home would help to describe the occurrence of symptoms and evaluate the effectiveness of interventions.

In the Rhodes et al. study, patients' pretherapy expectations of symptoms were associated with posttherapy symptom occurrence and distress. This points to the importance of assessing the patient's expectations about nausea and vomiting when the treatment is explained to the patient. The nurse should begin teaching at that time, to correct false assumptions and help the patient identify symptom control measures.

Finally, the Rhodes et al. study indicates that posttherapy anxiety is linked to posttreatment nausea and vomiting. Heretofore, many behavioral interventions have been used mainly to alleviate anticipatory nausea and vomiting. Behavioral interventions are nursing time intensive, and it may be advisable to identify patients with posttreatment anxiety and nausea/vomiting. Those symptomatic patients would be candidates for posttherapy antianxiety measures.

Rhodes et al. pose interesting questions for further study. For instance, clinical researchers could develop and test the effectiveness of relief measures targeted to specific patterns of nausea and vomiting, particularly antiemetic resistance patterns. Further research is also needed to determine what factors contribute to peak symptom occurrence during the hours immediately after treatment. Finally, since pretreatment expectations appear to be related to symptom occurrence, nurses should determine the impact of measures such as pretreatment teaching on expectations and subsequent symptoms.

Pregnancy-related nausea and vomiting were studied by DiIorio and van Lier and by Jenkins and Shelton. Both found that in many cases, symptoms were not limited to the classic morning time. In fact, peak periods of nausea and vomiting were identified, and often symptoms persisted throughout the day. It may be helpful to use a self-report tool such as the tool used by DiIorio and van Lier to help pregnant women identify their own patterns of nausea and vomiting as well as the effectiveness of relief measures. The nurse could then encourage women to schedule work/rest/activity periods around times when symptoms are most likely to occur.

Now that there are more data pointing to the effectiveness of certain measures to relieve pregnancy-related nausea and vomiting, perhaps nurses could develop a booklet on self-care of these symptoms. Rest and diet, in particular, appear helpful in reducing symptoms of morning sickness. Patients could be encouraged to incorporate short rest periods into their days, and nurses could collaborate with a nutritionist to write a booklet on a balanced diet with small frequent meals, possibly high in vitamin B.

Friends and relatives of pregnant women who themselves have experienced morning sickness are valuable sources of information and emotional support. Perhaps the clinician could sponsor a class for women in early first trimester, and each participant could bring along an "experienced" friend or relative and discuss ways to manage pregnancy-related nausea and vomiting. The wise nurse will also record suggestions mentioned in class and note those that are frequently identified as helpful.

Though the studies on nausea and vomiting in this volume do not focus on interventions, study results do lead us to consider the use of certain measures to manage these symptoms. Behavioral interventions such as progressive muscle relaxation, biofeedback, imagery, or music therapy may help to alleviate postchemotherapy anxiety, a significant factor in the Rhodes et al. study. Mast, Meyers, and Urbanski (1987) have written a series of articles on how to implement relaxation techniques, which may be a useful self-learning tool for the nurse. Women experiencing pregnancy-related nausea and vomiting may find relief by using these techniques as well. Many of these behavioral techniques can be initiated independently by the nurse, and if taught correctly, can give the client skills useful in other distressing situations. Nurses must remember, however, that behavioral interventions can be nursing time intensive and should perhaps be reserved for patients identified as at risk for symptom occurrence.

Another noninvasive, nonpharmacologic measure to consider in relief of nausea and vomiting is Transcutaneous Electrical Nerve Stimulation (TENS). A study by Saller, Hellenbrecht, Buhring, and Hess (1986) and a study in progress by this author indicate that TENS may be useful in alleviating chemotherapy-related nausea and vomiting, including delayed nausea and vomiting. Side effects from using TENS are negligible, and with further study it may prove to be an acceptable, helpful relief measure.

More research is needed to verify and expand upon the information generated by the studies on nausea and vomiting. To begin, the nurse clinician can take time to systematically document assessments of patterns of nausea and vomiting seen in the clinical area, and to report the effectiveness of interventions based on these assessments. I encourage nurses in the clinical area to link up with nurse researchers in developing studies of the work you do so well—promoting patient comfort.

References On Nausea

Abney, S. E. (1985). *Nausea and vomiting during pregnancy.* Unpublished manuscript.

Andrykowski, M. (1988). Defining anticipatory nausea and vomiting: Differences among cancer chemotherapy patients who report pretreatment nausea. *Journal of Behavioral Medicine, 11,* 59–69.

Armstrong, D., Pickel, V., John, T., Reis, D., & Miller, R. (1981). Immunocytochemical localization of catecholamine synthesizing enzymes and neuropeptides in area postrema and medical nucleus tratus solitarius of rat brain. *Journal of Complete Neurology, 196,* 505–517.

Beck, A. (1979). *Cognitive therapy and the emotional disorders.* New York: Meridian Co.

Bedell, C., Sowers, K., & Cotanch, P. (1988). *Anxiolytic effect of relaxation on chemotherapy side effects.* Unpublished manuscript, Duke University, Durham.

Biggs, J. S. G. (1975). Vomiting in pregnancy: Causes and management. *Drugs, 9,* 229–306.

Bouson, H., & Wang, S. (1949). Functional localization of central coordinating mechanism for emesis in cat. *Journal of Neurophysiology, 12,* 305–313.

Brandes, J. M. (1967). First-trimester nausea and vomiting as related to outcome of pregnancy. *Obstetrics and Gynecology, 30,* 427–431.

David, M. L., & Doyle, E. W. (1976). First trimester pregnancy. *American Journal of Nursing, 76,* 1945–1948.

DiIorio, C. (1985). First trimester nausea in pregnant teenagers: Incidence, characteristics, intervention. *Nursing Research, 34,* 372– 374.

Fairweather, D. V. I. (1968). Nausea and vomiting in pregnancy. *American Journal of Obstetrics and Gynecology, 102,* 135–175.

Frankenhaeuser, M. (1980). Psychobiological aspects of life stress. In S. Levine & H. Cuisen (Eds.), *Coping and health.* New York: Plenum Press.

Frankenhaeuser, M., Lundberg, U., & Forsman, L. (1980). Dissociation between sympathetic-adrenal and pituitary-adrenal responses to an achievement situation characterized by high controllability: Comparison between Type A and Type B males and females. *Biological Psychology, 10,* 79–91.

Fuller, S. S., Endress, M. P., & Johnson, J. E. (1978). The effects of cognitive and behavioral control and coping with an aversive health examination. *Journal of Human Stress, 4,* 18–25.

Grant, M. (1987). Nausea, vomiting, and anorexia. *Seminars in Oncology Nursing, 3*(4), 277–286.

Haylock, P. J. (1987). Breathing difficulty: Changes in respiratory function. *Seminars in Oncology Nursing, 3*(4), 293–298.

Jarnfelt-Samsioe, A., Samsioe, G., & Velinder, G. (1983). Nausea and vomiting in pregnancy—a contribution to its epidemiology. *Gynecologic and Obstetric Investigation, 16,* 221–229.

Karksu, S., Toth, L., Kiraly, E., & Jancso, G. (1981). Evidence of the neuronal origin of brain capillary acetylcholinesterase activity. *Brain Research, 206*(1), 203–207.

Kennedy, M., Packard, R., Grant, M., & Padilla, G. (1981). Chemotherapy- related nausea and vomiting: A survey to identify problems and interventions. *Oncology Nursing Forum, 8*(1), 19–22.

Klebanoff, M., Koslowe, P., Kaslow, R., & Rhoads, G. (1985). Epidemiology of vomiting in early pregnancy. *Obstetrics and Gynecology, 66,* 612–616.

Leventhal, H., & Johnson, J. E., (1983). Laboratory and field experimentation: Development of a theory of self-regulation. In Woolridge, Schmitt, Skipper, & Leonard (Eds.), *Behavioral science and nursing theory* (pp. 189–262). St. Louis: The C. V. Mosby Co.

Lundberg, U., & Frankenhaeuser, M. (1980). Pituitary-adrenal and sympathetic-adrenal correlates of distress and effort. *Journal of Psychosomatic Research, 24,* 125–130.

Mast, D. E., Meyer, J., & Urbanski, A. (1987). Relaxation techniques: A self-learning module for nurses: Units I, II, III. *Cancer Nursing, 10,* 141–147, 217–225, 279–285.

McCarthy, L., & Bouson, H. (1983). Animal models for predicting antiemetic drug activity. In J. Laszlo (Ed.), *Antiemetics and cancer chemotherapy.* Baltimore: Williams and Wilkins.

McCorkle, R. (1981). Non-obstructive measures in clinical nursing research. In R. Tiffany (Ed.), *Cancer nursing update* (pp. 20–26). London: Bailliere Tindal.

McCorkle, R, & Young, K. (1978). Development of a symptom distress scale. *Cancer Nursing, 1,* 373–378.

Minturn, L., & Weiher, A. W. (1984). The influence of diet on morning sickness: A cross-cultural study. *Medical Anthropology, 8,* 71–75.

Morrow, G. R. (1984). The assessment of nausea and vomiting: Past problems, current issues, and suggestions for future research. *Cancer, 53,* 2267–2278.

Morrow, G., Arseneau, J., & Ashbury, R. (1982). Anticipatory nausea and vomiting in chemotherapy patients. *New England Journal of Medicine, 306,* 431–432.

Myles, M. (1985). *Textbook for midwives* (10th ed.). Edinburgh & London: Churchill Livingstone.

Neely, C. A. (1980). Antepartal nursing care. In Aladjem (Ed.), *Obstetrical practice.* St. Louis: The C. V. Mosby Co.

Orem, D. E. (1980). *Nursing: Concepts of practice* (2nd ed.). New York: McGraw-Hill.

Orem, D. E. (1985). *Nursing: Concepts of practice* (3rd ed.). New York: McGraw-Hill.

Rhodes, V. A., & Watson, P. M. (1987a). Final Report of US PHS Grant #5 R01 NU01154-02.

Rhodes, V. A., & Watson, P. M. (Guest Eds.). (1987b). Introduction. *Seminars in Oncology Nursing, 3*(4), 241.

Rhodes, V. A., & Watson, P. M. (1987c). Symptom distress—the concept: Past and present. *Seminars in Oncology Nursing, 3*(4), 242–247.

Rhodes, V. A., Watson, P. M., & Hansen, B. (1988). Patients' descriptions of the influence of tiredness and weakness on self-care abilities. *Cancer Nursing, 11*(3), 186–194.

Rhodes, V. A., Watson, P. M., & Johnson, M. H. (1983). A self-report tool for assessing nausea and vomiting in chemotherapy. (Letter to the editor). *Oncology Nursing Forum, 10*(1), 11.

Rhodes, V. A., Watson, P. A., & Johnson, M. H. (1984). Development of reliable and valid measures of nausea and vomiting. *Cancer Nursing, 7*(1), 33–41.

Rhodes, V. A., Watson, P. M., & Johnson, M. H. (1985). Patterns of nausea and vomiting in chemotherapy patients: A preliminary study. *Oncology Nursing Forum, 12*(3), 42–48.

Rhodes, V. A., Watson, P. M., & Johnson, M. H. (1986). Association of chemotherapy-related nausea and vomiting with pretreatment and posttreatment anxiety. *Oncology Nursing Forum, 13*(1), 41–47.

Rhodes, V. A., Watson, P. M., Johnson, M. H., Madsen, R. W., & Beck, N. C. (1987). Patterns of nausea, vomiting, and distress in patients receiving antineoplastic drug protocols. *Oncology Nursing Forum, 14*(4), 35–43.

Rhodes, V. A., Watson, P. M., & Simms, S. (1985). *A cookbook of antiemetics: A preliminary report.* University of Missouri-Columbia.

Rhodes, V. A., Watson, P. M., & Simms, S. (1988). *The effectiveness of antiemetics in selected chemotherapy drug protocols.* Submitted for publication.

Saller, R., Hellenbrecht, D., Buhring, M., & Hess, H. (1986). Enhancement of the antiemetic action of metoclopramide against Cisplatin-induced emesis by Transdermal Electrical Nerve Stimulation. *Journal of Clinical Pharmacology, 26,* 115–119.

Scofield, R. P. (1980). *Patterns of illness behavior and patient perception of nausea during chemotherapy.* Unpublished doctoral dissertation, University of Arizona, Tucson.

Scott, J., & Huskisson, E. (1976). Graphic representation of pain. *Pain, 2,* 175–184.

Silverberg, E. (1988). Cancer statistics, 1988. *Ca–A Cancer Journal for Clinicians, 38*(1), 5–22.

Spielberger, C. D., Gorsuch, R., & Lushene, R. (1970). *STAI: Manual for the State-Trait Anxiety Inventory (Self-Evaluation Questionnaire).* Palo Alto, CA: Consulting Psychologists Press, Inc.

Tierson, F. D., Olsen, C. L., & Hook, E. B. (1986). Nausea and vomiting of pregnancy and association with pregnancy outcome. *American Journal of Obstetrics and Gynecology, 155,* 1017–1022.

Tursky, B., Jammer, L., & Friedman, R. (1982). The pain perception profile: A psychophysical approach to the assessment of pain report. *Behavior Therapy, 13,* 376–394.

Voda, A. M. & Randall, M. P. (1982). Nausea and vomiting of pregnancy: "Morning sickness." In C.M. Norris (Ed.), *Concept clarification in nursing* (pp. 133–165). Rockville, MD: Aspen Systems Corporation.

Watson, P. M., Rhodes, V. A., & Germino, B. B. (1987). Symptom distress: Future perspectives for practice, education, and research. *Seminars in Oncology Nursing, 3*(4), 313–315.

Wilson, J. N. (1984). *Crackers for morning sickness: A survey of self-care behaviors initiated by pregnant women for relief of the symptoms of morning sickness.* Unpublished manuscript.

Woolery, L. F. (1983). Self-care for the obstetrical patient: A nursing framework. *Journal of Obstetrical and Gynecological Nursing, 12,* 33–37.

Zenk, B. A. (1980). *The relationship of selected factors to nausea and vomiting in chemotherapy patients.* Unpublished doctoral dissertation, University of Arizona, Tucson.

Part V

COMFORT

[35]

Perceptions of Comfort
by the Chronically Ill
Hospitalized Elderly

Joan Hamilton

The elderly person who is hospitalized in a chronic geriatric setting may very well spend his or her remaining months or years in that institution. What are his or her needs and concerns? A review of the gerontological nursing literature reveals that most studies examine the needs of the elderly from the caregiver and expert perspectives (e.g., Havens, 1980; Heller, Bausell & Ninos, 1984; Talbot, 1985; Tilquin et al., 1980). Studies examining the comfort needs of institutionalized elderly from their perspective at this time in their lives are not found. What helps the institutionalized elderly become comfortable? What does "comfort" mean to them?

Researchers have developed their own definitions of comfort depending on the purpose of the research, and subjects have been asked about predetermined categories of comfort, based on how the researcher defined the word (e.g., Francis & Munjar, 1975; Freihofer & Felton, 1976; Hampe, 1975; Sohl, 1987; Strauss et al., 1984; Watson, 1979).

It is equally important to explore comfort from the patient's perspective. The nursing profession has only begun to explore comfort in this way. Very little research has been conducted from the patient's (Hamilton, 1985) or the consumer's (Morse, 1983) perspective. Thus, while comfort is a word nurses use in their daily practice to describe a nursing measure, an outcome, and a goal, from the patient's perspective its meaning remains vague and abstract.

The purpose of this study, therefore, was to explore the meaning and attributes of comfort as perceived by elderly patients in a chronic geriatric setting. Specifically, the elderly were asked what they meant by comfort, what contributed to or detracted from their comfort, and how they might become more comfortable. The goal was to identify the comfort needs of patients so that nurses would be better able to provide comprehensive comfort.

METHOD

The study was conducted in a 284-bed chronic geriatric hospital in southwestern Ontario, Canada. The sample included 30 patients located in all units throughout the hospital. All patients were over 65 and fluent in English. Only patients determined by the head nurses to be able to respond to interview questions were included as potential subjects. Interestingly, only 28% of the patient population met this criterion. This points to the possibility that the ideas and needs expressed by elderly who can communicate verbally with nurses are not necessarily the concerns of those who cannot.

This study was built on an earlier study of the meaning and attributes of comfort conducted with 14 terminally ill cancer patients in a palliative care unit (Hamilton, 1985). The findings of that study led the author to investigate other populations in different settings in order to determine if the dimensions of comfort were similar for them or if new dimensions emerged. The semistructured comfort interview guide designed for the previous study was used in this study, with one additional question (no. 4). The interview guide is given below.

Comfort Interview Guide

1. When someone asks you, "Are you comfortable?" what does that mean to you?
   Probes: To you, what does comfort mean?
   How would you define your comfort?
2. What kinds of things help you feel comfortable?
   Probes: What helps you get comfortable?
   What helps you become comfortable?
3. What gets in the way of your being comfortable?
   Probes: What interferes with your being comfortable?
   What hinders your being comfortable?

4. Keeping in mind that we want to learn how we can make living here better, what kinds of things do you think would help you become more comfortable?

   Probes: What kinds of things would help you get more comfortable?

   What kinds of things would help you feel more comfortable?

RESULTS

Five recurring themes emerged from the patients' responses to the four questions on the comfort interview guide; comfort was described in terms of disease process, self-esteem, positioning, approach and attitudes of staff, and hospital life (see Table 35.1).

Disease Process

Patients who discussed comfort in terms of their disease process talked about pain, bowel function, and disabilities. Several of them defined comfort in terms of the presence or absence of pain and reported that being in pain interfered with being comfortable. Pain medication was the only intervention that helped them get comfortable. They reported that better pain management would help them become more comfortable.

Most of the individuals who mentioned pain in discussing comfort also related comfort to other physical concerns such as bowel function. Regular bowel function, they said, helped them get comfortable. When asked what interfered with comfort, many subjects discussed their illnesses or the loss of function of legs, arms, hands, or eyes. Several patients described their physical losses as disabilities.

Self-Esteem

A number of patients defined comfort in terms of how they were feeling, their adjustment, or whether they felt they were independent and worthwhile. Faith in God, doing things themselves, feeling relaxed, and feeling useful aided them in being comfortable.

These elderly reported that being troubled and trying to go through changes in life interfered with comfort. They also reported being afraid—for example, being afraid of senility.

Patients believed that they would be more comfortable if they were able to make decisions about their lives and if they were better in-

TABLE 35.1 Patient-reported Dimensions of Comfort

	Contributing Factors	Detracting Factors	Proposed Factors That Would Increase Comfort
DISEASE PROCESS			
	Achieving pain relief	Physical disabilities	Better pain management
	Regular bowel function	Being in pain most of the time	
SELF-ESTEEM			
	Faith in God	Adjusting to change	Being informed
	Being independent	Being afraid	Taking part in decision making
	Feeling relaxed		
POSITIONING			
	Individually adjusted seating	Unsuitable wheelchairs	Returning to bed when requested
	Sitting correctly	Sitting too long	Better seating arrangements
	Independent movement in chair	Sliding down in the chair	
	Returning to bed on request	Being unfavorably positioned in bed	
APPROACH & ATTITUDES OF STAFF			
	Friendly, kind people	A lack of caring & understanding	Caring, understanding nurse encouraging patients to help themselves
	Empathetic nurses	Inaccessible nurses	
	Reliable nurses	Fragmented care	Continuity of staff
HOSPITAL LIFE			
	Homelike surroundings	Tolerating the system	New content in activities
	Social & family contacts	Boredom with activities	Continuation of personal aids
	Structured leisure activities	A lack of privacy	More enjoyable mealtimes
	Informal pastimes	Unpleasant mealtime atmosphere	Having some privacy
	Occupational & physical therapy		

formed about their care and better informed about who would be looking after them on the next shifts.

Positioning

A number of patients defined their comfort with reference to their position in bed, in the chair, and in the wheelchair, and on the basis of
whether they believed they were positioned correctly. A comfortable
position was defined as one from which they could carry out desired
activities.

When asked what helped them get comfortable, patients responded
that they often required the assistance of another person, most frequently the nurse, in order to get comfortable. Wheelchairs that fit, sitting up straight, being able to move about in the wheelchair to relieve
pressure, and being able to get back to bed all helped them get comfortable.

Factors detracting from comfort included wheelchairs that were too
big, too small, not functioning adequately, or difficult to manipulate;
and cushions and foot rests that were not properly placed. Patients
also reported that being kept up too long and not put back to bed
when they requested interfered with comfort. Patients also said that
slipping and sliding down in the chair and being positioned in bed on
a side that they did not want to be on interfered with comfort.

Factors they thought would increase their comfort included being returned to bed when requested and having improved chair and wheelchair positions.

Approach and Attitudes of Staff

Relationships with hospital staff, usually nurses, made up a large component of comfort. For many patients, their relationship with the nurse
was the only way in which they defined their comfort. These patients
defined comfort by descriptors that pertained to rapport with the nurse
and how they felt in the nurse's presence. Descriptors included feeling
cared for by the nurse, having a nurse who cared, and having a nurse
who showed interest and feelings toward the patient. Friendly, caring,
and kind people helped patients feel comfortable, as did empathetic
nurses, nurses who understood the patient's situation. Patients reported that some nurses were nicer, kinder, and more caring than
others.

The reliability of nurses—for example, following through on interventions, and doing what they said they were going to do—also helped the patient feel comfortable.

A lack of caring, understanding nurses frustrated and upset patients. They reported that some nurses lacked understanding of their situation and their basic physical care needs. Some patients said that nurses were inaccessible, they had to wait for them, and they were hard to get hold of. These elderly patients also suggested that care was fragmented: nurses would leave the room in the middle of bathing, changing, or positioning to respond to other requests.

It was clear from these responses that the nurse had a big impact on patient comfort. Proposed improvements included caring, understanding nurses, nurses who encouraged independence, and having the same nurse for a few days in a row.

Hospital Life

For some elderly, comfort reflected aspects of living in the hospital—feeling at home, being well fed, being able to wear their own clothes, having personal items in their room, and generally being in surroundings that were pleasant, enjoyable, and homelike.

Social and family aspects of hospital life, including going to the cafeteria for tea and talking socially with nurses, family, and friends, contributed to comfort. Patients reported that social interaction and family involvement were important components of comfort and said that structured leisure activities and informal pastimes also helped them feel comfortable. Interestingly, going to occupational and physiotherapy was noted by patients as helping them feel comfortable because this encouraged them and helped them feel they were improving.

Many patients reported that hospital life, inflexible routines, and boredom with repetitious structured activities interfered with their comfort. Many were fed up with sharing their personal space. Lack of privacy, inability to be alone at any time, and the necessity to cope with sharing were frustrating.

Food was an important aspect of life, and a number of these elderly reported dissatisfaction with meals—not with the food, but with the event.

Proposed ways to increase comfort included new structured leisure activities, ability to continue one's own hobbies and interests, more effective patient aids (e.g., an intercom system instead of a call bell system), improved efficiency and atmosphere at mealtimes, and more physical privacy as well as personal space.

DISCUSSION

It is evident from these findings that nurses have a great impact on patients' comfort, and the rapport nurses develop with patients can affect various dimensions of comfort. Many of the findings suggest that it is not hospital-wide interventions or complex changes that are needed to help the elderly get comfortable; rather, what matters are the one-to-one interactions between the nurse and the patient.

These are not new and startling ideas. They are common sense, reflecting the basic beliefs and practices of nurses. These findings indicate that nurses need to continue working to put our beliefs into practice.

The elderly in this study indicated that if patients in geriatric hospitals are to be comfortable, nurses need to be friendly, caring, and empathetic. It is clear from their descriptions that these people want a nurse who is gentle and kind with them, and who has an understanding of what they are experiencing. We need to try and look at life through the eyes of our patients so that we gain insight into what their needs mean to them.

The findings reinforce the idea that continuity and consistency of nursing staff are important to patients; these patients wanted to be told who their nurse would be in the shifts to come and if they would have the same nurse the next day. This emphasizes just how great an impact the nurse has on the patient's life.

The findings suggest that nurses working in this kind of setting need to develop patient assignments that provide consistent staff over time. Also, nurses should work with patients to identify needs and preferences, and organize their shifts and tasks so that they do not have to leave a patient in the middle of something. Identifying patient preferences and trying to accommodate them can also reduce a patient's sense of the inflexibilities of hospital routine.

These findings also indicate that nurses need to be more accessible. When patients call out or put on their call bells, nurses need to respond promptly. Although it was not articulated during these interviews, one wonders if the failure to get a quick response to a request was disturbing because it reinforced patients' feelings of powerlessness and helplessness.

Nurses need to set mutual goals and develop plans of care with patients. These elderly wanted to be better informed and more involved in their care and care planning. They wanted to make more decisions about their personal care and the home in which they now lived. Nurses can easily involve the patient in decision-making, especially about the patient's own care, though forgetful patients may need to be reminded of long- and short-term plans and goals.

The elderly's desire to be more involved in their care is closely linked to their need to feel independent and worthwhile. During the interviews, many of these elderly patients said that they would be more comfortable if the nurse worked with them to help them be more independent, and if the nurse encouraged them to do more for themselves. Encouraging patients to do things independently is often time-consuming and may be frustrating for both patient and nurse, yet we need to work harder to do this. These elderly also articulated a desire for the nurse to get them involved in hospital affairs so that they could feel more worthwhile. When we are organizing the Christmas party, when we are providing feedback about new meals and activities, or when a new bed is being considered for purchase, we need to ask ourselves how the patient can participate.

These elderly reported that they had very little social interaction with or acknowledgment from nurses on or off their units. This greatly interfered with patients' comfort, as the nurse's acknowledgment of them as people rather than as patients was very meaningful. Nurses can easily integrate this behavior into their practice. Instead of talking over the patient to another nurse about what happened on the weekend or what a grandson is doing in school, the nurse can talk directly to the patient. And, *each* time the nurse passes the patient in the hall, lounge area, or cafeteria, the nurse should address the patient, even though the nurse may have seen that patient several times during the day. This kind of acknowledgment is just as important when patients are alone as when they are with family and friends. The nurse should also recognize that sitting and talking with patients about their family, hobbies, or favorite soap opera can be meaningful.

Many patients in this study reported that a lack of privacy interfered with their comfort, and they were approached without consideration of their personal space. Patients wanted designated rooms and times so they could be alone and uninterrupted. Nurses need to remind themselves that these patients are rarely alone and they need some privacy and personal space. This may just mean leaving them uninterrupted for a period of time in the four-bed room. Acknowledging to the patient that he or she feels a need for time alone gives the patient permission to request it.

The elderly in this study reported that mealtime lacked a social atmosphere. Also, patients wanted to be out of bed and fed at their own pace. These findings suggest a need to identify regimes acceptable to both patient and nurse.

It was also not surprising to find that seating and positioning were important since the literature has referred to this association with comfort. Further investigations need to examine positioning practices and options. Why do the elderly want to lie down three hours after they get up? Do nurses believe the elderly should sit up in the same chair for most of the day? Are wheelchairs appropriately adjusted but not comfortable? Are assessment and evaluation of this aspect of care being communicated within the health care team? Seating and positioning concerns need to be investigated further so that nurses are better able to respond to individual needs.

The dimensions of comfort discussed here are key issues identified by the elderly. However, one must remember that the criteria for this study eliminated 72% of the hospital's population because they were not able to verbalize their needs and thoughts. Findings from this study cannot be generalized to those patients, for their needs and concerns may in fact differ.

When the findings of this study were compared to the findings of the initial study with terminally ill cancer patients, it was discovered that dimensions of comfort were very similar. Four major themes emerged from that study: patients spoke of comfort in terms of relationships with others, the illness and associated symptoms, feelings, and immediate surroundings. Positioning was discussed by a few cancer patients, but it did not emerge as a major theme as it did in the present study.

The clear message from this study is that comfort is multidimensional and it means different things to different people. Besides the physical component of comfort, the elderly view their comfort in terms of their relationships, environment, and feelings. Verifying patients' comfort needs from their perspective is imperative for meeting those needs. The nurse must clarify the meaning of comfort with the particular individual and individualize care.

Further studies could help to develop a concept of comfort that is precise and readily communicable. This study indicates that if we care enough to ask the questions, we can get concrete answers about comfort from patients, which expands the possibilities for appropriate nursing interventions.

[36]

Comforting the Child in Pain

Nancy Olson Hester

A primary responsibility of nurses is to alleviate children's pain. Sadly, however, nurses frequently respond inappropriately to children in pain, leaving them to suffer needlessly. Nurses fail to comfort children because they are missing information from an important source: the child. In a recent study by the author and a colleague (Hester & Barcus, 1986), children were asked to describe what they did to comfort themselves during pain experiences and what others could do to help them feel more comfortable. Interview excerpts from three children and two adolescents who participated in the study are presented here to illustrate what children use as comfort strategies and what they perceive as caring behaviors by others. Ways in which nurses can use this information to comfort children in pain are suggested.

METHOD

Twenty-eight child and adolescent informants (13 boys and 15 girls), ages 5 through 15, were interviewed about their pain experiences. The semistructured interview focused on building rapport with the child and asked about present and past pain experiences, the child's response to pain, and behaviors of others during the experience. Interviews were tape-recorded and then transcribed. In particular, children were asked, "What do you do when you hurt?", "What would you like to do when you hurt?" and "What do others do for you when you hurt?", "What would you like others to do for you when you hurt?", "What don't you want others to do for you when you hurt?"

290

COMFORT STRATEGIES: THE CHILD'S PERSPECTIVE

The comfort strategies described by these children and adolescents are illustrated by excerpts from interviews with five children: Mandy, David, Cindy, Jeffrey, and Alice.

Mandy Mandy, five years old (the youngest child interviewed for this study), was hospitalized for the insertion of a new stomach tube. She had had extensive experience with pain, having been hospitalized 35 other times. Mandy tried to alleviate her pain by taking medicine, telling her mother, "I'm hurting," being with her mother and father, and holding her teddy bear or her Cabbage Patch doll. Two of these strategies were under Mandy's control: she could tell someone she hurt, and she could hold her toys. However, she could not take medicine by herself, nor could she determine when her parents would be present. Hence, two implicitly caring behaviors were to give Mandy medicine when she was experiencing pain and to get her parents for her or have someone else stay with her. When asked what others could do for her, Mandy replied, "Hold my hand" and "Tell me to do something." Children of all ages in this study mentioned wanting someone to hold their hand. "Tell me to do something" is a distraction technique. While Mandy described this as something others could do to comfort her, older children in the study tried various forms of distracting themselves to alleviate pain.

David Hospitalizations were not new to David. By seven years of age, he had undergone 12 surgeries and approximately 30 hospitalizations. At the time of the interview David had been surgically treated for a bowel obstruction. An expert on pain, David said he cried when he hurt; he also would call for his mother. Although he said he would tell the nurses that he hurt, he said he couldn't tell the doctor. When asked why, he replied that he didn't have a doctor and added, "He never comes by."

David said that when he hurt he would throw his stuffed toys or blanket. But he quickly added that he would hold the special blanket he'd brought from home.

For David, nurses were the dispensers of medicine for his pain. Interestingly, like many of these children, David stressed that nurses could give him shots "through the IV" to relieve pain. A shot was acceptable only if it went through the IV; the children were frightened by intramuscular shots. One older girl described an IM shot as totally unacceptable and said she would consider it only if she were in really bad pain.

Like Mandy, David wanted someone to hold his hand; but he did not want anyone to poke him. Other children also perceived touching or poking places that hurt as noncaring behavior. Unfortunately, assessment techniques often include touching or poking painful areas.

Being involved in decision making was important to David. When asked to explain, he said, "They have things to make choices about and they decide things I don't like."

Most of the children emphasized, explicitly or implicitly, their desire to participate in decisions. Interestingly, following the interview with David, the doctor informed the interviewer that David would have surgery the next day—David had yet to be informed.

Cindy   Cindy, 10 years old, had broken her leg while skiing. This was her first hospitalization. Other than minor acute illnesses, knee scrapes, and cuts, Cindy had had little experience with pain. She described her reaction to pain thus: "Well, sometimes I can control myself and not cry too much. But if it's really bad, I do cry and I hold really tight to somebody's hand or a bar or something and squeeze real hard and pull it. . . ."

Later, she stressed the importance of holding her mother's hand. Cindy would press the call button to tell the nurse when her pain was bad. In Cindy's view, caring behaviors included "staying with me, bringing me presents, making me feel good, talking with me, and checking me." Cindy did not want others to make a "big fuss" about her. "I don't mind . . . if they check and ask me if I need something to drink or eat," she said. "But I don't like it when they stay and fuss . . . and say, 'Do you want more blankets and all that? Do you want this and that closer to you? Do you want the T.V. on?'"

But Cindy did not want to be ignored either: "I don't like it when people ignore me when I'm in pain, like if I buzz the nurse and she says 'Can I help you?' and I ask for a pain pill and she says 'Well, I don't think we should give you one because you're a child.'"

Cindy was particularly angry at one nurse who had rejected Cindy's request for pain medication simply because she was a child. "I've had them all the time . . . I can take them," said Cindy. "It makes me mad because (she) should have been informed that I am able to take up to two pain pills at one time and I can take them up to three times a day."

Cindy was a very take-charge individual. Her family situation provides some insight into this. "When I have pain," said Cindy, "it's hard on my mom because my dad has MS. She has to take care of him. . . . So when I get hurt, I feel guilty sometimes because that puts more pressure on my mom and she has to work a lot harder to take care of both of us."

When asked whether she ever talked to her mother about feeling guilty, Cindy replied, "Yes, I told her that I'll be all right. I can take care of myself. Just take care of my dad and just check on me once in a while and I'll be fine." Thus, Cindy didn't just take care of herself; she also tried to protect her mother from being overburdened both physically and emotionally.

Jeffrey Thirteen-year old Jeffrey was hospitalized for an infected hip. Medically, Jeffrey had had little experience with pain; however, he described extensive experience with pain as a football player. Jeffrey expressed a lot of anger about his pain experiences and how poorly he had been treated. When asked how he felt when he was hurting, he replied, "Like screaming. I get mad, I mean, I have a bad temper anyway and when I hurt, I want to get revenge . . . I want to grab my doctor's neck."

Jeffrey was particularly angry about how health care professionals had treated him: "They gave me valium and demerol to calm me down . . . but they gave me that too late." He perceived a lack of sensitivity and understanding on the part of his doctor. "A doctor," he said, "has no way of knowing what it's going to feel like," and added, "The doctor likes to inflict pain."

According to Jeffrey, others did not treat him in a caring way. They ignored his requests for medication and lacked sensitivity to his pain. When asked what nurses did for him, he said, "It depends on how nice of a nurse. They bring pain killers and stuff. Most of them try and understand but it's hard for somebody else to understand that you're in pain. . . ."

Alice Alice, a 15-year-old high school student and the oldest subject in the study, was hospitalized for pancreatitis for 45 days. The lengthy hospital stay was related to surgical complications, including a crash. Alice recounted vividly both the pain and crash experiences. Although she did things to comfort herself during pain, she was very dependent on others to comfort her during most of her hospital stay. Alice told others when she had pain, and when she was on the respirator she wrote notes to the nurses about her pain and asked nurses for pain medication. Despite her age, holding a stuffed toy comforted Alice. Looking back on her hospitalization, she remembered, "I had a pink bear . . . he was there for me the whole time . . . he was my best friend . . . I slept on him . . . He was like a security blanket. . . . They let me take him into the operating room until they put me under . . . and when I woke he was there again and that was so nice."

Alice wanted lots of love and comfort from others, and especially wanted her mother with her. "Once in a while," she remembered, "I would ask my mom, 'Can I have a shot? Will you stay here while I go to sleep? Please stay here and don't leave until I've fallen asleep.' I want that secure feeling that someone's there for me just in case I can't sleep or I need somebody to talk to for a while."

Alice's mother did stay with her most of the time. Her mother, a nurse, also taught Alice to use imagery. "When I was going to sleep," said Alice, "she would help me think about the beach or . . . being in sunny weather or some comforting ideas that . . . helped me sleep. It helped me relax. . . ."

After learning to use imagery, Alice used it on her own. Alice nicely summarized what others could do to comfort her: "I'd say just mostly be there for you, talk to you, give you positive things to think about before you sleep. I mean you don't want to tell somebody that they're going to die now or anything. I think a good night's rest and a little loving are what you need, because when you have that feeling of love, the pain will go away."

Alice did not see her doctors as particularly helpful with her pain. They never talked to her about pain even though that was the reason why she entered the hospital. She didn't know which doctor had done one of her surgeries. She named one doctor "the phantom," which epitomized her perception of the doctors.

Alice did not like the feeling of being crowded by people or machines when she was in pain: "I had three IVs. I had my respirator machine. I had the EKG and all that. . . . The machines were so big and my room was so crowded . . . I couldn't stand all the machines around. . . . What really bugged me was the noise . . . when you're in pain, the last thing you want to hear is those beepers going off."

DISCUSSION

The interviews with these five children illustrate how children comfort themselves (see Table 36.1) and what they think others should and shouldn't do to comfort them (see Table 36.2). This information can be useful to nurses in comforting the child in pain.

Using a brief questionnaire such as the Pain Experience History (see Table 36.3), the nurse can gain information about a child's experience of pain and potential comfort strategies. Additionally, employing the interview technique (see Table 36.4), the nurse can identify characteristics of the child that might be important in dealing with the pain. For example, Mandy, one of the children in this study, was a fairly quiet child, who probably would not seek others when she was hurting.

TABLE 36.1 Child-initiated Comfort Strategies[a]

Age Range	Strategies
5-15	Take medicine Tell others Be with someone Hold hand or stuffed toy
6-7	Throw something or hit something
6-13	Do nothing
7-12 (Female)	Don't show it
7-13	Rub it, blow on it Wish it away Take charge or be in control
7-15	Talk to someone or stuffed animal Rest, lie down, or sleep Cry, scream, yell, say ouch Try and get my mind off it Think about hurt
10-12	Breathe deeply
10-13	Get bandaid or bandage Look at it
10-15	Try to relax Picture in my mind Feel sad, mad, unhappy, scared
11-15	Find a comfortable position

[a]Hester (1987, March & August)

Thus, in caring for Mandy, the nurse would need to initiate a conversation about the presence of pain. In contrast, Cindy, who was very much in charge of her situation, would seek out others and tell them what she wanted done.

From such an interview, the nurse can also identify how self-reliant a child is. Mandy, for example, was dependent on others, especially her mother, for comfort. She only identified a few comfort strategies and only two of these she did on her own. The nurse would need to observe a child like Mandy frequently, particularly when her mother was not present. In contrast, David preferred to be involved in decisions about his pain; in this study the nurse facilitated this by offering David realistic alternatives from which to choose. For example, the changing of his abdominal dressing was very painful. To engage Da-

TABLE 36.2 Children's Reports of Caring and Noncaring Behaviors for their Pain[a]

Caring Behaviors

Someone is with me.
Someone holds my hand.
They give me hugs and lots of loving.
They give me medicine.
They ask me how I feel.
They bring me things (presents, liquids, blankets).
They pay attention to me.
They ask me what I want.
They tell me to do something.
They put ice on it or rub it.
They come to visit.
They do things (such as take off bandage) so they don't hurt.
They feed me when I can't.
They talk to me.
They stay with me until I fall asleep.
They let me have my choice.
They try to understand.
They listen.
They make me do what I need to, to get better.
They calm me down.
They let me participate.
They comfort me.
They turn the lights down and/or keep it quiet.
They get my mom.
They have different ways of helping me.
They tell the nurse I hurt.
They prepare me for what will happen.
They come to check me.
They treat me.
They allow me privacy.
They try to help.
They cheer me up.
They give me hope.
They help me through the crisis.
They celebrate with me when I'm better.

Noncaring Behaviors

They don't do anything.
They weren't here (particularly "Mom").
They poke or touch me where it hurts.
They say I can't have a pain pill when I can.

They don't give me medicine or they give it too late.
They move me around and it hurts.
They ignore me.
They don't know what is going on.
They shout at me.
They tell me to relax.
They tell me "Boy, you're tough."
They get mad at me.
They take a long time to do a procedure.
They think they know when they don't.
They don't try to understand.
They lie.
They cut me down.
They give me shots (IM).
They don't let me participate.
They make a big fuss over me or they shower me with gifts.
They don't keep the noise down.

[a]Hester & Ray (1987, March & August).

TABLE 36.3   Pain Experience History[a]

Tell me what pain is.
Tell me about the hurt you have had before.
What do you do when you hurt?
Do you tell others when you hurt?
What do you want others to do for you when you hurt?
What don't you want others to do for you when you hurt?
What helps the most to take away your hurt?
Is there anything special that you want me to know about you when you hurt?
   (If yes, have child describe.)

[a]From "Assessment and management of pain in children," by N.O. Hester and C.S. Barcus, 1986, *Pediatrics: Nursing Update, 1*(14), pp. 1–8. Copyright © 1986 by Continuing Professional Education Center, Inc. Reprinted by permission.

TABLE 36.4   The Pain Interview[a]

Tell me about the hurt you're having now. (Elicit descriptors, location, cause.)
How much hurt are you having? (A little? A lot? The most you've ever had?)
What would you like me to do? (e.g., give medication, be with you).

[a]From "Assessment and management of pain in children," by N. O. Hester and C. S. Barcus, 1986, *Pediatrics: Nursing Update, 1*(14), pp. 1–8. Copyright © 1986 by Continuing Professional Education Center, Inc. Reprinted by permission.

vid's participation, the nurse gave David a choice between two types of dressing.

From the information gleaned in the interview, the nurse can identify strategies that the child already uses and that others can use. For example, Alice wanted her mother to be with her until she fell asleep. If Alice's mother were unavailable, the nurse could arrange to be with Alice or have another staff person or even a volunteer stay with her. For children like Mandy, who don't identify many ways to attain comfort, the nurse might try the strategies listed in Table 36.2 or teach the child one of the strategies listed in Table 36.1.

When the nurse observes the child using strategies identified in the interview, the nurse should then determine if the child is using that strategy to relieve pain. For example, when Cindy, in this study, pulled at the bars on her bed, the nurse checked to see if she was in pain.

The questionnaire and pain interview can be used to verify the presence of pain and to determine how the child wants others to intervene. Thus, the nurse can check out the use of a particular strategy with the child ahead of time. For example, Jeffrey definitely wanted medication for pain. For a child like this, prior to a procedure, the nurse could confirm the desire to have medication, describe the medication he would receive, and discuss what he should do if the medicine did not work.

The nurse should validate the effectiveness of the strategies used. One of the problems described by Jeffrey was ineffectiveness of his medication. Sometimes the medication was not effective because it was given just before the procedure. And sometimes the dose was too low for Jeffrey. A larger dose or a different medication might have solved Jeffrey's problem.

Success in comforting the child in pain requires a partnership between nurses, child and family. Nurses and families must acknowledge the presence of pain and be willing to comfort the child. Often children in pain are lonely, bewildered, and frightened. They have told us how to comfort them and now nurses must do so.

[37]

Fatigue, Pain, Depression, and Sleep Disturbance in Rheumatoid Arthritis Patients

Leanna J. Crosby

A constellation of objective and subjective symptoms accompany rheumatoid arthritis (RA). Nearly everyone is familiar with the objective symptoms, which include swollen and frequently deformed joints or joints that are flaccid or rigid. However, the subjective symptoms of RA are less well known. They include joint tenderness, joint pain, fatigue or physical exhaustion, and emotional depression.

The fatigue associated with RA does not appear to be associated with physical activity (Rodnan, McEwen, & Wallace, 1973). A recent study reported that of 101 RA patients, 52 indicated that they lacked energy, 66 said that they tired quickly, and 34 reported that they could not function for more than four hours without resting (Crosby, in press).

Several factors seem to contribute to the fatigue experienced by RA patients, including the physical effort required to accomplish activities of daily living, the relentless nature of joint pain, and the lack of sleep due to joint discomfort. In fact, poor sleep quality and quantity are frequent problems experienced by RA patients. Some explain that their sleep is affected by painful joints and inability to get comfortable in bed. Others say that even when their joints are not painful, they continue to experience difficulty in sleeping, suggesting, perhaps, a habitual poor sleep architecture that may develop after weeks or months of fragmented sleep. It also may suggest that these patients are experiencing an emotional disturbance such as depression. Depression has been reported to be significantly higher in RA patients than in osteoarthritis patients (Pancheri, Thedori, & Aparo, 1978). Likewise, altered electroencephalogram (EEG) sleep variables and patterns of sleep organization have been demonstrated in clinically depressed individuals; i.e., there is a reduction in Stage 3 and 4 non-REM sleep, sleep that has been labeled restorative (Baker & Brewerton, 1981).

The altered sleep quantity and quality, fatigue, pain, and depression experienced by RA patients appear to be related and should be investigated as a constellation of variables. The purposes of this research, therefore, were to determine by electrophysiologic methods the overnight EEG sleep variables and sleep patterns of RA patients, and further, to assess the relationships among fatigue, depression, pain and EEG sleep variables of RA patients.

METHOD

The convenience sample was obtained through physician referrals and television advertisements. All subjects had to be nonsmokers and take no tranquilizers, chemical stimulants, sleep medications, steroids, or pain medications beyond aspirin, Tylenol, or ibuprofen. Fifteen RA patients, 11 females and 4 males, and 12 age and gender matched control subjects, 9 females and 3 males, were monitored for one night in a sleep laboratory. All RA subjects were confirmed to have the disease by a physician. However, they were not selected based on RA disease activity or complaints of sleep problems or fatigue. The mean age of the subjects was 44 years.

Several days prior to the monitoring night, all subjects were oriented to the sleep environment and sleep monitoring equipment. The subjects were encouraged to bring a family member to the orientation session in the hope that anxiety on the part of either party could be reduced.

The evening of the sleep study, seven standard monitoring electrodes were affixed to the subject's scalp according to Jasper's (1958) 10–20 system. All electrodes were affixed for at least three hours before the subject went to bed to allow for sensory accommodation.

During the three-hour period, subjects completed the Pearson Byars Fatigue Feeling Checklist, a visual analogue scale for fatigue, the Beck Depression Inventory, the Modified McGill Pain Inventory, and a visual analogue scale for pain. RA disease was evaluated through the use of an instrument designed to assess clinical parameters of disease activity. Items evaluated included the patient's assessment of the duration of morning stiffness in hours, functional ability measured in hours, and subjective assessment of present disease activity. Items were scaled categorically producing a numerical score that reflected RA disease activity. The scores indicated that the RA patients in this study could be split into two groups—RA disease in flare (acute group) ($n = 5$) and RA disease in nonflare (mild group) ($n = 10$).

Subjects were allowed to watch television or read until they were ready to go to bed. The sleeping environment was quiet and well ventilated. All monitoring leads were passed through a wall port and attached to a Grass Model 78 Instrument Polygraph. Time-lapse videotape recording of the subject during sleep was obtained through the use of an infrared video camera suspended above the bed to facilitate body movement count.

The subjects were allowed to sleep as long as they wished. The room was without light cues and did not contain a clock. All EEG records were scored by the investigator according to the criteria of Rechtschaffen and Kales (1968).

RESULTS

The mean sleep efficiency (time asleep/time in bed) for the control group was 84%, for the RA group in flare 61%, and for the RA group in nonflare 78%. There was no significant difference between the RA flare and nonflare groups or between the nonflare and control group. However, there was a significant difference in sleep efficiency between the RA flare and control groups [$t(15) = -4.3$, $p < .01$].

Within the RA group, sleep efficiency and fatigue were negatively correlated ($r = -.324$, $p = .151$); although not significant, this does indicate that the lower the sleep efficiency, the higher the fatigue level. Sleep efficiency and pain within the RA group were also negatively correlated ($r = -.250$, $p = .184$). Again, although not significant, this indicates that the lower the sleep efficiency, the greater the pain.

Pain and depression were positively correlated ($r = .70$, $p = .002$). Additional analysis (ANOVA) indicated that as a group, the RA patients were significantly more depressed than the control group [$F(1, 25) = 13.1$, $p < .001$]. Furthermore, those whose disease was in flare were more depressed than those whose disease was not in flare. The mean Beck Depression Inventory score for the acute group was 13; the mild group score was 6, with the control group scoring 3.

Pain and clinical parameters of disease activity were also positively related. The correlation between the number of words checked on the McGill Pain Inventory and RA disease activity was $r = .65$ ($p = .004$).

DISCUSSION

Several important conclusions can be drawn from these findings. First, RA patients in this study whose disease was in flare had significantly less sleep efficiency than other subjects. Second, the sleep of all RA patients in the study was fragmented due to frequent awakenings and reduced time spent in various sleep stages.

Other variables investigated in this research included fatigue, pain, and depression. Depression emerged as a dominant variable. The level of depression in the RA flare group was such that psychological assistance would have been an appropriate intervention for these patients. In addition, pain and depression were significantly correlated, which leads one to speculate that if the pain were treated, the depression might be reduced.

It was interesting that fatigue was not greatly related to sleep efficiency, pain, or depression. However, the type of fatigue experienced by RA patients may differ from the fatigue experienced by normal subjects. The subjective nature of fatigue may require the development of more sensitive instruments to capture subtle differences in this variable.

As nurses, we must consider the subjective symptoms of RA to be equal in significance to the objective symptoms. It is very easy to become distracted by the twisted and inflamed joints or the new medication protocol. If we do not indicate that we are aware of subjective symptoms, patients will rarely offer complaints. They have frequently been conditioned by family, friends, and health care providers to suppress the subjective symptoms or, at least, not to complain.

The first step is to make fatigue, pain, sleep, and depression a part of our nursing assessment. Second, we must be prepared to acknowledge that these are very real problems in the lives of RA patients. Third, interventions must be developed and used—for example, teaching the patient to rest and stressing that rest is often as important as medication. Finally, RA patients should be encouraged to join or form arthritis support groups.

This study was designed not only to gain understanding of the basis of a human response pattern such as fatigue, but also to gain understanding of physiologic and psychologic manifestations that may occur simultaneously. Discovering such relationships could provide direction for therapeutic nursing interventions to enhance the quality of life of the rheumatoid arthritis patient.

[38]

The Effects of Home Care on Patients' Symptoms, Hospitalizations, and Complications

Ruth McCorkle, Jeanne Q. Benoliel,
and Fotini Georgiadou

Lung cancer is now the leading cause of cancer deaths in both adult men and women. In spite of the poor outlook for lung cancer, it is not uncommon for patients to receive complex chemotherapy regimens and radiation therapies throughout their illness. Often these continuing treatments are done on an outpatient basis. As a consequence, more people are receiving aggressive and complex care outside the hospital environment, but ambulatory care for these patients may be fragmented, with various specialists failing to support patients and family members during critical periods of adjustment (Holland, 1979).

The prevalence and severity of patients' problems and needs increase as the disease progresses (McCorkle & Benoliel, 1983; Mor, Gaudagnoli, & Wool, 1987; Weisman & Worden, 1977), and patients become less and less able to meet their daily living and treatment-related needs independently (Houts, Yasko, Kahn, Schelzel, & Maroni, 1986). Most needs of cancer patients are met by family members; but as the disease progresses, treatment becomes more intense, and caretak-

Supported in part by grant number NU 01001, Division of Nursing, Bureau of Health Professions, Health Resources and Services Administration, U.S.P.H.H., 1983–1986.

ing burdens grow, many patients begin receiving formal home health services (Liu, Manton, & Liu, 1985).

Although home care services by nurses have been used to improve care and decrease health care costs, the efficacy of home care by oncology nurses for patients with progressive lung cancer has not been documented. This clinical trial was undertaken to test the effects of three home care treatment regimens on the psychosocial responses and outcomes of patients with lung cancer.

METHOD

Data for this study were collected as part of a larger study to evaluate the management of lung cancer patients through home care treatment (McCorkle, Benoliel, Donaldson, & Goodell, 1987). The current study focused on the effects of home care on patients' symptoms, number of hospitalizations, and medical complications over a 24-week period.

Subjects

Subjects included in the study were at least 40 years old, with a recent lung cancer diagnosis of any histological type, of stage II or greater. Subjects were identified through pathology reports and cancer registries at 19 hospitals and one outpatient facility. Eligible subjects were approached about the study by an intermediary aligned with their primary physician's office. Once consent was obtained, subjects were interviewed in their homes at six week intervals on five occasions, a baseline interview and four follow-up interviews. Within one week after the baseline interview, subjects were randomly assigned to one of three groups; two were home care programs and one was an office care control group. Two alternative home care trials were used since specialized or standard home care programs may vary in the intensity of services delivered to patients.

Treatments

The treatment groups were the following:

• *Specialized Oncology Home Care Program (OHC)*. Home care services were provided primarily by master's prepared community oncology nurse specialists. The emphasis was on providing skilled nursing care, assisting patients in making choices about treatment and source of care, and making smooth transitions through multiple care settings. Interventions generally included patient and family education and counseling, symptom control and monitoring, and coordination of health services. A high level of service intensity was expected as a function of 24-hour service availability and advanced preparation of nurse providers.

• *Standard Home Care Program (SHC)*. These multidisciplinary home care services represented standard Medicare reimbursed services available within the community. SHC services were generally limited to scheduled visits reimbursed by third party payers. The primary emphasis was on provision of skilled nursing care, rehabilitation and social services, and coordination of multiple home services. Nurses providing primary care were baccalaureate degree prepared without advanced training in community-based oncology care.

• *Office Care (OC)*. Nursing care was provided primarily through the office of the patient's physician. Subjects randomly assigned to OC did not receive home care and were thus treated as the control group.

Measurement of Variables

Home Care Treatment

To measure home care treatment, procedures for accessing home care records were established with both home care agencies. A record review instrument, the Home Care Record Audit Form, was used to collect systematic information about the care activities/interventions reported on the patient records of subjects assigned to the two home care agencies. The 32 nursing interventions identified by Mulhern (1981) served as the basis for the audit form, which records three types of information: (a) number of actual contacts with patient/family by nurses and other health care providers; (b) kinds of recorded assessments about the status of patient and family; and (c) kinds of recorded activities/interventions related to six types of work by providers (communication/coordination among providers; observation/symptom management; counseling; teaching/discussion interventions; execution of procedures and technical activities; activities/ interventions by providers other than nurses and utilization of other community resources). The form includes a total of 59 items and is scored by summing the items by categories. The validity of the measure has been discussed elsewhere (McCorkle et al., 1987).

Variables analyzed to compare the effectiveness of the two types of home care and office care were symptom distress, number of hospitalizations, complications, and baseline demographic characteristics.

Symptom Distress

Symptom distress was defined as the degree of discomfort from specific symptoms reported by the patient. Distress was not differentiated according to whether it resulted from the disease itself or from the treatment. The original scale developed by the investigators contained 10 symptoms: nausea, mood, appetite, insomnia, pain, mobility, fatigue, bowel patterns, concentration, and appearance (McCorkle & Young, 1978). The scale was subsequently modified in content and format (McCorkle & Benoliel, 1983) and the final version contained 13 symptoms. The additions were dyspnea, outlook, and cough.

Each symptom was placed on a 5 x 7 inch card, and at each interview, subjects were asked to identify the degree of their distress from the symptom using a 5-point Likert-type scale ranging from 1 (normal or no distress) to 5 (extensive distress). There were descriptive words for each point on the scale. Subjects were handed the 13 cards and asked to circle the number corresponding to their experience for that day. Total symptom distress was considered to be the sum of the 13 scales, a value that could range from 13 to 65. Validity and reliability of the scale were established on 60 patients with chronic illnesses (McCorkle & Young, 1978). The scale has demonstrated face and content validity for specific symptoms. The reliability coefficient alpha has been reported between 0.79 and 0.89.

Number of Hospitalizations

Number of hospitalizations was defined as the sum of admissions to a hospital during the study period. Subjects were asked at each interview if they had been hospitalized, received medical treatment, or visited their physician within the last six weeks. This information was used as a guide to identify the institutions in which medical records were to be reviewed. A Medical Record Review Instrument was used to collect systematic information about the utilization of services and other pertinent information at the participating hospitals.

Complications

Complications were defined as medical consequences of the disease or treatment effects by the physician documented on the patient's medical record at the time of admission. Nineteen potential complications were identified by a panel of medical oncologists and included on the Medical Record Review Instrument.

Audits of both the home care and medical records of the subjects were done over the entire 24 weeks of treatment by trained research assistants.

RESULTS

The sample consisted of the 78 patients who completed interviews on four occasions. (Data from the fifth interview were not analyzed because by that time attrition of subjects was considerable, leaving only a small sample.) The mean age was 59; 89% were Caucasian, 59% were male and 63% were married. Chi-square tests indicated no statistically significant group differences in sex, race, employment, living alone, insurance, histology, primary physician specialty, surgical resection, or death within the study period.

Home Care Treatment

Home care treatment by specialized oncology nurses was more intensive, as is evident in the significantly longer mean duration $[t(49) = 2.08, p = .04]$ of treatment for this group (mean = 11.2 weeks) than for the standard home care group (mean = 6.1 weeks) (see Table 38.1). For patients receiving OHC, actual weeks of home care treatment ranged from 1 week ($n = 7$, 29.2%) to 24 weeks ($n = 7$, 29.2%). For patients in SHC, weeks of home care treatment also ranged from 1 week ($n = 11$, 40.7%) to 24 weeks ($n = 1$, 3.7%). However, six subjects remained in OHC for the full 24 weeks whereas only one received SHC for the full 24 weeks. Reasons patients were dropped from home care services included decisions by the agency to close the case (primarily at recertification) or decisions by patients or family members to cease home care.

For the 24 subjects assigned to OHC, the total scores on the number of home care treatment interventions over 24 weeks ranged from 3 to 288 with a mean score of 62.7. For the subjects on SHC, the total home care treatment scores for 24 weeks ranged from 2 to 279 with a mean score of 50.9. Overall, subjects in OHC and SHC had similar levels of weekly total home care interventions (see Table 38.1).

To evaluate the characteristics of home care, the individual items in the various categories of intervention were analyzed. Subjects in the specialized (OHC) treatment group received fewer home visits (mean = 6.75) on the average than the standard treatment group (SHC) (mean = 8.62), but they received more telephone calls (OHC, mean = 4.54) than the standard care group (mean = 3.92). Both groups used the same proportion of home health aides. There were noticeable differences in the amount of coordination of services, counseling, procedures, and use of other disciplines between the two groups although none of these differences were statistically significant (see Table 38.1).

TABLE 38.1 Mean Number of Home Care Treatments by Treatment Group

	Treatment Group			
	OHC n = 24		SHC n = 24	
Home Care Treatment	Mean	s.d.	Mean	s.d.
Weeks of Home Care	11.24	10.01	6.12*	6.90
Total Home Care Treatments	62.73	77.90	50.90	74.02
Contacts				
Home Visits	6.75	10.69	8.62	15.37
Phone Calls	4.54	6.51	3.92	5.54
Assessments				
Patient Assessment	17.50	23.24	15.92	19.77
Family Assessment	1.54	2.98	1.08	2.31
Interventions				
Coordination	3.17	4.98	4.12	6.99
Counseling/Teaching	8.42	16.29	5.62	7.48
Procedures	1.75	2.40	3.14	4.32
Home Health Aide	2.83	9.71	3.15	8.79
Other Disciplines	.88	2.03	2.96	6.49

*$p < .05$

Symptom Distress

Multivariate analysis of variance was used to determine the effects of home care treatment on symptom distress over time. When the means for symptom distress were plotted by occasion, it was apparent that the groups differed notably on the first occasion, with the OHC group tending to do better on most of the variables. Because subjects had not been assigned to groups at Occasion 1, the pretreatment interview, mean differences cannot be attributed to group assignment. In an attempt to adjust for these differences, data from Occasion 1 were treated as covariates when analyzing scores on Occasions 2, 3, and 4. Thus, the principal analyses pertain to three occasions adjusted for Occasion 1—as if the groups had in fact been equal at Occasion 1. Although this kind of adjustment can be questionable when there is reason to believe that the covariate and treatment are confounded, the present conditions are precisely those that minimize this danger: since Occasion 1 *preceded* group assignment, there is every reason to believe that the initial differences were due to chance sampling error.

The major finding was that the office care group (OC) experienced increased symptom distress about 6 weeks sooner than either the oncology home care (OHC) or the standard home care (SHC) groups [$F(1, 60) = 5.01$, $p = .03$]. Moreover, the levels of distress of the two home care groups (OHC and SHC) were quite similar, suggesting that which home care treatment group patients were assigned to had little effect on symptom distress. Assignment to office care, however, resulted in significantly earlier distress. The easiest way to see this effect is to compare the office care line with the heavy line representing the mean of the OHC and SHC groups in Figure 38.1.

The means of individual symptom distress items were examined to identify differences between the two home care groups' ability to manage symptoms. Overall, both groups were able to manage nausea, appetite, fatigue, bowel patterns, and appearance. The primary difference between the two was that the specialized oncology nurses were able to assist patients with their insomnia and dyspnea whereas the standard care group was not. Neither group was successful in managing pain. Many of these patients had metastatic disease and it may be unrealistic to expect to eliminate patients' pain in the presence of progressive pathology.

Number of Hospitalizations

Hospital admissions for the sample were obtained from the record audits completed at participating institutions, and the numbers are considered conservative. They do not include hospitalizations at insti-

FIGURE 38.1. Adjusted symptom distress by group and occasion.

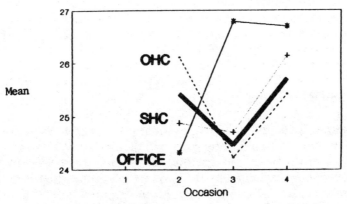

tutions not participating in the study. There were a total of 194 hospitalizations over the 24 weeks. Although the differences were not significant, the OHC group had fewer hospitalizations than the other two groups: the OHC group had a mean of 2.08 hospitalizations, SHC had 2.82, and OC had 2.62. Hospitalizations per person ranged from 0 to 11.

Reasons for hospitalization were grouped into several general categories: cancer treatment, palliation, diagnostic work-ups, other medical conditions, or complications such as bleeding or infection. The primary reason patients were admitted was to receive cancer treatment, specifically chemotherapy. Other reasons included management of respiratory problems, gastrointestinal symptoms, pain, anemia, and thrombocytopenia. Patients were generally admitted for active treatment, other medical problems, or complications, rather than for palliative care or diagnostic work-ups.

Medical Complications

Patients experienced over 130 complications, which were grouped into seven categories. Although all three groups had similar complications, the frequency of particular complications differed in different groups. Patients in the office care group were admitted for pain and respiratory difficulties. Patients in the standard home care group had more problems with respiratory symptoms and infections, whereas those with oncology nursing care had problems with pain and the gastrointestinal system. Although the difference was not statistically significant, the OHC group had fewer complications than the other two groups. This is not surprising since the home care oncology nurses were specialists in monitoring and managing symptoms related to lung cancer and its treatment, especially problems associated with infections, low blood counts, and respiratory distress. However, as the number of complications increased, patients in all three groups were more likely to be admitted to the hospital ($p = .002$).

DISCUSSION

In this study, patients who were randomly assigned to the office care group experienced significantly more symptom distress 6 weeks sooner than either of the home care groups. We assume that it was the home care interventions provided by the two nursing groups that maintained symptom relief 6 weeks longer than for the group who did not receive home care. Even though overall symptoms were less in both the home care groups, there were differences in the symptoms managed. Both groups managed nausea, appetite, fatigue, bowel patterns, and appearance; but only the nurses with specialized oncology training were able to manage patients' insomnia and dyspnea. Neither group had success in reducing the patients' pain.

Through audits of the home care records, we looked at specific nursing care provided at home in order to see whether and what differences existed between the two nursing groups, though the effects on patients' symptoms were similar. We found that the specialized nurses group (OHC) paid fewer home visits but more frequent telephone calls to patients, did less coordination and communication with other providers, but saw patients over a longer period. Both groups reported doing more assessments than specific interventions, and both groups talked with patients and clarified information about their disease and treatment and their responses to the disease. The oncology nurses were more likely to talk to patients about their personal concerns and solve problems with them than were the SHC nurses. The SHC nurses helped patients to plan for emergency help, but the OHC nurses rarely reported this intervention. The SHC group charted more procedures than the OHC group. Both used home health aides similarly, but the SHC used more providers from other disciplines, primarily medical social workers.

These differences in the characteristics of the home care interventions probably reflected philosophical differences in the home health agencies. It was not surprising that nurses with specialized knowledge in oncology (OHC) were able to manage a wide range of symptoms related to cancer and the effects of treatment, including dyspnea and insomnia. Findings indicate that the nurses in the SHC group were not as skilled in managing patients' symptoms and as a result more often called the physician for assistance, who in turn more often admitted the patient.

Subjects in the specialized home care group tended to show somewhat different patterns of hospital use from those in the standard home care group. Though the two groups had similar hospital admissions for active treatment of lung cancer, subjects receiving specialized home care had relatively fewer hospital admissions for symptoms and complications of the malignancy. The specialized home care providers may have been able to prevent certain symptoms and complications or to substitute for some types of inpatient care in a way that standard care providers could not. Patients in all three groups were admitted for pain and respiratory problems.

Although the findings from this study warrant further analysis with larger samples, there appear to be enough "clinically relevant" differences to offer some recommendations. There is beginning evidence that targeting a high risk patient group such as lung cancer patients in the early months after diagnosis improves the effectiveness of home care interventions in reducing their symptoms. However, home care by nurses without specialized knowledge seems to increase hospital use. It appears unlikely that master's prepared clinicians with advanced knowledge in oncology will be employed by home health agencies to provide direct care to patients with cancer because of the high cost of home care. Other possible mechanisms to increase staff's ability to assess and manage problems of patients with disease-related symptoms are standardized education programs and consistent utilization of clinical nurse specialists as consultants. Given the revolutionary changes in the home care industry today, it may be more realistic for nurses to assess and monitor patients through ambulatory clinics. The evidence demonstrates that nurses can improve the quality of living with progressive illnesses such as cancer, but additional work is needed to determine the most cost-effective ways.

[39]

Patient Comfort: The Nurse's Imperative

Charles E. Schunior

I am an assistant head nurse of an oncology research unit at Duke Medical Center. What I do most of the time is bedside nursing, that is, I attempt to provide comfort and healing to people suffering painful, disfiguring, usually terminal disease. For such an ordinary nurse to discuss the work of researchers might in the past have seemed daunting, surprising, strangely unwelcome, like Banquo's ghost at Macbeth's banquet. But congratulations are due to the editors of this volume for fostering a positive and productive model of clinical and research collaboration. My mandate is to examine the work presented here from a clinical perspective—that is, how does it contribute to the fundamental raison d'être of our profession, the care of patients in real nursing settings? Or, as we say in the South where I grew up, will these dogs hunt?

Hamilton's interactionist perspective is impressive. This dog will definitely hunt! Hamilton reminds us that comfort is not a commodity that can be prepackaged and administered in a standardized fashion. No matter how minutely behaviors are measured, no matter how fine the focus, one fundamental question will always escape objective measurement: the meaning of the situation to the actor. Comfort is a variable as heavily freighted with individual occult meaning as any we could study. As the chapters in this section emphasize, comfort is a social-psychological construct that requires the sensitivity of an anthropologist or a nurse to elicit. In one sense, this perspective complicates the study of comfort, but in a broader sense it opens windows of opportunity that may help the nurse to optimize comfort for patients. From another perspective—physiological monitoring—Crosby has shown that sleep, a major component of comfort, is fragmented in patients with rheumatoid arthritis. Further, says Crosby, these patients are depressed and in pain, but unless asked will rarely complain about their subjective symptoms.

The bad news from hospitals is that design factors and professional and institutional inertia mitigate against comfort. The good news is that nursing, which is wont to deplore its powerlessness, has substantial power to enhance comfort, though by and large nurses avail themselves of this power only partially and inconsistently.

Each comfort parameter identified in the papers presented here lies firmly within the domain of nursing—even within our present highly flawed institutions, and even with our severely depleted ranks. Let me comment on a couple of issues. First, comfort for each of us and each of our patients is an arcane private language, usually spoken best among families. Families are the logical and in some cases necessary adjuncts of nursing care—indeed, as many have asserted, the true locus of care. And yet, by means of hospital design and our own professional inertia and insecurity, we often segregate families, stripping their support for patients as we strip them of their clothing. Nurses typically have decisive power in this area. In most institutions, nurses are the gatekeepers to the patients' rooms; the sacred visitation rules are usually rules only we enforce. In the coronary care unit where I formerly worked, we encouraged the nurses to make family visitation an aspect of the care plan. Where appropriate, patients' privacy was enforced, but generally the extended presence of families was deemed therapeutic and our own informal measures of patient comfort and therapeutic outcomes confirmed the rightness of this policy. On the oncology ward where I currently work, families typically stay with patients overnight, assisting with many aspects of their care. Knowing they will not be bereft of the comforting insulation of family enables our patients to return without the fear and trembling commonly associated with hospital admission. Care that is home based affords maximum involvement of family, and as McCorkle and colleagues have shown, home care results in significantly less symptom distress for oncology patients.

Comfort is not usually a function of sophisticated interventions. In most cases it is the result of a highly complex informal language spoken among people who have shared much experience. Knowing when the lights are too bright, the room too cold, the music too raucous, knowing which parts of the body to touch and which not to, which subjects to avoid, which foods to bring or request: this is the learning of a lifetime. An empathetic nurse can provide many imaginative comfort measures, but it is a gross waste of resources not to maximize family involvement.

Second, I am an enthusiastic advocate of biofeedback, visualization, hypnosis, and music therapy, and as nurses we do not have to wait for the millennium when doctors will be holistic practitioners whose standard orders will include these interventions. Nurses can organize training sessions in techniques of relaxation, repaint patient rooms in non-institutional colors, hang prints on the walls, and procure cassette players and an extensive library of tapes. For many of our CCU patients the music that appeared to open the endorphin floodgates was Southern Gospel music. I have seen many a pacemaker or Swan insertion tolerated with a beatific smile as the patient listened to the sensuous harmonics of the Sensational Nightingales.

Nevertheless, I have little doubt that for the foreseeable future, drugs will remain the most widely used and potentially effective pain relief measures. Ironically, this area, arguably the greatest success story of medical science, is relegated to insignificance by many physicians and is closely studied by few. Nursing, in our scramble to define an independent scope of practice, leaves it to the physicians. And Hester's stories of abusive and neglectful pain control are by no means limited to the pediatric population. Nurses in fact are the only health care workers who communicate closely enough with patients and can

monitor effect closely enough to adequately administer analgesics. As
Donovan has reminded us, physicians have woeful misconceptions
about the appropriate use of narcotics, and yet, in my experience, they
are only too glad to defer to nursing judgment in this area. For example, when a doctor writes a prescription for Percocet, 1–2 tablets q.
4–6 hours, he or she in effect is devolving power to the nurse, who
abandons that power if she or he merely relegates the narcotic to the
amorphous category of prn, and proceeds to wait for the patient to call
out in pain.

Nurses must be encouraged to elicit pain histories and use our
knowledge of pharmacology as well as multifactoral etiology, to ration-
ally and effectively treat pain. When we document our case for more
effective dosage and scheduling or selection of analgesics, only in the
rarest instance will the physician not defer to our judgment.

Providing comfort for distressed humanity is the raison d'être of
nursing, and yet in an age of "medical miracles," hospital proliferation,
and enlightened autonomous nursing, the art and science of comfort is
widely lacking, and perhaps less available to the typical patient than it
was 50 years ago. The research presented in this volume represents
tools of great utility but only if grasped and put to work. As nurses we
have the training and sensitivity to elicit the patient's own private language of comfort, and we have the power and training to optimize it.
Why that power is not used, why that sensitivity is blunted, is, I hope,
the subject of much future investigation.

References On Comfort

Baker, G., & Brewerton, D. (1981). Rheumatoid arthritis: A psychiatric assessment. *British Medical Journal, 282*, 2014.

Crosby, L. (in press). Stress factors, emotional stress, and rheumatoid arthritis disease activity. *Journal of Advanced Nursing.*

Francis, G. S., & Munjar, B. (1975). *Promoting psychological comfort.* Iowa: Wm. C. Brown.

Freihofer, P. S., & Felton, G. (1976). Nursing behaviors in bereavement. *Nursing Research, 25*, 332–337.

Hamilton, J. (1985). *Comfort on a palliative care unit: The client's perception.* Unpublished manuscript, McGill University, Montreal, Quebec.

Hampe, S. (1975). Needs of the grieving spouse in a hospital setting. *Nursing Research, 24*, 113–119.

Havens, B. (1980). Differentiation of unmet needs using analysis by age/sex cohorts. In V. Marshall (Ed.), *Aging in Canada.* Ontario: Fitzhenry and Whiteside.

Heller, B., Bausell, R., & Ninos, M. (1984). Nurses' perceptions of rehabilitation potential of institutionalized aged. *Journal of Gerontological Nursing, 10*(7), 22–26.

Hester, N. O. (1987, March). *Child participation in the pain experience.* Paper presented at the International Conference on Research and Maternal Child Nursing, Montreal, Quebec, Canada.

Hester, N. O. (1987, August). *Child participation in the pain experience.* Poster presented at the Sigma Theta Tau International Nursing Research Congress, Edinburgh, Scotland.

Hester, N. O., & Barcus, C. S. (1986). *The human experience of pain for hospitalized children.* Paper presented at the International Nursing Research Conference, Edmonton, Alberta, Canada.

Hester, N. O., & Ray, M. A. (1987, March). *Assessment of Watson's carative factors: A qualitative research study.* Paper presented at the International Conference on Research and Maternal Child Nursing, Montreal, Quebec, Canada.

Hester, N. O., & Ray, M. A. (1987, August). *Assessment of Watson's carative factors: A qualitative research study.* Paper presented at the Sigma Theta Tau International Nursing Research Congress, Edinburgh, Scotland.

Holland, J. (1979). The emotional impact of breast cancer and the question of premorbid personality. In A. Smith and C.A. Alvarez (Eds.), *Advances in Medical Oncology, Research, and Education, Vol. 2: Cancer Control.* Oxford: Pergamon Press.

Houts, P., Yasko, J., Kahn, S., Schelzel, G., & Maroni, K. (1986). Unmet psychological, social and economic needs of persons with cancer in Pennsylvania. *Cancer, 58*, 2355–2361.

Jasper, H. (1958). Ten-Twenty system of EEG electrode placement. *Electroencephalography and Clinical Neurophysiology, 10*, 371–375.

Lee, E. T. (1980). *Statistical Methods of Survival Data Analysis*. Belmont, CA: Lifetime Learning Publications, 395–403.

Liu, K., Manton, K. G., & Liu, B. M. (1985). Home care expenses for the disabled elderly. *Health Care Financing Review, 7*, 51–58.

McCorkle, R., & Benoliel, J. Q. (1983). Symptom distress, current concerns, and mood disturbance after diagnosis of life threatening disease. *Social Science and Medicine, 17*(7), 431–438.

McCorkle, R., Benoliel, J. Q., Donaldson, G., & Goodell, B. (1987). *Evaluation of Cancer Management*. Final Report of Project Supported by the Division of Nursing, Bureau of Health Professions, Public Health Service, Grant No. NUO1001, 1983–1986.

McCorkle, R., Packard, N., & Landenburger, K. (1984). Subject accrual and attrition: Problems and solutions. *Journal of Psychosocial Oncology, 2*(3/4), 137–146.

McCorkle, R. & Young, K. (1978). Development of a symptom distress scale. *Cancer Nursing, 1* (October), 373–378.

Mor, V., Gaudagnoli, E., & Wool, M. (1987). An examination of the concrete service needs of advanced cancer patients. *Journal of Psychosocial Oncology, 5*(5), 1–17.

Morse, J. (1983). An ethnoscientific analysis on comfort: A preliminary investigation. *Nursing Papers, 15*, pp. 22–26.

Mulhern, P. (1981). *Identification of nursing interventions delivered to terminal care patients at home*. Unpublished Master's thesis. University of Washington, Seattle.

Pancheri, P., Thedori, S., & Aparo, U. (1978). Psychological aspects of rheumatoid arthritis vis a vis osteoarthritis. *Scandinavian Journal of Rheumatology, 7*, 42–48.

Rechschaffen, A., & Kales, A. (1968). *A manual of standardized terminology, techniques and scoring system for sleep stages of human subjects*. National Institutes of Health Publication No. 204. Washington, DC: US Government Printing Office.

Rodnan, G., McEwen, C., & Wallace, S. (1973). *Primer on Rheumatic Diseases, 224*(5), 1–140.

Sohl, R. (1987). How to comfort and guide the family. *Nursing 87, 17*, 63–64.

Strauss, A., Corbin, J., Fagerhaugh, S., Glaser, B., Maines, D., Suczek, B., & Wiener, C. (1984). *Chronic illness and the quality of life*. Toronto: The C.V. Mosby Co.

Talbot, D. (1985). Assessing needs of the rural elderly. *Journal of Gerontological Nursing, 11*(3), 39–43.

Tilquin, C., Sicotte, C., Paquin, T., Tousignant, F., Gagnon, G., & Lambert, P. (1980). The physical, emotional and social conditions of an aged population. In V. Marshall (Ed.), *Aging in Canada*. Ontario: Fitzhenry and Whiteside.

Watson, J. (1979). *Nursing: The philosophy and science of caring*. Boston: Little, Brown and Company.

Weisman, A. D., & Worden, J. W. (1977). *Coping and vulnerability in cancer patients*. Project Omega, Boston: Harvard Medical School.

Part VI

RESEARCH UTILIZATION

[40]

Strategies for Using Research in Practice

Linda R. Cronenwett

This chapter discusses practical strategies for using research, and is directed toward you, clinician. It is written keeping in mind the frenetic nature of most of your work environments and the other attention-demanding priorities you face.

MAKING NOTES

The strategies you adopt for using research will vary depending on the quality of the research supporting your innovation. A volume like this, focusing on a few distinct topics, is a tremendous help to those of us who are interested in using research in practice. We have summaries of the research on the care of patients and families who are coping with pain, fatigue, and nausea. In addition, some of the studies reported here represent the newest wave of knowledge in this domain.

After reading these studies, you may think of a promising new assessment strategy, imagine a way to alter the interventions or goals on one of your standardized care plans, note a new intervention you would like to evaluate, or jot down references to research you can use to convince others to bring their practice into line with your current standards. If you haven't made notes on your ideas, I encourage you to do so. It is amazing how the realities of the practice world can wipe out the concrete insights gained from reading interesting work.

When you have a list of ideas for using research in practice, take a realistic look at what you know about the research base for your ideas.

Did the work that inspired you summarize a group of studies from which findings converge to support your idea for a change in practice? Or did the author indicate that this was the first and only study with the reported findings? How similar were the characteristics of the people studied to the patients with whom you work? How similar was the study's environment to the setting in which you work? These are the kinds of questions you will be asked if you propose your idea to colleagues. You will assist your cause by thinking through what you learned and keeping notes.

PERSUADING OTHERS

Next, you will have to decide how much further effort to devote to evaluating the research base. Stetler and Marram (1976) described two areas you need to consider: feasibility and the basis for practice. Regarding the basis for practice, the two major questions are:

1. Do you have a theoretical or scientific basis for your current practice behavior?
2. How effective is your current method of practice in this area?

Your ideas for changes in practice will require significantly more evidence and evaluation if the current practice is (or is believed to be) already based on scientific or theoretical rationale.

In considering the feasibility of your innovation, you need to think about four questions regarding risk, resources, and readiness (Stetler & Marram, 1976):

1. What degree of potential risk would be associated with the change in practice?
2. What level(s) of the organization would need to be involved in this change in practice?
3. Given the level(s) that would be involved, what is the degree of readiness for such a change in practice?
4. What amount of resources would be needed to implement such a change?

Obviously the effort needed to make the case for a change in practice will differ depending on the answers to these questions.

An innovation that involves minimal or no risk that you can implement all by yourself with no additional resources is unlikely to meet with opposition. On the other hand, if your innovation is perceived as risky, if it involves withholding care that is currently considered standard practice, if implementation would require changes in policies, procedures, or documentation systems, if new equipment or supplies would be required, or if implementation would be impossible without the support of physicians—if any of these are true, then greater effort needs to be made to collect and evaluate data and present a case for the quality of the research base that supports your innovation.

We know from a large body of work on innovation diffusion by Everett Rogers (1983) that five perceived characteristics of innovations have a significant impact on the rate of adoption of an innovation. These five characteristics will be important when you're trying to persuade others that your idea is worth trying. According to Rogers, the rate of adoption of your innovation will depend on:

1. Relative advantage—the degree to which the innovation is perceived to be better than the idea it supersedes. The greater the relative advantage in terms of economics, social prestige, convenience, satisfaction, or any form of positive comparison, the greater the likelihood of a positive attitude toward its use.
2. Compatibility—the degree to which the innovation is perceived as being consistent with existing values, past experiences, and/or the needs of adopters. The greater the extent of compatibility with prevalent norms and values of the social system, the more positive will be the attitudes toward use.
3. Complexity—the degree to which the innovation is perceived as difficult to understand and use. The greater the complexity, the less the chance of a positive attitude toward use.
4. Trialability—the degree to which the innovation can be experimented with on a limited basis. The greater the ease of trialability, the greater the likelihood of a positive attitude toward use of the innovation.
5. Observability—the degree to which results of an innovation are visible to others. Greater observability stimulates peer discussion and, again, positively influences your ability to persuade others.

Once you have evaluated your ideas for changes in practice using Stetler and Marram's (1976) questions on feasibility and basis for practice and Rogers' (1983) characteristics of innovations that influence persuasion, you will have some idea of the amount of resistance you are likely to encounter as you attempt to change practice. The CURN (Conduct and Utilization of Research in Nursing) Project (1983), using many of the same principles, developed a "Probability of Adoption Assessment Guide" that you may also find useful. You are now ready to make an appropriate plan for evaluation of the research base.

EVALUATING THE RESEARCH BASE

Most authorities on research utilization emphasize the importance of evaluating the research base before proposing a change in practice (Haller, Reynolds, & Horsley, 1979; Krueger, Nelson, & Wolanin, 1978; Stetler & Marram, 1976). To do this, you must know enough about research to critique individual studies. Further, you must have access to library resources in order to gather the articles that must be examined to see if there is sufficient evidence for the practice innovation being considered.

Integrating a body of research literature into a coherent argument for a practice innovation is no small task. If you have had training to critique a research base as a part of your education and you have some flexibility in how you spend your work time, I encourage you to conduct your own review and critique of the literature. In our society in particular, nothing establishes expertise on a topic as well as intimate familiarity with the research base. By reviewing the literature yourself, you also have the advantage of being exposed to other ideas, other nuances of the same idea, or other strategies or suggestions for practice that perhaps haven't yet occurred to you.

However, many people feel uncomfortable with their ability to find or critique a research base. Does that mean you can't use your ideas for changing practice? No—you just choose different strategies for this phase of the process. Here are some ideas:

1. Find a colleague in your setting who is responsible for reviewing research and proposing research-based innovations—a clinical nurse specialist, a director of research, the chair of your practice or standards committee, a staff development instructor, or a nurse with advanced education who works on your unit. Share your ideas with this person and request help in evaluating the research base. Offer to call the investigator whose study set you thinking about change to speed the process of finding the studies that deserve consideration. Ask the person to lead a discussion of the articles with you and other nurses on your unit.

2. Contact a faculty member in your specialty at your local school of nursing. See if you can set up a process whereby a student is assigned to assist in evaluating a specified research base as part of the requirements for a research course. If that's not possible, maybe the faculty member would do the evaluation for you in return for your giving one or two lectures to his or her students.

3. If you have no access to nursing colleagues who are capable and willing to assist you in the review process, do the best job you can to

collect all the pertinent articles related to the innovation, and then ask a colleague from another discipline to validate your understanding of the implications for practice to be derived from this research base.

4. If none of these strategies are possible, return to your assessment of the risk of implementation and your basis for current practice. If there is no obvious risk associated with your innovation and there is no better rationale for the current practice than the rationale in the studies in this volume, go ahead and try your idea. You try practice innovations now based on logic, common sense, and problem solving. If there is no conflicting research base, try out your idea as you would any nonresearch-based innovation.

Evaluation of the research base will lead you to draw conclusions about what is required to use new research-based ideas. You are likely to make one of three decisions:

1. The research base is sound and the findings are generalizable to the type of patients with whom you work. You are ready to attempt to change your practice, and if necessary, change the standards of practice in your organization.

2. The research base is adequate, but the study populations or the study environments are different enough from your patients and setting to warrant an evaluation of the innovation at your site.

3. Further research is needed. You might be able to use some ideas without risk or great expense, but replication or extension of the work is needed before changes in practice are proposed.

Obviously, the strategies you use in the next step of research utilization will differ depending on which of these conclusions you draw after you evaluate the research base. Let's take each scenario separately, understanding that you're trying to influence others, not just your own practice.

WHEN THE RESEARCH BASE IS SOUND

First, let's consider the strategies you might use if the research base is sound and the practice innovation has been tried in a number of settings with successful results. You have a number of decisions to make about strategies. One of the first questions is: Who are you going to have to convince and what will convince them? Although the focus of this volume is on using research findings as a basis for practice and I've spent a good deal of time emphasizing the importance of evaluating the research base, the reality is that not too many people will care

about your research critique. As scientists testing Rogers' (1983) innovation diffusion theories discovered, people tend to adopt innovations
that their friends adopt and innovations that are compatible with previous hunches or values. Only a few people in your organization, then,
may actually want to evaluate the science from which your idea came;
however, you need to have the information ready. In fact, you might
consider compiling booklets that contain:

1. The original articles that form the research base.
2. A 1–2 page summary of the findings that bear on your innovation
   and the outcomes that might be expected if a change in practice
   occurred.
3. Relevant letters of support from whatever authority figures might
   be involved.
4. A clear, succinct statement of your protocol or innovation with an
   accompanying plan for implementation.

When you have these materials ready, it is time to consider the people you need to persuade. Again, from Rogers' work, there is a consistent pattern of five adopter categories into which your colleagues are
likely to fit. Rogers (1983) labels these "innovators," "early adopters,"
"early majority," "late majority," and "laggards." Innovators tend to be
active information seekers. They have a lot of mass media exposure,
wide interpersonal networks, and are able to cope with high levels of
uncertainty. In the same vein, early adopters tend to be more empathetic, less dogmatic, better able to deal with abstractions, more rational, and more intelligent than the early and late majorities and laggards. They are people who hold more favorable attitudes toward
change, education, and science. Early adopters also have higher
achievement levels and higher aspirations, are more interconnected in
their social systems, and have greater social participation, more change
agent contact, and greater exposure to the mass media. You get the
idea. The individuals on your unit who fit the above descriptions are
the people most likely to be interested in the research base. They are
also the people most likely to try a change in practice.

So that you won't be discouraged in the process of trying to achieve
change, please know that Rogers (1983) and his colleagues have also
shown that the rate of adoption of an innovation appears on a graph
like an S curve. One generally finds very few adopters at first; then,
following adoption of the innovation by innovators and early adopters,
there is a surge in the adoption rate as the early majority pick up the
innovation, followed by a leveling off as the late majority come on
board, and a plateau as the laggards finally embrace the change.

One other concept to keep in mind is the fact that social structure also affects diffusion of an idea or innovation (Rogers, 1983). Formal patterns of communication are important; therefore, you are likely to benefit from the support of the people to whom you report, or the people who are responsible for formalizing policies and standards, or local content specialists—for instance, the director of the pharmacy if you're changing to a system where patients will take their own medications.

Informal patterns of communication are also important. If you're going to attempt to change practice in a way that will affect whole units of nursing staff, you need to acknowledge or find out who the opinion leaders of the unit are. Any of us who work in hospitals know that opinion leaders can vary considerably in their openness to change. Opinion leaders are rarely members of the "innovator" adopter category. Innovators tend to be too different and too threatening to be informal leaders of the majority. Your change process will differ tremendously, however, depending on whether the opinion leaders on the unit in question are early adopters or laggards. If the opinion leaders can't be convinced of the value of an innovation, you are going to have a hard struggle to change practice. In order to maximize your chances for success, you might choose the unit for the trial of your innovation based on the qualities of both the formal and informal leaders.

If you are up against a group of colleagues who are members of the late majority or laggards, a final strategy is to determine who is the reference group for the people involved. Most of us can readily identify the nurses whose reference groups are physicians or administrators rather than nurses. People tend to adopt innovations that their reference groups adopt; therefore, if physicians are the reference group for the opinion leaders on your unit, a good strategy is to enlist the support of the relevant physicians. For many health professionals, patients may also be an important reference group. If your innovation is visible and valued by patients or their families, you may be able to enlist them to help you convince colleagues to try the innovation.

To summarize the strategies to consider if you're ready to attempt to change practice:

1. Have your evaluation of the research base ready for those to whom the quality of the research base is important. Be clear about what you want to do.
2. Carefully consider the social structure of the group of professionals you are trying to persuade. Plan strategies to persuade both the formal and informal leaders.
3. Enlist the support of reference groups, when needed, to create more positive attitudes towards change.

WHEN CLINICAL TRIALS ARE NEEDED

Now let's consider appropriate strategies when the research base is adequate to propose an innovation, but the change in practice requires a "clinical trial" or evaluation with the patients in your own setting. Clinical trials represent a step in the use of new information in which "planned change processes and research methodologies are used to implement the innovation on a small (pilot) scale and evaluate its effectiveness in solving a patient care problem" (CURN Project, 1983). Clinical trials serve many purposes. For instance, clinical trials limit the opportunity for misuse of research findings by identifying problems with an innovation prior to large scale implementation. Clinical trials may also decrease resistance to the innovation. A pilot change is less permanent and other affected parties can be reassured that permanent changes will not be made unless the data show that the innovation is a success (CURN Project, 1983).

There isn't sufficient space here to discuss all the strategies and methods for planning clinical trials. But here are a few general thoughts:

1. If you can try the innovation yourself first, do so. Figure out what the problems will be. Solicit the initial reactions of patients, families, nursing leaders, and medical staff. Think about what outcome measures would be appropriate indices of the success or failure of the innovation. Keep track of the time involved in using your innovation. Does it save time? Add time? Use the insights you gain to develop plans for the clinical trial.

2. If you do not have a background in research methods, find a partner who does. The methods used in clinical trials are research methods. You want to evaluate your innovation in a manner that will convince others, be publishable, and, most of all, give you the information you need. Much time will be saved if at least one member of the planning team has research expertise.

3. Even if you never thought about instrument development before, the studies in this volume indicate the complexity involved in measurement. If you can't find help for any other part of your trial, at least find help in determining what to measure and how to measure it. Again, the researchers represented here are the logical people to call if you have no one with the expertise you need nearby.

4. Use Chapter 6 of the CURN Project (1983) book, *Conducting a Clinical Trial and Evaluation of the Innovation*, as another helpful reference.

5. Avoid discouragement by giving yourself sufficient time for the whole process. Set a realistic timeline with someone who knows how long these projects take.

6. Seek funding for time for data collection, coding, computer entry, and data analysis costs, if needed.

7. Publish the results of your evaluation! If you cannot envision a full article, try writing a shorter piece, such as for the "Consider This" column in *JONA* or a letter to the editor of a specialty practice journal.

8. By all means, report your results to nurse researchers who have a program of research in the area of your innovation. Your findings will be extremely interesting to them. Share your hunches about why something didn't work with a particular group of patients. In addition, share the ideas you gained for further research.

FURTHER RESEARCH OR REPLICATION IS NEEDED

The important point here is that clinicians are a vital link in *generating* as well as using research. You need not bear the burden for conducting research projects alone; however, if you are interested in contributing to the generation of new knowledge, you offer something of real value to the profession. As I review nursing research articles for potential summaries for *Research Review: Studies for Nursing Practice*, I am impressed to see how often I select studies that have been done either by scientist-clinician teams, by researchers who spend a significant amount of time in practice settings, or by clinicians who have committed time and energy to mastering the methods of a particular research project.

If you are a clinician without much research experience or a researcher without much current clinical time or expertise, I urge you to consider the benefits to be gained from creating clinician-researcher teams. The complementary resources offered by researchers and clinicians include these:

Clinicians	Researchers
Are constantly exposed to practice	Are constantly exposed to literature
Know the pragmatics	Know theory
Can gain onsite cooperation	Have more experience in writing proposals and articles
Have access to subjects	Have access to library resources
Can oversee data collection	Can guide planning of research design
Can assume some data collection costs	Can assume some analysis and secretarial costs
Can offer strong clinical interpretations of data	Can offer strong theoretical and statistical interpretations of data.

Certainly, many nurses have some or even all of both sets of resources described above. More often than not, however, these complementary but different strengths develop by virtue of our place of employment and the nature of our daily work. If you are primarily a clinician, I want you to recognize the importance of what you have to offer. The nursing profession has much to gain from scientist-clinician teams in terms of both the quality and relevance of our science.

If collaboration with a scientist to generate the further knowledge you need is not an option, here are some final strategies to consider:

1. Consider replicating the original study. Replication is important to the establishment of the research base, yet you do not have to develop the research design, instruments, or plans for data analysis. The original investigators are likely to be interested in your desire to replicate their study and may therefore provide consultation if needed.

2. Make systematic observations about your ideas and hunches that have yet to be validated by research findings. Build a case for further research in this area and present this case to faculty, doctoral students, or researchers you meet at conferences.

3. Alert your librarian, clinical nurse specialist, director of research, and administrator to your interest in a particular line of research. Ask them to notify you when they come across new studies on your topic.

The most important activity is one in which you are already engaged, that is, *thinking* about your practice. Through sharing your ideas and hunches, you will stimulate other nurses to think about and evaluate their practice as well. Even if this outcome is the *only* way you use the research you have read here, the results will be valuable.

If you *are* thinking about your practice in light of the studies in this volume, my guess is that you also will use this research in a number of other informal ways. I doubt that any of us will care for a child in pain in the same way that we did before reading the studies on pediatric pain. If nothing else, our assessment of a child's pain should be keener and our consideration of options for pain management broader. In the same manner, we cannot help but be impressed by the pervasiveness of fatigue among all kinds of patients. Certainly, this sensitivity will result in attempts to provide patient care environments that are more conducive to rest and sleep. Finally, whenever I read studies that capture patients' lived experiences, as many of the studies here do, I feel a desire to listen better, to hear more. All of these informal ways that we "use" research are important.

Nursing practice is fascinating when there is time and an impetus to think about it. The result of all the thinking shared in the volume produces a collective high. Each of us can share the excitement in our own setting. Whatever the ideas or strategies you have formed in your mind, I challenge you to follow up on them. If everyone extends the generation or use of our knowledge in one small or large way, the contributions to nursing will be felt as a ripple effect through hospitals and schools of nursing across the country.

BIBLIOGRAPHY[1]

ANA Commission on Nursing Research. (1981). *Guidelines for the investigative function of nurses.* Kansas City, MO: ANA.

Barnard, K. E. (1980). Knowledge for practice: Directions for the future. *Nursing Research, 29,* 208–212.

Brett, J. L. (1987). Use of nursing practice research findings. *Nursing Research, 36,* 344–349.

Breu, C., & Dracup, K. (1985). Implementing nursing research in a critical care setting. *Journal of Nursing Administration, 6* (12), 14–17.

Buckwalter, K. C. (1985). Is nursing research used in practice? In J. C. McCloskey & H. K. Grace (Eds.), *Current issues in nursing* (2nd ed., pp. 110–123). London: Blackwell Scientific Publishers.

Connelly, C. E. (1986). Replication research in nursing. *International Journal of Nursing Studies, 23,* 71–77.

Crane, J. (1985). Research utilization—nursing models. *Western Journal of Nursing Research, 7,* 494–497.

Crane, J. (1985). Research utilization: Theoretical perspectives. *Western Journal of Nursing Research, 7,* 261–268.

Cronenwett, L. R. (1988). Disseminating research to clinicians. *CNR* (Newsletter of the ANA Council of Nurse Researchers), *15* (1), 1,3.

Cronenwett, L. R. (1986). Research contributions of clinical nurse specialists. *Journal of Nursing Administration, 16* (6), 6–7.

Cronenwett, L. R. (1987). Research utilization in practice settings. *Journal of Nursing Administration, 17* (7–8), 9–10.

CURN Project (Horsley, J. A., Crane, J., Crabtree, M. K., & Wood, D. J.). (1983). *Using research to improve nursing practice: A guide.* New York: Grune and Stratton.

Goode, C. J., Lovett, M. K., Hayes, J. E., & Butcher, L. A. (1987). Use of research-based knowledge in clinical practice. *Journal of Nursing Administration, 17* (12), 11–18.

Haller, K. B., Reynolds, M. A., & Horsley, J. A. (1979). Developing research-based innovation protocols: Process, criteria, and issues. *Research in Nursing and Health, 2,* 45–51.

Havelock, R. G. (1969). *Planning for innovation through dissemination and utilization of knowledge.* Ann Arbor: Center for Research on Utilization of Scientific Knowledge, ISR, University of Michigan.

Horsley, J. A. (1985). Using research in practice: The current context. *Western Journal of Nursing Research, 7,* 135–139.

Horsley, J. A., Crane, J., Crabtree, M. K., & Wood, D. J. (1983). *Using research to improve nursing practice: A guide.* New York: Grune & Stratton.

Ketefian, S. (1975). Application of selected nursing research findings into nursing practice: A pilot study. *Nursing Research, 24*, 89–92.

King, D., Barnard, K. E., & Hoehn, R. (1981). Disseminating the results of nursing research. *Nursing Outlook, 19*, 164–169.

Kirchhoff, K. T. (1983). Should staff nurses be expected to use research? *Western Journal of Nursing Research, 5* (3), 245–247.

Kirchhoff, K. T. (1982). A diffusion survey of coronary precautions. *Nursing Research, 31*, 196–201.

Krueger, J. C., Nelson, A. H., & Wolanin, M. O. (1978). *Nursing research: Development, collaboration and utilization.* Germantown, MD: Aspen Systems Corporation.

Lobiondo-Wood, G., & Haber, J. (1986). *Nursing research: Critical appraisal and utilization.* St. Louis: C.V. Mosby.

Loomis, M. E. (1985). Knowledge utilization and research utilization in nursing. *Image, 17* (2), 35–39.

Mallick, M. (1983). A constant comparative method for teaching research critiquing to baccalaureate nursing students. *Image, 15*, 120–123.

Miller, J. R., & Messenger, S. R. (1978). Obstacles to applying nursing research findings. *American Journal of Nursing, 78*, 632–634.

Notter, L. E., & Hott, J. R. (1988). *Essentials of nursing research* (4th ed.). New York: Springer Publishing Co.

Roberts-Gray, C., & Gray, T. (1983). Implementing innovations: A model to bridge the gap between diffusion and utilization. *Knowledge: Creation, Diffusion, Utilization, 5*, 213–232.

Rogers, E. M. (1983). *Diffusion of innovations.* New York: Free Press.

Stetler, C. B. (1985). Research utilization: Defining the concept. *Image, 17*, 40–44.

Stetler, C., & Marram, G. (1976). Evaluating research findings for applicability in practice. *Nursing Outlook, 24*, 559–563.

Stokes, J. E. (1981). Utilization of research findings by staff nurses. In S.D. Krampitz & N. Pavlovich (Eds.), *Readings for nursing research.* St. Louis: C.V. Mosby.

---

[1]A full bibliography on research utilization is included here for those wishing to learn more about moving research into practice.

Subject Index

Subject Index